Clinical Research in Complementary Therapies
Principles, Problems and Solutions

For Churchill Livingstone:

Publishing Manager, Health Professions: Inta Ozols
Project Development Manager: Katrina Mather
Design: George Ajayi

Clinical Research in Complementary Therapies
Principles, Problems and Solutions

Edited by

George Lewith MA DM FRCP MRCGP
Senior Research Fellow and Honorary Consultant Physician,
University of Southampton, Southampton, UK

Wayne B Jonas MD
Director, Samueli Institute for Information Biology,
Associate Professor,
Department of Family Medicine,
Uniformed Services University of the Health Sciences,
Bethesda, Maryland, USA

Harald Walach Dip Psych PhD
Director of Research, Institute of Environmental and Hospital Epidemiology,
University Hospital Freiburg, Freiburg, Germany

Foreword by

HRH The Prince of Wales

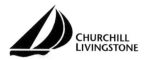

CHURCHILL
LIVINGSTONE

EDINBURGH LONDON NEW YORK PHILADELPHIA ST LOUIS SYDNEY TORONTO 2002

CHURCHILL LIVINGSTONE
An imprint of Harcourt Publishers Limited

© Harcourt Publishers Limited 2002

✑ is a registered trademark of Harcourt Publishers
Limited

The right of George Lewith, Wayne B Jonas and Harald
Walach to be identified as editors of this work has been
asserted by them in accordance with the Copyright, Designs
and Patents Act 1988.

First published 2002

ISBN 0 443 06367 2

British Library Cataloguing in Publication Data
A catalogue record for this book is available from the British
Library

Library of Congress Cataloging in Publication Data
A catalog record for this book is available from the Library
of Congress

Note
Medical knowledge is constantly changing. As new
information becomes available, changes in treatment,
procedures, equipment and the use of drugs become
necessary. The editors and contributors and the publishers
have taken care to ensure that the information given in this
text is accurate and up to date. However, readers are
strongly advised to confirm that the information, especially
with regard to drug usage, complies with the latest
legislation and standards of practice.

The
publisher's
policy is to use
**paper manufactured
from sustainable forests**

Printed in China

Contents

Contributors

Honor M Anthony MBCHB
Specialist in Allergy and
Environmental Medicine, Adel,
Leeds, UK

John Brazier BA MSc PhD
Sheffield Health Economics Group,
University of Sheffield, UK

Alan C Breen DC PhD
Director, Institute for Musculoskeletal
Research and Clinical Implementation,
Anglo-European College of
Chiropractic, Bournemouth, UK

Carlo Calabrese ND MPH
Research Institutes of Bastyr
University, Bothell, WA, USA

Edzard Ernst MD PhD FRCP (Edin)
Director, Department of
Complementary Medicine, School of
Postgraduate Medicine and Health
Sciences, University of Exeter, UK

Tiffany Field PhD
Director, Touch Research Institutes,
University of Miami Medical School,
Department of Pediatrics, Miami,
Florida, USA

Mike Fitter BSc PhD CPsychol
Research Director, Northern College of
Acupuncture and Consultant
Organizational Psychologist,
Foundation for Traditional Chinese
Medicine, York, UK

Richard Grimm MD MPH PhD
Director, Berman Center for Outcomes
and Clinical Research, Minneapolis
Medical Research Foundation,
Minneapolis, MN, USA

Wayne B Jonas MD
Director, Samueli Institute for
Information Biology,
Associate Professor, Department of
Family Medicine, Uniformed Services
University of the Health Sciences,
Bethesda, Maryland, USA

Irving Kirsch PhD
Professor of Psychology, University of
Connecticut, Storrs, Connecticut, USA

Willem Kramers MD PhD
Senior Lecturer, Department of
Medicinal Chemistry, Utrecht
University, The Netherlands,
Visiting Professor, University of
Witten/Herdecke, Germany

George Lewith MA DM FRCP
MRCGP
Senior Research Fellow and Honorary
Consultant Physician, University of
Southampton, UK

Klaus Linde MD
Senior Researcher, Center for
Complementary Medical Research,
Department of Internal Medicine,

Simon Mills MA FNIMH MCPP
Secretary, European Scientific
Cooperative on Phytotherapy
(ESCOP), Exeter, UK

Anne Morgan B Bus MSc
Research Associate, Sheffield Health
Economics Group, University of
Sheffield, UK

Rebecca W Rees MA MSc
Research Officer, EPPI-Centre, Social
Science Research Unit, Institute of
Education, University of London, UK

Elisabeth Targ MD
Director, Complementary Medical
Research Institute, California Pacific
Medical Center, San Francisco,
California, USA

Kate Thomas BA MA
Deputy Director, Medical Care
Research Unit, University of Sheffield,
UK

Roeland van Wijk PhD
International Institute of Biophysics,
Neuss, Germany

Andrew J Vickers D Phil
Assistant Attending Research
Methodologist, Integrative Medicine
Service, Memorial Sloan-Kettering
Cancer Center, New York, USA

Harald Walach Dip Psych, PhD
Director of Research,
Institute of Environmental and
Hospital Epidemiology,
University Hospital Freiburg,
Freiburg, Germany

Fred Wiegant PhD
Senior Scientist, Department of
Molecular Cell Biology,
Utrecht University, The Netherlands

Werner W Wittmann PhD
University of Mannheim, Faculty of
Social Science, Chair for Psychology,
Mannheim, Germany

Adrian White MA BM BCh
Senior Lecturer, Department of
Complementary Medicine, School of
Postgraduate Medicine and Health
Sciences, University of Exeter, UK

Foreword

From His Royal Highness, the Prince of Wales

ST. JAMES'S PALACE

The urgent need for more research into complementary and alternative medicine has been highlighted by the House of Lords' Select Committee on Science and Technology. Conventional medicine is working towards provision of "evidence-based medicine", which means that complementary medicine will have to meet the same exacting requirements of research evidence to stand any chance of being integrated into public health provision.

Within complementary medicine there is a lack of capacity in research. There are thought to be up to 50,000 complementary practitioners in the UK, yet this is not reflected in the number of researchers, research projects undertaken or published reports. Complementary medicine provides some challenges to research methodologists and to researchers looking to evaluating treatments.

I am sure this book will inspire some of those interested in research in complementary medicine to enquire further, to become involved and undertake research not only for their own benefit, but to further the evidence base and, hence, choice and availability of complementary medicine to the public. The contributors represent a wide range of experience and perspectives of research into complementary medicine. This book will be a valuable resource not only to those in complementary medicine, but also to conventional researchers perhaps seeking a different approach to a research problem.

"Clinical Research in Complementary Therapies" is most welcome – as a tool for researchers, a guide for practitioners contemplating research and hopefully as a catalyst for high quality investigations into complementary medicine.

Preface

This book reflects the progress that has been made in the last six years in our intellectual and financial research investments in the field of complementary therapy research. Section 1 deals with the strategic issues raised by complementary and alternative medicine (CAM) research: How should we phrase the questions we need to ask in this area of medicine, and what are the practical issues that face us in researching complementary and alternative medicine? These range from attempting to develop an evaluative culture within our practices (clinical audit) through to multicenter, randomized, controlled trials. How do we select patients for clinical trials within CAM? Is the benefit perceived by patients receiving CAM simply a sophisticated and non-specific therapeutic response, and, how do we evaluate the placebo in the context of a CAM clinical trial?

We have been overwhelmed with systematic reviews within CAM, many of them based on very poor primary research: How do we interpret these reviews? CAM practitioners claim that they can maintain health, and also that many of their treatments are cheaper, safer and sometimes more effective than conventional interventions. We need to understand the economic implications of providing CAM to large populations and we need to test these assumptions. The first section therefore raises these issues and suggests strategies that may allow us to address them across various therapies. We certainly do not have all the answers, but at least we are beginning to understand how we may ask thoughtful and intelligent research questions. As a consequence the first section of this multi-author text raises as many questions and issues as it answers.

The second section translates the issues raised in the first into a variety of specific therapies. For instance, in herbal medicine the evidence base is probably greater than that for many other CAM interventions, but issues of safety, good manufacturing practice and therapeutic claims are of great importance to both the public and the various legislative bodies involved. Homeopathy, on the other hand, raises fundamental issues about the credibility of CAM, largely because the idea that homeopathic medicines 'might work' seems so improbable, particularly as we have no understanding of what the underlying mechanisms might be. There is no doubt that, as a general rule, we have very limited evidence about the clinical effectiveness of many of the therapies discussed in Section 2. These therapy-based chapters provide a narrative review of some of the important research to date and clear suggestions as to how a research strategy, with respect to a particular therapy, might progress over the next 10 years.

We do not see this research methodology book as either endorsing or rejecting any specific complementary medical intervention. Rather, it provides a forum for debate of the current issues that face us in integrating an evidence-based complementary medical approach to illness, into conventional care, to the benefit of both patients and doctors so that the treatments we prescribe are both safe and effective. We have embraced the full extent of the philosophy and concepts within complementary medicine in Sections 1 and 2 and it will be apparent that a number of the authors contributing to this book are quite deliberately not medically qualified. We therefore believe that we have made an attempt to represent the complete CAM constituency rather than a medicalized view of CAM.

George Lewith
Wayne Jonas
Southampton 2001   Harald Walach

Methods and strategies

This section addresses the general principles of research with specific reference to the evaluation of the clinical effects of complementary and alternative medicine (CAM). How can we evaluate CAM? Is it really different from conventional medicine? Should we phrase our research questions differently in CAM as compared to conventional medicine? Is CAM safe and cost effective and how can we address these specific issues? CAM research presents an intellectual challenge for the interested clinician; it is possible but difficult to evaluate scientifically. Randomized controlled trials of specific medications are much easier to construct and deliver than similar studies in fields such as acupuncture, homeopathy and manual medicine. The tactics and strategies of clinical research in the field of CAM present a series of conceptual challenges that we have begun to address in this section but that will take many years to answer fully.

Thoughts

An article entitled 'what is CAM"?

a) many conventional.
b) many unconventional.
c) many a different system

1

Balanced research strategies for complementary and alternative medicine

George Lewith   Harald Walach   Wayne B Jonas

Complementary and alternative medicine (CAM) is a significant subset of health-care practices not integral to conventional Western care but used by patients in their health-care decisions. CAM practices are not new. They have been an important part of the public's health care for thousands of years but notice of their use has recently increased. CAM encompasses a number of diverse health-care and medical practices, ranging from dietary and behavioural interventions to high-dose vitamin supplements and herbs, to ancient systems of medicine such as Ayurvedic medicine and traditional Chinese medicine. CAM practice is not a fad so reliable information on its safety and effectiveness is needed. This is the role of clinical research. In this chapter we review the main types of information needed for CAM (or conventional) decisions in medical practice and how we can organize research methods into logical strategies to obtain and synthesize that information.

THE AUDIENCE FOR CAM RESEARCH

One of the striking features of the current interest in CAM is that it is a publically driven trend. The audience for CAM use is the public. Surveys of unconventional medicine use in the United States have shown that CAM use increased by 45% between 1990 and 1997. Visits to CAM practitioners are over 600 million per year, more than to all primary care physicians. The amount spent on these practices out of pocket is $27 billion, on a par with conventional medicine out-of-pocket costs (Eisenberg et al 1998). Conventional medicine has usually been antagonistic to CAM but it is now embracing it. Two-thirds of medical schools teach about CAM practices (Wetzel et al 1998), many hospitals are developing complementary and integrated medicine programs and more and more health management organizations include alternative practitioners and service benefits (Pelletier et al 1997).

The mainstream is also putting research money into these practices. For example, the budget of the Office of Alternative Medicine at the US National Institutes of Health rose from $5 million to $89 million in 7 years and it then became the National Center for Complementary and Alternative Medicine (NCCAM) although the conventional research leadership resisted (Marwick 1998). Because the public has been at the forefront of the CAM movement, questions about clinical investigation methods, what evidence they provide and who that evidence serves have naturally arisen.

HUMAN VALUES AND EVIDENCE

Two crucial issues that arise in developing appropriate evidence are the rigor and relevance of the information. Rigor refers to the management of biases that threaten the valid conduct and interpretation of data. Relevance addresses the use to which information will be put by specific audiences. Relevance involves values placed on different types of information, even when valid. When deciding whether or not to use a therapy, everyone wants to know if there is evidence that the therapy will work. While audiences are often curious about all types of information, groups will differ over which type of information is most important for their use. These differences involve values, not science. An ethical approach to scientific investigation will seriously consider the populations it serves. Failure to consider different group values when designing and conducting research risks 'methodological tyranny' in which we become slaves to rigid research hierachies that serve only a few rather than using research as a tool for broad service. Research strategies must start with the goals and purposes of information, before deciding on what information to collect and how to collect it. For whom is the information meant and for what purpose? How do the values of patient, practitioner, scientist and provider infuse research?

Patients

Patients who are ill or their family members may want to hear details about other individuals with similar illnesses who have used a treatment and recovered. If the treatment appears to be safe and there is little risk of harm from it, evidence from these stories may be sufficient for them to decide to use the treatment. This type of evidence is called anecdotal or case reports.

Practitioners

Doctors may want a different type of evidence. They realize that what works in one case may not work in another and need more than a few patient recovery stories to recommend a therapy. They often want to know what the likelihood or probability is that a patient will recover based on a whole series of similar patients who have received the treatment in actual practice. For example, out of 100 patients with the condition who received a treatment, did 20% or 80% improve? They also want to know about the complications and complexity of using the therapy, including its cost and inconvenience. This type of evidence is called clinical outcomes data, systematic case series or practice audit evidence.

Clinical investigators

Scientists may only accept a different type of evidence. They often want to know how much improvement occurred in a group who received the treatment compared to another group who did not receive it. If 80% of patients who received a treatment got better, do 60% of similar patients get better just from coming to the doctor? This is comparative or clinical trials evidence. Some scientists will only accept comparative evidence for a treatment if it has come from an experiment in which detailed methods, such as blinding and randomization, have been followed. This is clinical experimental evidence.

Laboratory scientists

Basic science investigators often only accept clinical evidence if laboratory experiments also support or can explain the effects or identify what in a treatment is causing the effect. This is basic science evidence.

Providers

Those in charge of determining public laws and policy often need definitive 'proof' that a practice is safe and effective. They require evidence in which a high degree of confidence can be placed since errors made in policy can adversely affect millions. This type of evidence comes from extensive evaluation and synthesis of several research reports through systematic reviews, metaanalyses and consensus reports of expert panels.

There is no shortage of people who are willing to believe almost anything based on a single story. There are also people who do not care about scientific evidence, preferring to rely solely on faith or intuition to make decisions, and there are those who are trying to profit from claims about products they sell. Conversely, there are people who are not willing to believe anything unless it can be explained with a specific theory they accept. Likewise, there are always those who will never accept something as real, even after the evidence for it on all levels is overwhelming.

Fortunately, most people fall somewhere in between and unfortunately, most evidence also falls somewhere in between. When a patient is sick, they need to make a decision about treatment based on the evidence available now. In many areas of medicine, conventional and alternative, there is often little good evidence of any kind available.

KNOWLEDGE DOMAINS: BUILDING BLOCKS OF A RESEARCH STRATEGY

What are the elements of a research strategy? How can we build an evidence house that has both rigor and relevance? In the diverse areas that CAM encompasses at least six major knowledge domains are relevant. Each of these domains has its own goals, methodology and quality criteria (Fig. 1.1).

Mechanism and basic biological effects on and in living systems

This domain is investigated through basic science and laboratory techniques and asks the questions 'what happens and why?'. Basic research can provide us with explanations for biological processes that are required to refine and advance our knowledge in any therapeutic field.

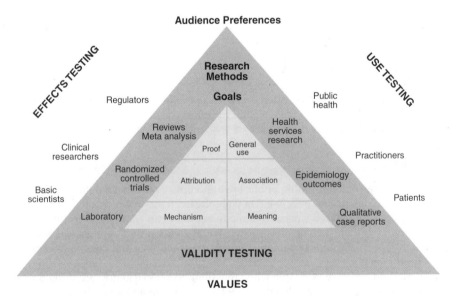

Figure 1.1   The audience, evidence, relevance interface.

Meaning and the examination of the subjective

This information comes through stories, anecdotes and descriptions of case reports and interviews. Quality research in this area, however, requires detailed qualitative evaluation methods. This knowledge domain provides information about whether our efforts are taking the correct focus by incorporating patient-centered outcomes and patient preferences which reduces the risk of outcomes substitution when a therapy is applied.

Attribution

In clinical research, this is termed 'efficacy' and is best obtained through research methods such as the randomized controlled trial. This domain looks for cause-and-effect evidence of proof and is useful when information is needed about how parts of a therapeutic system affect certain outcomes in a clinical condition. This is what those involved in conventional medicine mean when they are trying to determine whether a treatment 'works'.

Associations

When the identification of cause-and-effect links is impractical, unethical, unreasonable, impossible or misleading, information on associations is needed. In clinical medicine this is known as 'effectiveness' and involves such research methods as epidemiological and outcomes research. This is best applied when one is evaluating complex, long-term or chronic conditions where narrow selection and treatment criteria are inappropriate. The evaluation of complex systems is needed for traditional medicine and the utility of specific therapies when applied in the delivery (not study) environment. This type of knowledge is useful when indications are the goal and when one is seeking knowledge about adverse effects that have not been previously expected or which occur rarely.

Confidence

This knowledge domain is studied through peer review, systematic reviews and metaanalysis of scientific literature. Its purpose is to refine and determine whether definitive proof of a phenomenon exists. It is part of, but not the whole of, the validation process and requires a wide peer review process. This area, like all others, requires an objective, systematic, explicit and comprehensive approach to providing valid information.

Generalizability

This area involves evaluation of the practice in action. It is desirable when the goal is the acceptance and adoption of particular practices. This area deals with the evaluation of so-called 'external (to the trial) validity' criteria such as access, feasibility, use, etc. The type of research that provides information in this knowledge domain is health services research or health technology assessment.

From the clinical perspective, the ultimate goal of all these domains of knowledge is the identification of optimal medical management and the selection of diagnostic or therapeutic strategies that warrant direct comparative trials. From the basic biomedical perspective, the ultimate goal of all these domains is the understanding and control of the fundamental processes of life. From the practitioner and patient perspective, these domains seek to determine what 'works' or at least is appropriate.

The progress of a practice from clinical observation through investigation and evaluation to validation requires a research strategy with a balanced portfolio of methods feeding all of these knowledge domains. Excessive emphasis on one domain to the neglect of others (e.g. only pursuing anecdotal information or randomized controlled trials) will impede progress toward full validation and will neglect important sectors of the population. Not only do research strategies need to be balanced but the methods applied within each domain must be rigorous. The 'rules of evidence' for determining the internal validity, external validity and model fit of any research strategy must be applied in a careful, comprehensive and rigorous way. This is what is meant by rigor in research.

Unrecognized biases give us false information, leading to harm when that information is then applied in error. It is quality science that provides the 'level playing field' called for in these areas and prevents undue influence by a few audiences (advocates or skeptics, payers or the public). Screens that increase the likelihood that bias will be reduced in the evaluation of these areas are an important element in applying good science to complementary and alternative medicine. Such biases occur among patients, practitioners and scientists and threaten the validation of any practice. These biases, and ways to address them, are discussed in the rest of this chapter.

RESEARCH EVALUATION PRINCIPLES IN MEDICINE

Scientific methods in medicine

Research on alternative medical practices requires the same rigorous methods developed for conventional medicine. In addition, there are often added requirements because of the variety and implausibility of some CAM practices. The application of scientific methods to medicine is a relatively recent phenomenon. Rigor in biomedical research examining cellular functioning, the genetic regulation of life, the mechanisms of infectious disease and environmental influences on disease has developed only in the last 100 years. The randomized controlled clinical trial (RCT) is even younger, being only 50 years old and its details are still being worked out. It has been the standard for the acceptance of new drugs for only about 25 years and is still not the standard for many procedures in conventional medicine (Jadad 1998). Many statistical principles and techniques have also only recently evolved. Distinct types of research methods have evolved corresponding to the six knowledge domains discussed previously. These methods include laboratory techniques, observational methods, randomized controlled trials, metaanalysis, qualitative research methods, health services research and health technology assessment.

The research spectrum relevant to CAM

Figure 1.1 also illustrates six types of research methods and how they correspond with the knowledge domains. While there are variations within certain designs (e.g. a RCT can be controlled with standard care, placebo or no treatment, etc.), each of these methods captures distinct goals.

Laboratory methods

Laboratory and basic science approaches examine the basic mechanisms of CAM practices. In vitro (cell culture, intracellular, e.g. with gene technology) and in vivo (testing in animals) are now extensively used and expanding into the molecular realms.

Qualitative research

Qualitative methods include detailed case studies and interviews that describe medical approaches and investigate patient preferences and the meaning they find in their illness. Qualitative methods are extensively developed in anthropology and nursing and are increasingly common in primary care.

Randomized controlled trials

Randomized controlled trials (RCTs) seek to isolate specific effects of different treatments on outcomes. RCTs usually assign patients to one treatment group or another with a random method which ensures that groups are comparable on all factors that influence outcomes except for the treatment. Various methods are used such as random number tables or computer-generated random assignment. The treatment may or may not be delivered or evaluated blind but the best approach is to conceal knowledge of which patients get which treatment (allocation concealment).

Observational methods

Observational and outcomes studies (including practice audit, epidemiological research, outcomes research, surveys and other types of observational studies) describe associations between interventions and outcomes. Practice audit is monitoring all or a selected sample of patients that receive a treatment with before and after outcome measures. These studies may or may not have a comparison group or their comparison groups may be samples of patients not treated with the intervention of interest.

Reviews

Metaanalysis, systematic reviews (the most rigorous of the review methods) and expert (peer) review and evaluation are methods for judging the accuracy and precision of research. Methods of expert review and summary of research have evolved in the last decade by using protocol-driven approaches and statistical techniques. These are increasingly used along with subjective reviews to improve confidence that the effects in clinical research are accurate and robust.

Health services research

Health services research (and health technology assessment) explore the utility and impact of interventions in actual delivery settings. This evaluates factors such as access, feasibility, costs, practitioner competence, patient compliance, etc. for its interaction with proven treatments. Often this type of research may use surveys or sample groups receiving an intervention and look at quality and costs or other factors. Random sampling may be used but not random assignment to treatment.

Balanced research strategies

Note how there is a dialectic between research designed to isolate specific effects and mechanisms (laboratory, RCTs, metaanalyses, etc., all on the left side of Figure 1.2) and research designed to identify the utility, public impact and patient relevance of a practice in the real world (qualitative, observational and health services, etc., all on the right side of Figure 1.2). One can rarely address more than one knowledge domain in a single research project adequately. Thus, designing research that attempts to provide both specific (left side) and pragmatic (right side) information simultaneously is often problematic.

A research strategy can be balanced by applying orchestrated research methods so as to gain information about both specificity and utility. Without balanced strategies interpreting individual research studies is incomplete and so subject to error or misapplication. Developing decision rules that provide balanced research strategies is an important quality criterion for development of science-based medicine (Eddy 1996). If balance is the key feature of an appropriate research strategy combining research designs, rigor is the key feature of any one method. Rigor is assured by applying quality criteria within each of the evidence domains in Figure 1.1.

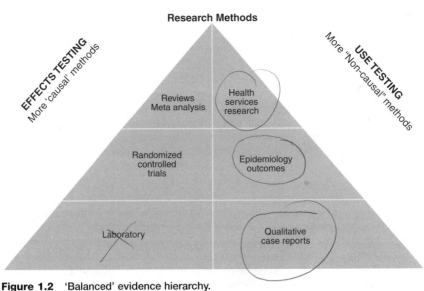

Figure 1.2 'Balanced' evidence hierarchy.

Comprehensive research quality criteria are increasingly available for evaluating the quality of any study and are discussed below (Jonas 1993).

Quality criteria for clinical research

The evaluation of research quality in CAM uses the same approach as that in conventional areas but there are additional items relevant to specific CAM areas. For example, the validity of RCTs assessed with quality criteria testing 'internal validity' or the likelihood that observed effects in the trial are biased. High-quality observational trials use quality criteria for 'external validity' or the likelihood that the observed effects will occur consistently in a range of appropriate clinical environments. A number of 'quality rating' systems are used for the evaluation of clinical research. The CONSORT group has produced a widely adopted set of quality reporting guidelines for RCTs (Begg et al 1996, Moher 1998). These criteria focus on the importance of allocation concealment, randomization method, blinding, proper statistical methods, attention to drop-outs and several other factors. They include internal and some external validity criteria. Table 1.1 lists the criteria in the most recent version of the CONSORT guidelines. Other guidelines are published for judging the quality of metaanalyses, observational trials and diagnostic tests (Egger et al 2000, Stroup et al 2000). These guidelines cover the basic quality items useful for any clinical research, including those on CAM.

Table 1.1 CONSORT checklist of items to include when reporting a randomized controlled trial (adapted from Begg et al 1996)

Heading	Subheading	Descriptor
Abstract		How participants were allocated to their interventions (e.g. random allocation, randomized or randomly assigned)
Introduction		The scientific background and specific trial objectives and hypotheses
Methods	Setting	The trial population: (a) inclusion and exclusion criteria; (b) the setting(s) and location(s) where the data were collected
	Design	The interventions administered to each trial group and who administered them
		Operationally define the primary and secondary outcome measures and, if applicable, any methods used to enhance the quality of measurements (e.g. use of multiple observations, training of assessors)
		How sample size was determined and, if applicable, details of any planned interim analyses or stopping rules
	Allocation	Method used to generate the random allocation sequence (i.e. sequence generation). Any additional details on restriction (e.g. stratification)
		If and how the randomization scheme was concealed (or not), until assignments were made (i.e. allocation concealment)

Table 1.1 (Continued)

Heading	Subheading	Descriptor
		Who generated the allocation sequence, who enrolled participants and who assigned participants to trial groups
	Blinding (masking)	Whether or not trial participants, those administering the interventions, those who assessed the outcomes and those who analyzed the data were masked to group assignment. If known, to what degree masking was successful
	Statistical methods	The statistical methods used to compare trial groups for primary outcome(s); methods for additional analyses, such as subgroup analyses and adjusted analyses, indicating which were prespecified
Results	Participant flow	Flow of participants through each stage of the trial: specifically, report the number randomly assigned to each group and the number analyzed in each group at the end of the trial (a diagram is strongly recommended). The number of participants in each trial group who completed the planned protocol
		The beginning and ending dates of the period of recruitment
	Analysis	The baseline demographic and clinical characteristics of each trial group
		Number of participants (denominator) in each group included in each analysis and whether the analysis was by 'intention to treat'
		The estimated effect size and a measure of its precision (e.g. 95% confidence interval). Any subgroup and adjusted analyses
		All clinically important adverse events or side effects, by trial group
Discussion comment		Interpretation of the results of the trial, taking into account sources of potential bias or imprecision
		The generalizability (external validity) of the trial findings
		General interpretation of the results of the trial in the context of current evidence

Model validity

Additional criteria besides internal and external validity are needed for CAM research. CAM research also requires evaluation for 'model validity' which assesses the likelihood that the research has adequately addressed the unique theory and therapeutic context of the CAM system. Many CAM systems arise outside developed countries. Clinical research requires expertise in the CAM system under investigation (Jonas 1997). Some CAM practices are investigated in populations where the practice is integral to the culture. Even standardized treatments can produce marked variations that may be culture specific. Results from one laboratory (culture) may not always translate to another (Moerman 2000). Finally, the informed consent procedure can influence outcomes significantly (Bergmann et al 1994, Kirsch 1999). Table 1.2 lists the main quality criteria for evaluating internal, external and model validity. These are summarized in an approach called the

Table 1.2   The Likelihood of Validity Evaluation (LOVE) guidelines ©WB Jonas; K Linde, 9/99

Dimension	Main criteria
Internal validity How likely is it that the effects reported are due to the independent variable (the treatment)?	**Randomization** (was subject assignment to treatment groups done randomly and in a concealed manner?) **Baseline comparability** (Were gender, age and prognostic factors balanced?) **Change of intervention** (Was there loss to follow-up, contamination, poor compliance?) **Blinding** (Did the patients, practitioners, evaluators, analysts know who got the treatment?) **Outcomes** (Were the objectivity, reliability and sensitivity of the outcome assessed?) **Analysis** (Was the number treated large? Were p-values significant? Were multiple outcomes measured and analyzed?)
External validity How likely is it that the observed effects would occur outside the study and in different settings?	**Generalizability** (Was there a range of patients as would be seen in practice or were there multiple or narrow inclusions and exclusions? Was the study done at several sites with similar results?) **Reproducibility** (Was what was done clear? Were confidence intervals reported? Was the treatment transferable to other practitioners?) **Clinical significance** (Was the effect size big enough to make a difference? Is the condition in need of this type of treatment? Were any preferences determined? Was adherence good?) **Therapeutic interference** (Was there flexibility in varying the treatment? Was feedback on the outcomes available? Is the treatment feasible in most (or your) practice settings?) **Outcomes** (Were the outcomes clinically relevant? Were the outcomes checked for importance with the patients? Were any important outcomes missing?)
Model validity How likely is it that the study accurately reflects the system under investigation?	**Representativeness/accuracy** (Were the therapists well trained and experienced? Was the treatment strategy adequate? Was the treatment clearly described?) **Informed consent** (Was the informed consent comprehensive? Was it effective – did patients understand it? Did it generate expectations different from practice?) **Methodology matching** (Were the goals of the study clear and limited? Did the investigators select the correct research method to achieve the goals? See the citation categories)

Table 1.2 (Continued)

Dimension	Main criteria
	Model congruity (Were the patients classified, was the treatment determined and were the outcomes assessed according to the system of the practice being assessed?) **Context/meaning** (Did the patients/practitioners believe in the therapy? How well was the intervention adapted to the culture, family, meaning of the patient?)
Reporting quality How likely is it that the report accurately reflects what was found in the study? How clear and accurate is the information presented?	**Comprehensive** (Can you address the above criteria?) **Clarity** (Could you reproduce this study?) **Conclusions** (Were the conclusions and reporting format (e.g. relative vs absolute improvement rates, strength of wording) appropriate to the data collected?)

Likelihood of Validity Evaluation (LOVE) system and have been applied to the evaluation of several areas of CAM research.

ISSUES FOR CLINICAL RESEARCH ON CAM

While research methods are fundamentally no different for complementary and alternative medicine and conventional medicine (Levin et al 1997, Vickers et al 1997), there are certain conceptual and contextual issues that the investigator should be aware of when conducting and evaluating CAM topics (Eskinaski 1998). These include:

- differing diagnostic classification
- ensuring adequate treatment
- the interaction of placebo and non-placebo factors
- selection of theory-relevant or patient-relevant outcomes
- the risk of premature, hypothesis-fixed standard practices
- assumptions about randomization
- non-locality
- blinding and unconscious expectancy
- learning and therapeutic growth
- and the nature of 'equipoise' in CAM
- risk stratification and levels of proof.

In addition, when summarizing CAM research, reviews should also explicitly consider the level of risk and cost of certainty in making recommendations.

Diagnostic classification

When 'homogeneous' groups collected for a clinical trial are evaluated from the perspective of another medical tradition, the groups may not be homogeneous.

The differing diagnostic taxonomies of CAM systems must be addressed on creation of a research population.

For example, the diagnosis of osteoarthritis may represent over a dozen classifications when evaluated by traditional Chinese medicine (TCM). A 'standardized' treatment may approximate the 'average' syndrome and it simplifies the treatment strategy which may turn out to be suboptimal treatment and so produce 'false-negative' results in the trial. This is poor model validity but it is rarely evaluated in research since it requires at least three arms in a clinical trial. For example, in a study of patients with irritable bowel syndrome, one-third of the patients were treated with individualized TCM, one-third with a standardized Chinese medicine approach and one-third received placebo. Subjects treated with the TCM model improved for longer than those given a standardized approach and both groups did better than the placebo group (Bensoussan et al 1998).

In addition to a three armed trial as an approach to the different diagnostic taxonomies in alternative medical systems, a double selection design can be used in which group selection is done according to both Western medicine and the alternative system. This double selection adds considerable complexity to the study and increases the likelihood of trial ambiguity. However, failure to carry out double classification may also result in false negatives. For example, Shipley tested the homeopathic remedy *Rhus toxicum* on a 'homogeneous' group of osteoarthritis patients without careful homeopathic classification and reported no effect of *Rhus toxodendron* over placebo (Shipley et al 1983). Fisher, in a follow-up study, used double selection for testing *Rhus tox.* that provided both good internal validity and model validity. Patients met criteria for fibromyalgia *and Rhus tox.*, producing a group 'homogeneous' for both medical systems. Those treated with *Rhus toxi.* did better than those given placebo (Fisher et al 1989). Double classification studies are more complicated and may require more resources than standardized studies but are more valid.

Adequate treatment

[handwritten annotation: The trial of PMT (Yakir) did this ... must show intervention at its best —]

Pilot data should always be obtained to ensure adequate treatment is being tested in a clinical trial. For example, a study of acupuncture for HIV-associated peripheral neuropathy published in the *JAMA* reported negative results although many acupuncturists report good results in this condition (Shlay et al 1998) but with considerably more treatments. Acupuncture is more like surgery than drug therapy, being applied with different styles and by practitioners with different skills. A treatment being tested must be optimal or at least representative for a defined group of providers and piloted for that condition. Rarely is adequate pilot work done in acupuncture research. For example, a review of 15 randomized trials of acupuncture for asthma found different treatment approaches in almost all of them (Linde et al 1996). Only two trials used the same points.

The interaction of placebo and non-placebo factors

It is typical to see 70–80% effectiveness reported from practices in both conventional and alternative medicine (Jonas 1994, Roberts et al 1993). Traditional medicine systems and various mind/body and spiritual approaches attempt to induce self-healing often by manipulating the context and meaning of illness. Effects arising from the context and meaning of a treatment are, by definition, the placebo element of treatment and interact with non-placebo elements of therapy in complex ways (Bergmann et al 1994, De Craen & Moerman 1996, Moerman 2000). Arthur Kleinman's classic study on why healers heal illustrates the importance of these contextual issues for all medicine (Kleinman et al 1978). The 'specific' and 'placebo' aspects of medicine effects is an area in need of focused research (Moerman & Jonas 2000).

A number of examples from CAM research illustrate the importance of being clear about conducting research and interpreting and labeling research results. Imprecision or general terminology (such as simply saying a treatment 'works' or does 'not work') is a red flag for biased interpretation. For example, research on acupuncture treatment of smoking cessation shows clear evidence that acupuncture acts similarly to several types of 'placebo' acupuncture (White & Rampes 1997, White et al 1997). There is no difference in smoking cessation rates between acupuncture and most sham acupuncture but there is also no difference between acupuncture and many proven smoking cessation treatments (White & Rampes 1997). Thus, acupuncture can be said to 'not work' (being no better than placebo) and 'work' (being equally effective as a proven conventional treatment)! The introduction of placebo controls and blinding (to increase rigor and 'internal validity') both clarifies and confuses the interpretation of acupuncture research. What is a 'good' placebo for acupuncture? Is it stimulation of non-acupuncture points, points thought not to be indicated, with superficial needling or with switched-off devices using ultrasound, electrical or laser stimulation? Deep needling techniques are probably not inert and may be required for optimal acupuncture treatment. No needling methods are likely to be distinguishable.

What matters most to patients? Is it whether a specific acupuncture technique is better than a questionable placebo technique or whether acupuncture helps patients more than no treatment or adds to standard treatment? The answer to these questions can radically affect how we design and interpret research yet one rarely, if ever, sees detailed patient input of this information into the developmental phase of research. Again, without patient input, model validity may be poor.

Outcomes selection

A related issue is the selection of outcome measures. For ease of study conduct, an outcome that is easy to measure is often used instead of more difficult patient-oriented, subjective outcomes. Eric Cassel has pointed out that because of an overemphasis on finding a 'cure', researchers (and others) are moved away from gaining knowledge that may help in healing the illness, a core goal of medicine (Cassel 1982). There is a higher risk of this when the investigator, in the name of 'rigor', tries to maximize internal validity by using objective measures instead of measures that have more external and model validity. As with control group selection, the selection of outcomes irrelevant to patients is more likely when there is inadequate patient input into study design.

This is not a unique issue for CAM but is one of the main reasons for CAM's popularity. Cassidy documented interviews with over 400 patients visiting acupuncturists (Cassidy 1998a,b). Most patients did not have a 'cure' of their Western diagnosis but they continued acupuncture treatment because of other factors such as an improved ability to 'manage' their illness and a sense of well-being. Such outcomes are not easy to measure objectively in clinical trials and are often avoided in clinical research. Measuring these outcomes may require adding persons and processes such as qualitative research methods.

Hypothesis testing

Hypothesis-focused research is how investigators identify cause-and-effect relationships in medicine. When properly conducted, it is a powerful method for confirming or refuting theories about treatment–outcome links. However, a downside of hypothesis testing is that by focusing on a particular theory-driven causal link, we risk prematurely fixing our conclusions about the value of a therapy which restricts investigation of other, possibly better therapies (Heron 1986).

Once treatments are established from a single perspective they become the 'standard of care'. After this, alternative treatments are ethically more difficult to investigate. Lifestyle therapy for coronary artery disease (CAD) is an example. Current standard-of-care treatments for CAD are oriented around an anatomically based hypothesis about the etiology of CAD. Coronary artery bypass grafting (CABG), balloon angiography and stents are all established treatments of coronary artery disease based on the anatomic hypothesis. An extensive industry has developed around these procedures. Lifestyle therapy can also successfully treat CAD but it is based on a non-anatomical hypothesis of CAD etiology. It may be that lifestyle therapy is better than CABG for treatment of CAD given its low cost, preventive potential, reduction in fatigue and improvement in well-being (Blumenthal & Levenson 1987, Haskell et al 1994, McDougall 1995, Ornish et al 1998). The comparison of CABG with lifestyle therapy is often challenged because perceptions and resources are already committed to CABG. We do not know which hypothesis about the cause of CAD is correct because they cannot be tested in placebo-controlled trials. We often assume CABG has specific effects and that lifestyle therapy has effects mostly because of belief and placebo. However, in the 1950s, sham surgery of internal mammary ligation was reported to be as effective as CABG produces are today (Cobb et al 1959). We know that placebo effects of surgery are large (Beecher 1961, Johnson 1994), yet sham surgery cannot be done for CABG today, so we do not know how much of the effects of CABG are placebo.

Acceptance of the anatomic hypothesis in CAD is a double-edged sword. It drives our research in a particular direction and inhibis it in other directions. Revealing partial causes runs the risk of preventing the discovery of what may be more beneficial therapies for chronic disease. Research strategies for chronic disease need to have the flexibility to test multiple hypotheses (Coffey 1998, Gallagher & Appenzeller 1999, Harwitz 1987).

Assumptions about randomization

Randomization is the sacred cow of clinical testing. When the results of observational and randomized studies are different it is assumed the randomized study is more valid. However, this dogma has recently been challenged by an increasing number of articles claiming that properly done observational studies do not differ from those that are randomized. In some clinical situations, randomization assists in revealing true effect sizes. In behavioural medicine interventions, it may obscure or have no effect on outcome (Lipsey & Wilson 1993). Some complex traditional or alternative systems believe that randomization can interfere with a therapy (by eliminating choice) and obscure our awareness of how bias affects it. For example, traditional Chinese science is based not on linear cause-and-effect assumptions but on an assumption that 'correspondences' occur between system levels (biological, social, cosmic, etc.) (Porkert 1974). In Chinese medicine, to influence one level is to affect all other levels. Thus, linear causes can change and may be less important for an individual case than to establish accurate correspondences, for example between the body ailment and a seasonal imbalance (Unschuld 1985). From this perspective extensive efforts to establish precise causal links between intervention and outcome (as done in RCTs) are of less interest than in Western medicine (Lao 1999).

Non-locality

In conventional medicine, adequate blinding is assumed to control for any effects of intention or preference on outcome. Intention has no direct effects as participants are blinded. However, in many CAM systems intention and consciousness have effects both directly and indirectly and can influence apparent chance phenomena (Dossey 1999). If this is true, the implications for researchers are of three types. First, what are the effects of intentionality on the randomization process of RCTs? Metaanalyses of RCTs often have effect size variability similar to that seen in experiments of mental intention on random systems in general (Counsell et al 1994, Radin & Ferrari 1991). Second, do negative intention, skepticism or positive intention such as enthusiasm or compassion block or enhance effects? Most in conventional science believe they cannot. Some alternative systems assume they can. Finally, is it ethically acceptable to interfere with beliefs that can have a major impact on patient outcome? If assumptions about the non-local effects of mental intention are significant, then the interaction of bias and randomization is more complex than we currently assume in traditional statistics (Jahn 1996, Radin & Nelson 1989). In some clinical situations, randomization may assist in revealing true effect sizes. We don't know if experimenter intention is directly relevant to medical research. These issues are probably significant only when the results of high-quality trials are contradictory. The significance of these influences can only be determined when rigorous research methods are used.

Blinding and unconscious expectancy

Blinding or masking is primarily used to control for expectation effects in clinical studies. Although there is no foolproof method to ensure successful blinding, it is still an important part of quality research (Begg et al 1996). Some alternative treatments, such as certain herbal preparations and superficial acupuncture techniques, can be at least partially blinded. Special attention is needed to match smell and taste in herbal products. When giving acupuncture, the practitioner cannot be completely blinded except with special types of acupoint stimulation, such as with ultrasound. Homeopathy is more easily double blinded than most conventional drugs. Complex behavioral or lifestyle programs cannot be delivered blind. Controlling for time and attention can be done and it is possible to code groups and so blind those measuring outcomes and doing the analysis. For example, equal time and the presence of a sham therapist can be incorporated into studies of therapeutic touch (Gordon 1998). In most traditional medical systems such as Ayurvedic or Native American medicine, a deep connectivity to all information about a therapy is assumed to exist and overt blinding cannot eliminate this, whether conscious or not. These systems assume that expectation has effects even when unconscious (Rigby 1988). In fact, a therapy in a traditional system may even try to enhance these unconscious expectation effects by manipulation of 'spirits' or 'energy' forces (Jonas 1999). From this perspective masking and sham interventions simply eliminate our awareness and conscious discussion of expectation effects rather than eliminating the effects themselves. If unconscious expectancy is an important part of the therapy it may be counterproductive to the therapy. There is evidence that autonomic and physiological effects occur unconsciously (such as reactions to music when under anesthesia), something many traditional systems would predict (Bennett 1986, Blankfeild 1991, Radin 1997). Unconscious expectancies may influence outcomes in clinical trials. For example, the physiological effects of 'active' placebos (drugs that produce 'side effects' but not the therapeutic effect) in studies of antidepressants can influence outcomes even under double-blind conditions (Greenberg et al 1992, Kirsch & Sapirstein 1998). These unconscious effects may mask detection of drug effects (Moerman 2000).

The assumptions of many CAM systems about intuitive access to information and direct effects of mental intention on random processes are the only two substantial challenges to current Western scientific methods, if they are true. These concepts need more study. However, CAM investigators should be aware of the complex relationships between expectation, awareness, physiological processes and outcomes when designing clinical studies. In addition, researchers should be sensitive to the fact that some CAM systems may not share the basic assumptions (of locality and no direct interaction of consciousness and outcomes) that are required for rigorous experimental design. These assumptions should not be used as an excuse for conducting or accepting poor-quality research, however, for rigorous research criteria also apply to non-experimental (e.g. observational) studies.

Learning and therapeutic growth

Many CAM therapies involve learning such as biofeedback, mediation, imagery and hypnosis. These practices produce progressive improvement over time as skill improves. Lifestyle therapies are also in this category. Blinding in a clinical trial of these therapies is usually not possible but if it were it would reduce the very processes upon which they are based. Some physiological reactions may change, even during a single therapeutic episode, and so the degree of blindness may also change, altering expectation effects and the relative efficacy of the 'active' treatment. Increasing a patient's awareness of unconscious processes, the goal of many of these therapies, enhances self-efficacy on multiple levels. Hand-warming biofeedback, for example, is used to treat a variety of conditions, not just to increase microcirculation of the extremities (1996). Meditation interventions such as 'mindfulness' and Transcendental Meditation influence a variety of conditions (Alexander 1988, Epstein 1999, Kabat-Zinn 1996).

The nature of equipoise in CAM

Preferences have important consequences for clinical research, especially in CAM. Randomization is ethical only when true equipoise exists between treatment groups. This can occur when efficacy is truly ambiguous and there are not strong preferences for one or another therapy. Equipoise is present when new drugs are tested, especially if no established therapy exists, and placebo controls are ethically acceptable. This situation often does not exist in alternative medicine. If patients are using or avoiding CAM therapies it is often because of strong preferences (Furnham & Kirkcaldy 1996).

Recruitment to RCTs is problematic in these cases and good clinical studies have either been abandoned or their randomization dropped because of refusal of patients to enter such a study. Randomization processes in conventional studies have been subverted by well-meaning health-care practitioners, a problem that may also happen in CAM research (Schulz et al 1995). In addition, research may be contaminated when subjects use alternative therapies that interact with the treatments being tested. For example, over 16% of patients in clinical trials at the US National Institutes of Health Clinical Center were using herbal therapies not reported to the investigators (Sparber et al 2000). Preferences must be carefully considered when managing clinical research on CAM.

Risk stratification

Most therapies, conventional or alternative, become used and often accepted before good evidence on their effectiveness is collected (Eddy 1990). Acupuncture provides a current CAM example of this. There is a growing acceptance of acupuncture in general, even in the absence of proof for its effectiveness for most conditions. The clear safety of acupuncture make many (including the NIH acupuncture consensus panel) willing to recommend it with less evidence than other higher risk interventions. This type of risk stratification is a useful step in deciding on what type of evidence is needed for balancing rigor and relevance in evidence-based medicine (Jonas et al 1999). There is a need for observational studies before extensive, controlled trial research is conducted. For many therapies and conditions observational research may be sufficient for clinical decisions. For example, few patients or physicians would recommend against the use of a low-cost and inexpensive therapy (e.g. mind-body or homeopathic treatment) for a non-life threatening disease (e.g. seasonal allergies) if outcomes data indicated that it benefited patients. Practice outcome studies can help guide both practice and research (Linde & Jonas 1999).

DEVELOPING RESEARCH STRATEGIES FOR CAM

Matching goals and methods in clinical research

A theme in research is the importance of clearly defining what information is needed and how it will be used, the questions that can help obtain that information and the appropriate research methods used to answer those questions (Feinstein 1989). Of the many types of research methods, each has its own purpose, value and limitations. The quality of these methods should be judged in relationship to the research goals and the purpose to which the answers will be put. For example, when defining concepts, constructs and terms and when assessing the relevance of an outcome measurement, qualitative methods, with their in-depth interviews and content analysis, are the most appropriate strategy. When seeking associations of variables, surveys, cross-sectional or longitudinal studies with methods that allow for factor analysis are the most useful. When trying to measure the overall impact of a complex intervention delivered in a clinical context, pragmatic trials and outcomes methods should be applied. When attempting to isolate and prove that there are specific effects of treatment on selected outcomes, randomized controlled trials are clearly the method of choice.

In Figure 1.3 we have outlined a CAM research strategy map that illustrates the relationship between study goals, the type of information being sought on a therapy and the type of methodology that will be most appropriate. An important part of clinical research evaluation in CAM is checking to see that the questions asked and the methods selected are appropriate for each other (Linde & Jonas 1999). Of course, once selected, a research method must be used in a rigorous and quality manner.

Choosing research strategies in CAM

How does this guide us when choosing research strategies in CAM? Figure 1.3 provides a step-wise guide for mapping out an appropriate research sequence for the type of information needed. One begins first by clarifying who will primarily use the resulting information and for what purpose. The decision to pursue a particular approach depends on a number of factors including:

- the complexity of the condition and therapy being investigated
- the information sought (causal, descriptive, associative, etc.)
- the purpose for which the information will be used
- the methods of that are available, ethical and affordable.

Figure 1.3 illustrates how these factors flow. The main audience and the use for which a research project is undertaken are the anchoring factors in determining the best method. For example, in multimodality practices that are often not well described (e.g. spiritual healing, lifestyle therapies) and where the interest is on impact on chronic disease, outcomes research or pilot trials are the best initial approach (domain 3A). In well-described modalities that are safe and not expensive where effectiveness (not efficacy) is the main interest (e.g. acupuncture, homeopathy), outcomes data coupled with decision analysis may provide the best strategic approach (domain 3B) (Dowie 1996). In many natural products, where the active or

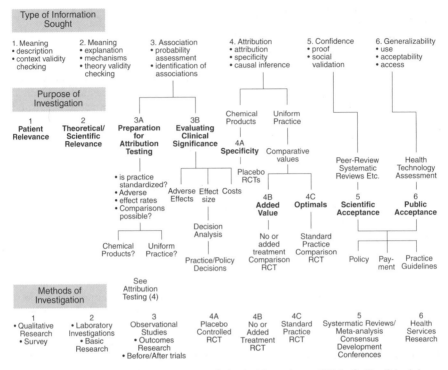

Figure 1.3 CAM research strategy map. (adapted from Jonas WB in Gallin: Principles and practice of Clinical Research)

standard constituents are variable, basic science work (e.g. laboratory characterization and safety data) is needed before controlled clinical research is done (domain 2). Products that are well characterized but have potential direct adverse effects may need RCTs provided their public health implications warrant such an investment. Placebo studies of natural products are more useful for making regulatory decisions (e.g. product marketing and claims, etc.) than for individual decisions (domain 4A). The US National Institutes of Health's study of the efficacy of St John's wort for depression, using a large, three-armed, multicentered, placebo-controlled trial, is an example of this latter approach. It is a widely used treatment, has significant potential drug–herb interactions (through the P450 system) and is treating an important, common clinical condition (domain 2).

Practice audit may be more useful than RCTs for individual decisions. For example, a physician considering referral of a patient with back pain for acupuncture will want to know what kind of patients local acupuncturists see, how they are treated, whether these patients are satisfied with treatment and what the outcomes are. This type of data comes from practice audit (observational research), surveys and qualitative research (domains 3B and 1) (Cassidy 1998 a,b). Information from local practice audits is more valuable than relying on the results of small (or large) placebo-controlled trials done in other countries where the practitioners and populations are quite different from those in US populations. Data collection, monitoring and interpretation of observational studies must be as carefully performed as experimental studies. Finally, when exploring theories and data that do not fit into current assumptions about causality (e.g. psychic healing, homeopathy, etc.) a carefully thought-out basic science strategy for investigator topics is needed. Given the public interest and the implications for science of these areas, it is irresponsible for the scientific community to completely ignore them (Jonas 1997). A balanced approach to exploring the spectrum of evidence presented here can justify and guide these types of studies.

Within RCTs (domain 4) there are several goals that determine which design and sequence of studies are most appropriate. If the goal is obtaining information on the specificity of molecular or procedural effects (e.g. drug effects), placebo controls are required (domain 4A). Placebo controls cannot, however, provide information about added value from a therapy (domain 4B), which requires a no treatment or alternative treatment control (e.g. hypericum vs antidepressant control), or about what is optimal therapy (e.g. is lifestyle better than bypass?), which requires a standard care control (domain 4C). Single sets of research (domains 1–4) do not provide enough evidence for public policy or public acceptance, however. Proof (domain 5) and generalizability (domain 6) require systematic review and health technology assessment, respectively. Examples of these two are the NIH Consensus Conference statement on acupuncture, which influenced public decisions on reimbursement for acupuncture and the Agency for Health Care Policy and Research's practice guideline on low back pain and manipulation and the subsequent establishment of chiropractic services in the US military.

Assuring the quality of research methods

Uniform criteria that define scientific rigor should be used to define 'quality' and not simply study design (Sackett et al 1991). For example, experimental, observational and research summary are three designs with published quality criteria (Begg et al 1996, Egger et al 2000, Moher 1998, Stroup et al 2000). These and others (e.g. qualitative research) are needed to investigate the validity and the value of CAM. Cross-tradition and cross-disciplinary research, involving experts in both conventional and CAM, is often required. The field of psychoneuroimmunology (PNI) arose because psychologists and immunologists began collaborative projects bringing together both laboratory and clinical research methods. Such exploration would allow us to develop a scientific basis for chronic disease management.

Rigor, relevance and realism

How do we balance rigor and relevance so as to provide good science and an ethical process? Evaluating effectiveness is complex. A handful of randomized trials will not answer even the primary questions posited by different audiences with different needs. CAM use continues to increase at a rapid rate and while research money is also increasing, it cannot provide data on all the pertinent areas of CAM. One cannot afford to fix on a single research method or hierarchy. The investigation of global medicine in all its diversity and mystery requires a spectrum of methods that collectively balance relevance, scientific rigor and feasibility. To remain ethical there are several different audiences that research must serve: patients; providers;

the scientific community; and policy makers. Each audience is usually interested in many types of information but they have different priorities (Fig. 1.1). These require a finite spectrum of research methods. Considering how each audience uses the research information can also help guide the design of research on CAM (Fig. 1.2).

CAM and evolution of the scientific method

Unconventional practices are often used as a testing ground for new research ideas and scientific methods. Fifty years ago, for example, blinding and randomization became parts of orthodox medical research only after they were first applied to unorthodox practices such as mesmerism, psychic healing and homeopathy (Kaptchuk 1998). It is likely that many therapies will never be fully 'scientifically established', in the sense that they will fill in all six evidence domains as described in this chapter. Decisions about what is 'sufficient' for particular audiences (individual, practice, regulatory, public health, etc.) require careful examination of the role of science in the management of chronic disease and in the investigation of alternative 'paradigms'. Science answers incremental and isolated questions and research can never answer all questions of interest. Skepticism about unorthodox practices is high and so rigorous evidence is often required before such practices are accepted. Such rigor is important and it should be applied in a balanced strategy, not dogmatically in the name of 'rigor'.

The march toward global medicine challenges us to explicitly define the terms 'rigorous research' or 'scientifically established' and demonstrate the evidence upon which those quality criteria are based (Moher 1998). Quality research in CAM helps us develop the decision rules for a strategic approach for medical research. The ongoing interaction between orthodox and unorthodox medicine is the opportunity for developing new research strategies and clarifying the appropriate role of science in the service of chronic disease treatment. A creative tension between the established and the frontier can advance scientific knowledge and help us understand both the benefits and limitations of the scientific process for medicine.

REFERENCES

1996 Integration of behavioral and relaxation approaches into the treatment of chronic pain and insomnia. NIH Technology Assessment Panel on Integration of Behavioral and Relaxation Approaches into the Treatment of Chronic Pain and Insomnia. Journal of the American Medical Association 276 (4): 313–318

Alexander CN 1988 Transcendental Meditation. In: Corsini RJ (ed) Encyclopedia of Psychology. Wiley Interscience, New York, pp. 1–5

Beecher HK 1961 Surgery as placebo. Journal of the American Medical Association 176: 1102–1107

Begg C, Cho M et al 1996 Improving the quality of reporting of randomized controlled trials. Journal of the American Medical Association 276: 637–639

Bennett HL 1986 Pre-operative instructions for decreased bleeding during spine surgery. Anesthesiology 65(3A): 245

Bensoussan A, Talley NJ et al 1998 Treatment of irritable bowel syndrome with Chinese herbal medicine. Journal of the American Medical Association 280: 1585–1589

Bergmann J, Chassany O et al 1994 A randomised clinical trial of the effect of informed consent on the analgesic activity of placebo and naproxen in cancer pain. Clinical Trials and Meta-Analysis 29: 41–47

Blankfeild R 1991 Suggestion, relaxation, and hypnosis as adjuncts in the care of surgery patients: a review of the literature. American Journal of Clinical Hypnosis 172–186

Blumenthal JA, Levenson RM 1987 Behavioral approaches to secondary prevention of coronary heart disease. Circulation 76 (1 Pt 2): 1130–1137

Cassel E 1982 The nature of suffering and the goals of medicine. New England Journal of Medicine 306(11): 639–645

Cassidy CM 1998a Chinese medicine users in the United States Part I: utilization, satisfaction, medical plurality. Journal of Alternative and Complementary Medicine 4(1): 17–27

Cassidy CM 1998b Chinese medicine users in the United States Part II: preferred aspects of care. Journal of Alternative and Complementary Medicine 4(2): 189–202

Cobb LA, Thomas GI et al 1959 An evaluation of internal-mammary-artery ligation by a double-blind technic. New England Journal of Medicine 260: 1115–1118

Coffey D 1998 Self-organization, complexity, and chaos: the new biology for medicine. Nature Medicine 4: 882–885

Counsell CE, Clarke MJ et al 1994 The miracle of DICE therapy for acute stroke: fact or fictional product of subgroup analysis? British Medical Journal 309(6970): 1677–1681

De Craen AJ, Moerman DE 1996 Gastrointestinal diseases and their treatment with placebo. OAM/NIH Conference on Placebo and Nocebo Effects: Developing a Research Agenda. National Institutes of Health, Bethesda, MD

Dossey L 1999 Reinventing medicine: beyond mind-body to a new era of healing. HarperSanFrancisco, New York

Dowie J 1996 Evidence based medicine. Needs to be within framework of decision making based on decision analysis [letter; comment]. British Medical Journal 313(7050): 170; discussion 170–171

Eddy DM 1990 Should we change the rules for evaluating medical technologies? In: Gelijns AC (ed) Modern methods of clinical investigation. National Academy Press, Washington DC, 117–134

Eddy DM 1996 Clinical decision making: from theory to practice: a collection of essays from Journal of American Medical Association. Jones & Bartlett Publishers, Boston.

Egger M, Davey SG et al 2000 Systematic reviews in health care: metaanalysis in context. British Medical Journal Books, London

Eisenberg DM, Davis RB et al 1998 Trends in alternative medicine use in the United States 1990–1997: results of a follow-up national survey. Journal of the American Medical Association 280: 1569–1575

Epstein RM 1999 Mindful practice. Journal of the American Medical Association 292: 833–839

Eskinaski DP 1998 Factors that shape alternative medicine. Journal of the American Medical Association 280: 1621–1623

Feinstein AR 1989 Models, methods and goals. Journal of Clinical Epidemiology 42(4): 301–308

Fisher P, Greenwood A et al 1989 Effect of homeopathic treatment on fibrositis (primary fibromyalgia). British Medical Journal 299: 365–366

Furnham A, Kirkcaldy B 1996 The health beliefs and behaviours of orthodox and complementary medicine clients. British Journal of Clinical Psychology 35: 49–61

Gallagher R, Appenzeller T 1999 Beyond reductionism. Science 284(79):

Gordon A 1998 The effects of therapeutic touch on patients with osteoarthritis of the knee. Journal of Family Practice 47(4): 271–277

Greenberg RP, Bornstein RF et al 1992 A meta-analysis of antidepressant outcome under 'blinder' conditions. Journal of Consulting Clinical and Psychology 60(54–551): 664–669

Haskell WL, Alderman EL et al 1994 Effects of intensive multiple risk factor reduction on coronary atherosclerosis and clinical cardiac events in men and women with coronary artery disease. The Stanford Coronary Risk Intervention Project (SCRIP). Circulation 89(3): 975–990

Heron J 1986 Critique of conventional research methodology. Complementary Medicine Research 1(1): 10–22

Horwitz RI 1987 Complexity and contradiction in clinical trial research. American Journal of Medicine 82(3): 498–510

Jadad A 1998 Randomized controlled trials: a user's guide. British Medical Journal Books, London

Jahn RG 1996 Consciousness, information and health. Alternative Therapies 2: 32–38

Johnson AG 1994 Surgery as placebo. Lancet 344: 1140–1142

Jonas WB 1993 Evaluating unconventional medical practices. Journal of NIH Research 5: 64–67

Jonas WB 1994 Therapeutic labeling and the 80% rule. Bridges 5(2): 1, 4–6

Jonas WB 1997 Researching alternative medicine. Nature Medicine 3(8): 824–827

Jonas WB 1999 Models of medicine and models of healing. In: Jonas WB, Levin JH (eds) Essentials of complementary and alternative medicine. Lippincott Williams and Wilkins, Philadelphia

Jonas WB, Linde K et al 1999 How to practice evidence-based complementary and alternative medicine. In: Jonas WB, Levin JS (eds) Essentials of complementary and alternative medicine. Lippincott Williams and Wilkins, Philadelphia

Kabat-Zinn J 1996 Mindfulness meditation: what it is, what it isn't, and its role in health care and medicine. Comparative and psychological study on meditation. Haruki, Y. Ishii and M. Suzuki. Eburon, Netherlands, pp. 161–170

Kaptchuk TJ 1998 Intentional ignorance: the history of blind assessment and placebo controls in medicine. Bulletin of the History of Medicine 72: 389–433

Kirsch I 1999 How expectancies shape experience. American Psychological Association, Washington DC

Kirsch I, Sapirstein G 1998 Listening to prozac but hearing placebo: a meta-analysis of antidepressant medication. Prevention and Treatment 1

Kleinman A, Eisenberg L et al 1978 Culture, illness, and care: clinical lessons from anthropologic and cross-cultural research. Annals of Internal Medicine 88(2): 251–258

Lao L 1999 Traditional Chinese Medicine. In: Jonas WB, Levin JS (eds) Essentials of complementary and alternative medicine. Lippincott Williams and Wilkins, Philadelphia.

Levin JS, Glass TA et al 1997 Quantitative methods in research on complementary and alternative medicine. A methodological manifesto. NIH Office of Alternative Medicine. Medical Care 35(11): 1079–1094

Linde K, Jonas WB 1999 Evaluating complementary and alternative medicine: the balance of rigor and relevance. In: Jonas WB, Levin JS (eds) Essentials of complementary and alternative medicine. Lippincott Williams and Wilkins, Philadelphia

Linde K, Worku F et al 1996 Randomized clinical trials of acupuncture for asthma – a systematic review. Forschende Komplementärmedizin 3: 148–155

Lipsey MW, Wilson DB 1993 The efficacy of psychological, educational, and behavioral treatment: confirmation from meta-analysis. American Psychologist 48(12): 1181–1209

Marwick C 1998 Alterations are ahead at the OAM. Journal of the American Medical Association 280: 1553–1554

McDougall J 1995 Rapid reduction of serum cholesterol and blood pressure by a twelve-day, very low fat, strictly vegetarian diet. Journal of the American College of Nutrition 14(5): 491–496

Moerman D, Jonas WB 2000 Toward a research agenda on placebo. Advances 16: 33–46

Moerman DE 2000 Cultural variations in the placebo effect: ulcers, anxiety, and blood pressure. Medical Anthropology Quarterly 14: 51–72

Moher D 1998 CONSORT: an evolving tool to help improve the quality of reports of randomized controlled trials. Journal of the American Medical Association 279: 1489–1491

Ornish D, Scherwitz LW et al 1998 Intensive lifestyle changes for reversal of coronary heart disease. Journal of the American Medical Association 280: 2001–2007

Pelletier KR, Marie A et al 1997 Current trends in the integration and reimbursement of complementary and alternative medicine by managed care, insurance carriers, and hospital providers. American Journal of Health Promotion 12(2): 112–123

Porkert M 1974 The theoretical foundations of Chinese medicine – systems of correspondence. MIT Press, Cambridge, MA

Radin DI 1997 The conscious universe: the scientific truth behind psychic phenomena. HarperEdge, San Francisco, CA

Radin DI, Ferrari DC 1991 Effects of consciousness on the fall of dice: a meta-analysis. Journal of Scientific Exploration 5(1): 61–83

Radin DI, Nelson RD 1989 Evidence for consciousness-related anomalies in random physical systems. Foundations of Physics 19(12): 1499–1514

Rigby BR 1988 New perspectives in medical practice: the psychophysiological approach of Maharishi Ayurveda. Modern Science and Vedic Science 2(1): 77–87

Roberts AH, Kewman DG et al 1993 The power of nonspecific effects in healing: implications for psychological and biological treatments. Clinical Psychology Review 13: 375–391

Sackett DL, Haynes RB et al 1991 Clinical epidemiology: a basic science for clinical medicine. Little, Brown, Boston

Schulz KF, Chalmers I et al 1995 Empirical evidence of bias. JAMA 273: 408–412

Shipley M, Berry H et al 1983 Controlled trial of homoeopathic treatment of osteoarthtritis. Lancet i: 97–98

Shlay JC, Chaloner K et al 1998 Acupuncture and amitriptyline for pain due to HIV-related peripheral neuropathy. JAMA 280: 1590–1595

Sparber A, Johnson E et al 2000 Biomedical research and patient utilization of natural herbal products: a case study. Cancer Investigation 18(5): 436–439

Stroup DF, Berlin JA et al 2000 Meta-analysis of observational studies in epidemiology. JAMA 283: 2008–2012

Unschuld PU 1985 Medicine in China. A history of ideas. University of California Press, Berkeley, CA

Vickers A, Cassileth B et al 1997 How should we research unconventional therapies? International Journal of Technology Assessment in Health Care 13(1): 111–121

Wetzel MS, Eisenberg DM et al 1998 A survey of courses involving complementary and alternative medicine at United States medical schools. JAMA 280: 784–787

White A, Rampes H 1997 Acupuncture in smoking cessation. In: Lancaster T, Silagy C (eds) Tobaccos addiction module of the Cochrane Database of Systematic Reviews. The Cochrane Collaboration. Update Software, Oxford

White A, Resch K et al 1997 Smoking cessation with acupuncture? A best evidence synthesis. Forschende Komplementarmedizin 4: 102–105

2

The role of outcomes research in evaluating complementary and alternative medicine

Harald Walach   Wayne B Jonas   George Lewith

INTRODUCTION

Randomized controlled trials (RCTs) are the gold standard for evaluating new treatments and are required for the approval of new medicinal products (CPMP Working Party 1995). Unfortunately, randomization is often used to overcome poor methodology, when randomization itself is simply a tool to balance the groups being studied (Feinstein 1989).

The methodological superiority of the RCT stems from its capacity to preclude several forms of bias: by randomizing patients to treatments, groups are made statistically equivalent at baseline, at least in theory, such that observed differences at the end of the trial can be attributed with more confidence to the intervention instead of group differences. By blinding patients, doctors, evaluators and biometricians, bias stemming from expectations and knowledge is precluded, as well as the possibility of fraud or subconscious preference on the part of raters, nurses or statisticians. Therefore RCTs, if possible double blind, seem to be the most rigorous methodological standard available for evaluating complementary and alternative medicine (CAM) (Ernst 1995, 1997, Ernst et al 1998). We do not know enough about CAM interventions and therefore have to employ methodologies which give us the highest possible certainty about the conclusions that we can draw from clinical studies. Internal validity is high and less likely to be challenged in RCTs, while other studies are often considered to be poor science, producing irrelevant results (Ernst 1998a).

While we do not question the accepted high internal validity produced by RCTs, we would nevertheless like to illustrate some of the weaknesses of the argument that RCTs are the primary design of choice for many types of medicine, including CAM. The main weakness derives from the fact that RCTs make presuppositions which often are not met in CAM interventions. We would also like to delineate where RCTs are the method of choice and where they are not. We argue for a staged and complementary methodological approach in evaluating CAM and finally we present some examples of outcomes research as a valuable tool in CAM evaluation.

THE PLACE OF RANDOMIZED CONTROLLED TRIALS IN THE EVALUATION OF MEDICAL INTERVENTIONS

Randomization and blinding, two procedures often combined in RCTs, are two methodological steps taken to enhance internal validity. Internal validity is usually defined as the certainty with which inferences from a study can be drawn because of its methodological soundness and rigor (Cook & Campbell 1979). In other words, internal validity reflects the fact that the method of a study makes the results reliable. Clinical trials usually attempt to enhance internal validity at the expense of external validity (Cook & Wittmann 1998, Wittmann 1985, 1988). External validity is often translated into generalizability, but it comprises much more than that. In social science external validity is sometimes referred to as ecological validity, i.e. the study should be valid in terms of the 'real world'. Not only should study results pertain to the specific population studied but they should also be applicable to a broader range of patients. The more a study is tailored to be internally valid – by randomizing patients to interventions, by blinding patients, practitioners and evaluators, by homogenizing patients using stringent inclusion and exclusion criteria – the less externally valid it becomes (Chen & Rossi 1981, 1983, Rossi & Freeman 1982).

Thus, there is a tension in any study between attempts to control internal validity, and so increase the accuracy of conclusions, and attempts to maximize external validity, and so increase generalizability: that is, the usefulness of the study information for practice. Ideally, it is best to attempt to maximize one or the other. Studies that mix the goals of security of conclusion and generalizability often give ambiguous information for either purpose (Feinstein 1989). These different goals for different types of clinical research information are reflected in the US Agency for Health Care Research and Policy's definitions of 'efficacy', which seeks to maximize internal validity, increase attributional value of a specific intervention and almost always requires RCTs, and 'effectiveness', which seeks to maximize external validity and obtain information about actual effects in broad practice (Gatchel & Maddrey 1998, Weeks 1997). A number of investigators have usefully applied this conceptualization to the research information on several conditions and therapies, including CAM (Gatchel & Maddrey 1998, Melchart et al 1997, Raskin & Maklan 1991, Schuck et al 1997, Standish et al 1997).

With this in mind, we can proceed to understand the place of RCTs in the evaluation of medical interventions. RCTs were formally introduced into the arsenal of research methodology at the Cornell Conference on Therapy in 1945 (Conferences on Therapy 1946, 1954), following Fisher's introduction of randomization as a statistical procedure to estimate bias in 1935 (Kaptchuk 1998, Kiene 1993). Blinding as a methodological procedure to eliminate observer, patient or doctor bias or all of them has a history dating back at least to 1784, when in France blinded experiments on Mesmerism were conducted, followed by the first trials of homeopathy in 1834 in Paris and 1842 in Nuremberg (Kaptchuk 1998).

Randomization is a statistical technique. In order to be able to randomize patients to treatment and control conditions, blinding to group assignment and randomization were usually employed conjointly, because only group assignment blinding made it possible to have confidence that balanced groups were obtained. In addition, blinding to the treatment received was also usually employed, not because this impacts group assignment but because patients would have known that they were not being treated and so might object. These procedures were deemed necessary because the psychological effects of being treated within a medical context had become obvious, acknowledging that pharmacologic effects always act in conjunction with the psychological effects of expectation, hope and knowledge (Kleijnen et al 1994). Blinding, therefore, usually became a corollary of RCTs in order to better ensure that the purpose of randomization was attained.

The expansion and subsequent broad application of RCTs were a consequence of the modern pharmaceutical era, where efficacy of a treatment is either not immediately obvious or unclear and small, compared to the effects attributable to the natural course of the disease or the therapeutic relationship. Thus, RCTs are typically used to evaluate a single component of an intervention, usually a new (or old) drug or, rarely, a surgical or medical procedure and its effects on a single aspect of the disease, usually an easily measured outcome. They are designed to find out whether an intervention has a specific effect over and above the non-specific effect of treatment and patient care. If we hypothesize that an intervention has a specific and additive (non-synergistic) effect in a certain condition, then an RCT can tease out this effect. An RCT answers one particular question and this question is always related to the specific efficacy of a particular intervention on a particular outcome over and above the contextual effects of the treatment in general or in comparison to another treatment.

From this, it becomes easier to identify when the application of a RCT is most likely to be useful and when it is not. RCTs can most likely achieve their goal when attribution and internal validity are most easily achieved and when precise measurement of specific causality is required. Attribution of causality is more easily achieved with RCTs when the diagnosis is discrete, easily defined and measured, the persons involved are in agreement as to what the most important outcome measure is, the intervention is simple, short and content based (as compared to process based), the outcome is easily defined and measured, certainty about the intervention must also be sufficiently lacking that providing alternative interventions becomes ethically acceptable and when the determination of the specific effect attributable to the intervention is essential (for example, when the intervention is high cost or risky or will be used to make large-scale population and public health decisions) and when it is reasonable to assume that the effect of the intervention is additive. Under these circumstances it is more likely that an experimental approach (such as a RCT) can usefully be employed. These conditions are most often met when a disease occurs over a short period of time and involves single domains so that multiple confounding factors have little time to influence the outcome. This type of research design best fits the biomedical model assumptions inherent in drug testing where tight cause-and-effect links can be measured under blind conditions.

THE PROBLEM OF EVALUATING CAM INTERVENTIONS

Problems with RCTs in CAM

It is important to ascertain whether a certain CAM intervention has a specific effect or not but this is quite a different task from the problem of evaluating a new, single pharmaceutical substance. Typically, in CAM we have a whole array of possible interventions or strategies for a given disease, which in most cases are applied with detailed individualization. This application is usually based on a disease assessment and classification different from those usually selected for homogeneity in clinical trials. For instance, in classical homeopathy, the target of treatment is not the nosological or diagnostic entity but a set of complex characteristics of the patient and all of their symptoms. Therefore, two patients with two different diseases end up with the same prescription because their symptom pictures are similar; on the other hand, two patients suffering from the same disease may receive different remedies. The same is true for acupuncture and indeed for many other types of CAM interventions.

While this does not preclude RCTs (Walach et al 1997a), it makes them more difficult and by the same token more sensitive to problems of external and internal validity (Walach 1996). To be considered well designed, a blinded RCT has to ask a single, very simple question, namely the question about specific efficacy and that frequently relates to a single intervention or a package of interventions. The question about specific efficacy of homeopathy, for instance, can and has been asked and answered in a series of well-conducted RCTs (Reilly & Taylor 1985, Reilly et al 1986, 1994) and in a recent metaanalysis of RCTs on homeopathy (Linde et al 1997). The results of these studies are that homeopathy does not appear to be a placebo, although not everybody in the field would go along with these conclusions (Ernst 1998b, Walach 1999). But what do these studies tell us about the effects of homeopathy in the real world? The particular intervention tested by Reilly, a variant of homeopathy called isopathy, is not representative of homeopathy as practiced by most doctors; rather, it was chosen because of its simplicity for testing using blinded RCT methods. And even if we know from these studies that isopathy in patients with allergic rhinitis and asthma is probably superior to placebo, we do not know whether it is a useful and effective treatment in a clinical context.

A similar situation exists when judging the value of acupuncture, where a recent consensus conference highlighted P6 acupuncture as having specific effects for nausea and vomiting (Lee & Done 1999). This conclusion arose because P6 acupuncture for nausea and vomiting meets most of the conditions listed above for the useful application of blind RCTs (simple intervention, clear outcome measure, short-term follow-up, blindability, etc.). However, acupuncturists rarely use P6 acupuncture alone for control of nausea and vomiting as it is felt to act synergistically with other points.

CAM practice usually involves an array of interventions, many with synergistic interactions, and we do not have the means to submit every single component and combination of components to RCTs in order to test their specific efficacy. Isolated RCTs usually provide a small amount of evidence at high cost. RCTs alone cannot provide the information which users, purchasers, providers, the medical profession and the public seek in relation to CAM. Such information can be useful for all these groups if the practice is high cost or high risk. However, for the majority of CAM practices that are low cost and low risk, this information is primarily of use for those involved in policy, payment and public health (population) decisions and is often of marginal value for individuals and practitioners making choices about therapies. This is because of the requirements previously outlined for obtaining accurate data from a RCT and because of some assumptions underlying RCTs that often do not exist in practice situations.

Problems with RCT assumptions

There are a couple of reasons why RCTs alone cannot provide the knowledge about CAM which is required.

RCTs as a research instrument designed to evaluate specific effects

With the design of an RCT to test a CAM intervention go several assumptions. These include the following:

- specific effects are the most valuable therapeutic effects an intervention can produce
- only the demonstration of specific effects over and above non-specific or synergistic effects defines a valid therapeutic intervention
- CAM interventions probably have such specific effects.

We would like to challenge all three of these assumptions.

While it might be true that it is necessary for new pharmaceuticals to prove superiority over and above non-specific effects of treatment such as hope, belief and expectation, it is by no means clear that the same applies to CAM. Pharmaceutical interventions are single interventions, usually derived from a more or less elaborate theory about pathology and detailed mechanisms. Pharmaceuticals are designed to influence usually one or more well-defined physiological systems in order to alleviate a specific symptom or cascade of reactions. Therefore, it is a fair question to ask whether a drug really has this purported or hypothesized action. This question can only be tested in a placebo-controlled RCT. In CAM we usually have a very complex theoretical model of disease, which demands complex interventions. The illness model itself fulfils the function of a treatment rationale and this is not validated by an RCT. While the model in itself could be outside the realm of empirical testing, as may be the case for much of CAM, it could well be that the actions inspired by it are safe and effective. Placebo-controlled RCTs are precise instruments designed to dissect a single hypothesis of pharmacological specificity. In CAM interventions the hypothesis is much more diverse.

There is the implicit assumption and scientific prejudice that only specific effects are of therapeutic benefit (Grünbaum 1985, 1989). The prejudice of specificity, as we might call it, is a consequence of the era of pharmacology and targeting single diagnostic or etiologic entities with single pharmacological (or surgical) interventions. It is the heir to Virchow's cellular pathology model of disease (Uexküll & Wesiack 1988). This model, however, has long since been superseded by the biopsychosocial model of disease and health (sometimes called the systemic or biosemiotic model) (Engel 1981, 1982, Uexküll 1995). As soon as one realizes that disease is a complex phenomenon which not only has a multifaceted causality but can also be influenced by a multitude of possible routes, pharmacological specificity being just one of them, the question of specific efficacy becomes only one of many possible meaningful questions. For instance, while pharmacological interventions seek to block or eliminate pathology, most naturopathic or CAM approaches try to influence the system as a whole, in theory relying on a self-regulation process. It could be hypothesized that CAM interventions instill hope, thereby influencing the psycho-neuro-endocrinological axis (Frank 1989), or that they redress a delicate balance of physiological systems.

The decisive point here is that CAM interventions usually have theoretical models that underpin their specific actions but they need not necessarily employ specific processes to achieve their goals. For example, specificity in the light of the CAM theory need not be specificity in terms of the therapeutic and physiological processes but in terms of whole-organism sensitivity and reactivity. Therefore, although CAM interventions are purportedly based on specific interventions, a variety of these theories might be incorrect. Most of what CAM practitioners do might relate to the non-specific and dynamic stimulation of a self-healing response. This, incidentally, might also be true for pharmacological interventions (Frank 1989). While specificity is theoretically the most powerful component, non-specific or synergistic effects might be the most therapeutically powerful in practice. If the questions we ask only relate to specificity, then non-specific and synergistic effects are overlooked.

Every therapeutic theory necessarily has a claim to make about specific effects. This applies to psychotherapy, pharmacological treatments and also to CAM interventions. While for psychotherapy this claim is all but empirically validated (Arnkoff et al 1993, Dawes 1994, Fischer et al 1998, Rosenzweig 1936, Strupp & Hadley 1979, Wampold et al 1997a, b, Weinberger 1993, 1995), it might also be true for pharmacological interventions that non-specific effects are more important than usually acknowledged (Moerman et al 1996). It is pure (and unnecessary) speculation to suggest that CAM interventions are specific and that this specificity is at the core of their therapeutic efficacy. Therapeutic interventions need theories about their specificity but it does not follow that therapeutic effects brought about by such an intervention are due to its hypothesized specific effects. The theory of specificity might be necessary to guide therapeutic action and to suggest therapeutic interventions which appear to be individual and specific, but which, in the end, might turn out to be nothing more than mechanisms designed to bring about non-specific effects. Moerman (1983) has shown that placebo responses in RCTs of cimetidine in duodenal ulcers demonstrate huge variation in non-specific effects which themselves determine the significance of a particular study. Its non-specific effects – comprising the effects of general care, circumstantial effects, dietary treatments, psychological effects, natural course of the disease – are approximately two-thirds of the therapeutic effect, while the pharmacological effect adds another third. There is no reason to presume that the outcome would be different for CAM.

Consider the following thought experiment (Fig. 2.1). Treatment A in xy-disease produces a positive response rate in 70% of the patients. After close scrutiny one finds out that 65% of this effect is non-specific. Treatment B, provided in the same disease and in the same type of patients and measured by the same outcome instruments, produces a response rate in 50% of the patients, 20% being due to non-specific

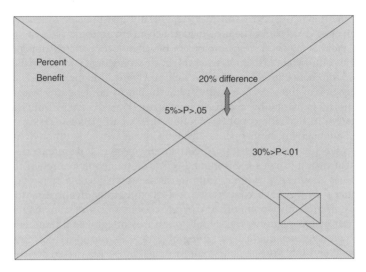

Figure 2.1   Consequences of differences in specific and non-specific effects in clinical trials.

and 30% to specific effects. The net effect in the first example is 5% specific efficacy, which probably would not be statistically or clinically significant, without very large numbers of subjects. The net effect in the second experiment would be 30% specificity, six times the effect of example A, and would likely reach statistical and clinical significance with a few subjects. Intervention A, however, might be more valuable from a practical point of view, since 70% of patients given it would get better while only 50% would get better with the proven intervention B. The point to emphasize is that if the standard of comparison is the magnitude of non-specific effects and if this standard changes depending on the nature of the intervention, then our measuring instrument is variable and results in changing standards of evidence for evaluation of a therapy by not adjusting for the nature of the intervention. We presume that this could be an issue in the evaluation of CAM.

Equipoise

RCTs presuppose that both doctor and patient are indifferent about the treatment options (Black 1996). This is termed 'equipoise' in clinical research and is considered a requirement for the ethical testing of a therapy in a RCT. Equipoise is usually present in new pharmaceuticals and so blinded RCTs are ethically the method of choice when evaluating new drugs. These preconditions are, however, rarely met with CAM. Usually the doctor has a long experience with and hence bias towards his intervention while patients also have strong preferences and are usually seeing a CAM practitioner for definite reasons (Furnham 1994, Furnham & Forey 1994, Furnham & Kirkcaldy 1996, Furnham et al 1995, Vincent & Furnham 1996). Therefore, if we want to evaluate CAM in a pragmatic environment that is provided by experienced practitioners and in patients with strong preferences, a RCT may not be the best option to produce the maximal therapeutic response and may be ethically questionable for many participants. However, CAM should be used in just such an environment if the study is to be externally valid. It may be a strong preference which induces patients to spend money, take risks and thus engage them in what might be an essential part of the therapeutic effect of CAM. These effects can never be captured by RCTs alone.

Probably one of the most internally valid studies of homeopathy was our own trial of classical homeopathy in chronic headaches (Walach et al 1997a). The results were negative in that homeopathy was not superior to placebo. This was subsequently challenged by homeopaths, even by those who co-authored the study, because patients had not chosen this treatment themselves but were recruited via a publicity campaign (Lowes & Springer 1997). The homeopaths argued that these patients were completely different from those seen by clinicians in everyday practice and that they were less cooperative and trusting, thus invalidating the results from an external validity point of view. While cooperation and trust may not be an integral part of homeopathic theory (although it is integral to a number of CAM systems), self-selection might be an integral part of its purported effectiveness. If this is true, then RCTs are less able to capture this purported preference-dependent effect.

While the above-mentioned points are unique problems in RCTs of CAM, there are serious problems of RCTs in general (Black 1996, Feinstein 1980, 1998).

- RCTs cannot be used for every intervention because of limited resources.
- Results of RCTs often are of limited practical usefulness because patients studied within RCTs are often not patients seen in everyday practice. Patients in real life are often co-morbid and pose several treatment problems which designers of RCTs try to avoid by tailoring exclusion criteria so that a homogeneous sample is studied.
- The methodological soundness of blinded RCTs can be challenged because often the blinding is broken by patients and doctors cheating or easily guessing the treatment group because of side effects in the active treatment. These well-described methodological shortcomings are rarely addressed when evaluating the evidence for a treatment (Melchart et al 1998).
- Publication bias is considerable, since funding often comes from the pharmaceutical industry which has the power to suppress unwanted results (Antonuccio et al 1999, Dickersin & Min 1993, Dickersin et al 1987). Thus, evidence synthesized in metaanalyses and systematic reviews may be positively biased.

Learning from psychotherapy research

Psychotherapy research (PTR) can serve as a good example. Few would challenge the overall effectiveness of psychotherapy (PT), although a number of problems remain to be resolved (Garfield & Bergin 1986, Grawe et al 1994). In a first phase, PTR modelled its methods according to the medical approach, until quasi-blinded and placebo-controlled studies were questioned. It became apparent that any intervention, even a placebo intervention, had therapeutic impact and thus could not serve as a control (Horvath 1988, Kirsch 1978, Wilkins 1985). In consequence, mainly randomized, but also non-randomized, and open comparison trials were conducted, many of them against waiting-list control groups. This, then, became a standard design in PTR, apart from single case research designs.

Seligman (1995) has argued that RCTs of PT were rarely, if ever, relevant to clinical practice (see above). He presented and advocated outcomes research as a means of evaluating PT. Of 22 000 people who answered a customer questionnaire, 7000 answered questions about mental health, of whom 4100 reported experience with mental health professionals. Out of these single items, the authors constructed a multivariate index of effectiveness, which yielded clearcut results. Of those who said that at the beginning of treatment their status was very bad, 87% reported improvement. Those with longer treatment improved more. Pharmacological treatment added to PT yielded no extra benefit. Trained professionals were more effective in the long run than paraprofessionals and freedom of choice and activity on part of the patient were associated with better results. These results were equally valid for various schools of PT. These results can all be challenged; the self-selection of the respondents and the uncontrolled design are issues that need to be addressed. However, the large number of respondents and comparatively long observation periods, added to the already existing evidence, enabled this method to fulfill an important function in the overall pattern of evidence available for PT. These data answer questions about overall effectiveness of PT in real life and therefore have great external validity.

THE PLACE OF OUTCOMES RESEARCH IN CAM

CAM is in a position similar to that of psychotherapy in the 1960s, when Eysenck had questioned its efficacy (Eysenck 1952). Everybody practicing PT was sure that it worked but proof was lacking. PT is a complex intervention and, as with CAM, it makes little sense to ask about specific ingredients. It is of great importance to learn from the early mistakes in PTR which enhanced internal validity at the expense of pragmatism and external validity. This created a monoculture, relying exclusively on RCTs to answer questions about effectiveness.

Without questioning the methodological validity and rigor of the RCT, we would like to challenge its role as the sole arbiter of effectiveness. There are evaluation problems in CAM, in which large-scale outcomes studies may be just as good as RCTs if certain boundary conditions are met (Black 1998). If, for instance, expected effects are large or very large, then RCTs are not necessary because effects are so obvious. Penicillin was never tested in RCTs because its effects were obvious. Careful observation was enough to ascertain the usefulness of this intervention. Secondly, if the natural course of a disease is known and its prognosis can be estimated or if the baseline status is fairly stable, then clear and lasting effects, documented over a long observation period, can be a very persuasive argument. This is the case in most chronic conditions, such as chronic pain, chronic atopic conditions, rheumatological diseases or chronic inflammatory bowel diseases. In all these instances patients and doctors are often desperately looking for interventions which are effective, be they specific or non-specific, because patients have a long history of often ineffective treatment.

While a single observed case does not add much to our knowledge, a large number observed over a long time period can provide strong evidence. Furthermore, if this is generated by a large number of different patients involving many practitioners, then a large-scale outcomes study yields more useful evidence than a RCT. It is not usually feasible, moreover, to conduct RCTs over prolonged periods of time, especially if blinding is important or a treatment preference exists. With the help of a good documentation system which documents sequential treatments without selection or with the cooperation of insurance companies (Walach et al 1996, 1997b) it is possible to compile large databases of treatment outcomes at comparatively moderate costs. These data can answer questions as to overall effectiveness of interventions in patients with chronic diseases. Apart from that and by virtue of the large number of patients, predictive regression and other analysis models can be used which relate prognostic characteristics of patients, treatment and doctors to outcome.

CRITERIA FOR OUTCOMES RESEARCH IN CAM

Outcomes research in CAM could be considered as an alternative to a RCT if the following conditions are met.

- The question is about general practical effectiveness rather than efficacy.
- The question whether effects are specific or non-specific is irrelevant (as it is when the intervention is patient oriented and practice guided or involves patient cooperation and learning or individualization and variability).
- The natural course and prognosis of the condition are well described.
- The patients to be studied have a well-documented history of their previous treatments.
- Effects are expected to be large from clinical experience.
- A large number of patients can be entered over long periods of time (years).
- The research covers at least the period which is known from the literature to be representative for the average time to relapse in recurrent or fluctuating diseases.
- A well-known, widely used and valid outcome measure, such as a visual analogue scale or SF-36, is used so that results can be seen and interpreted in relation to other studies in both CAM and conventional medicine.

If all these conditions are met, then an observational outcome study probably is the best and most cost-effective research option. There certainly are problems still to be solved in long-term observational studies, like the handling of patient attrition and missing data. The procedures to be used here do not differ from standard procedures in clinical trials (Curran et al 1998). Sensitivity analyses will have to be employed to estimate effects under different assumptions. In addition, decision analysis methods, with patient input, will need to be used when applying the results (a procedure that should also be used when applying RCT data to patient decisions).

A STAGED APPROACH TO CAM RESEARCH

Ultimately, outcomes research should be one step in a staged approach to CAM research. No single research methodology in itself yields all the knowledge necessary with respect to effectiveness, efficacy, safety and patient/doctor treatment preferences. Table 2.1 is an attempt to systematize methodologies according to research questions and the audience for which the information is most useful.

Table 2.1 Research questions, methods, addressees, shortcomings of methods and solutions

Question	Method	Addressee	Shortcoming	Solution
1 General effectiveness in normal practice	Prospective documentation, outcomes studies	General public, purchasers, practitioners, scientific community	Open to bias, only unspecific effects	Large numbers, long periods, well-documented baseline, chronic and severe problems
2 Cost effectiveness, effectiveness compared to conventional treatment in patients with preferences	Non-randomized, quasi-experimental comparisons	General public, purchasers, practitioners, scientific community	Comparability has to be achieved statistically	Good planning, statistical expertise
3 Effectiveness against natural course of disease	Open, waiting-list controlled RCTs	General public, purchasers, practitioners, scientific community	Only feasible for a limited time	Back results with outcome data
4 Comparative effectiveness without preference	Randomized, open comparisons of CAM vs conventional treatment	Purchasers, scientific community	Patient attrition due to preferences, low external validity	Back results with outcome data
5 Specific efficacy	Blinded, placebo-controlled RCT	Scientific community, purchasers	Low external validity, low relevance to patients	Back results with outcome and comparison data

Table 2.1 describes a hierarchy and circularity in method. What is generally agreed to be the gold-standard, blinded RCTs, appear last in our list, not because the evidence has the least value but because this type of evidence is the most difficult and expensive to obtain and because it presupposes knowledge about all the other types of questions, at least implicitly. Because the evidence for specific efficacy is usually achieved in artificial settings it has to be grounded contextually through outcome data in order to be practical and useful. The table therefore describes not only a hierarchy but also a circle. Methods of high external but low internal validity, like RCTs and outcomes study, are not mutually exclusive but complement each other (United States General Accounting Office 1992). Note that the primary audiences for which the information is most useful change. The question of specific efficacy is largely irrelevant to patients, who usually just want a fair chance to get better regardless of the underlying mechanisms or precision of attribution. It is most cherished by the scientific community because studies addressing this question have the highest scientific merit and lead to better planning of future research

and more efficacy in purchasing and public health policy. However, studies addressing the question of general practical effectiveness are not highly valued scientifically but are often more worthwhile from a practical, patient-orientated and political viewpoint. Thus, the implicit hierarchy can also be envisaged as a circle. Depending on the question and the individuals requiring the data, one could start anywhere, bearing in mind that no single method will solve all problems. RCTs and outcomes research can also be executed together, by nesting one within the other or following a RCT with a long-term observational phase (Linde & Jonas 1999).

A type of study which is nearly completely neglected in CAM research is the non-randomized or quasi-experimental comparison (Abel & Koch 1998, Cook & Campbell 1979). The great benefit of this type of research methodology lies in the fact that it works with natural groups, thus honoring patients' and doctors' preferences and being close to clinical practice. Studies of this type are often shunned by researchers because one rarely knows beforehand whether the respective groups will be comparable. In order to be able to balance the groups, one has to understand and document the relevant prognostic variables, which usually necessitates at least as much planning as that of a classical RCT. The statistical expertise needed to evaluate these studies is often greater than for RCTs, but such methods do exist (Rosenbaum & Rubin 1983, Rubin 1998).

An argument often raised against outcomes studies is that pure observation can only indirectly discern the effects of treatment from the effects of time. Although this should be less of a problem with stable or worsening chronic diseases and large numbers of patients, one needs to address this question. In this case a waiting-list controlled RCT with open treatment can be a solution. Our own experience with such designs in a study of healing was positive (Wiesendanger et al 2001). If the treatment is sought after by patients and the waiting period is not too long (in our study it was 5 months) patients will comply. At least the natural course of the disease can be controlled this way, although the length of treatment is necessarily limited by the feasibility of the waiting period, which for organizational and ethical reasons would not usually be extended beyond 6 months.

EXAMPLES

What knowledge is actually provided by outcomes studies? Our own ongoing documentation in collaboration with a German insurance company of 5000 patients seeking acupuncture or homeopathy shows a patient-reported improvement rate of roughly 70% after acupuncture treatments in patients with a mean disease history of 8 years (Güthlin et al 1998, Walach et al 1996, 1997b, 1998). These rates are reflected in a significant and clinically meaningful (Lydick & Yawn 1998) 10 to 20-point improvement in the SF-36. As yet we have not evaluated follow-up data so we do not know whether these results will remain stable over the 4-year follow-up. If they should turn out to be stable this would be a strong argument for the clinical usefulness of acupuncture and homeopathy. It certainly would not answer the question about whether these methods are specifically efficacious or only non-specifically effective. However, this would matter little to those patients seeking symptom relief for chronic illness in whom conventional medicine has frequently proved to be ineffective.

Experience from acupuncture trials shows that rates of effectiveness in uncontrolled practice can be quite high but drop within the context of controlled trials, although therapist and treatment style have remained the same. This points to the fact that clinical results are probably highly context dependent which argues in favor of a multistaged research approach (Dowson et al 1985, Lewith & Vincent 1996).

Between 1979 and 1982 one of us (GL) ran an open referral acupuncture clinic in the Department of Primary Care at the University of Southampton. Data on patients with headache were recorded at entry to acupuncture treatment and all patients followed up at 3, 6 and 12 months after treatment (Lewith & Machin 1981). On the basis of this uncontrolled outcome study, we established that 80% of our patients with migraine-like headaches did experience a 30% improvement 3 months after treatment. We therefore designed a RCT involving mock TENS as a placebo/control. This study involved the same doctors working in the same practice environment and setting as our open referral clinic. We entered patients with headache who had not previously received acupuncture but were prepared to enter our clinical trial as they had not responded effectively to conventional treatment. Our results suggest that no more than 50% of patients responded to acupuncture treatment in the context of a randomized controlled study, again measured as a 30% improvement on baseline 3 months after the completion of treatment. We have no real idea why our response rate dropped by 30% from an open referral clinic to an RCT, particularly when we consider that on both occasions the primary method of measuring outcome was patient-based questionnaires (Dowson et al 1985). We can only assume that some non-specific effect, introduced when patients were randomized and blinded, came into play. The available evidence is very confusing for a potential purchaser or public health official. Should they be guided by clinical outcome or an RCT and how do they judge the validity of the data? It is clear that in open practice, however, individual patients who seek out CAM for their migraine with these practitioners can expect the higher response rates.

Outcomes research can be a valuable tool in evaluating CAM interventions. It cannot replace controlled and well-established trial methodology but it can and should complement it in important ways. It adds the flavor of practical relevance and external validity to the otherwise detached research efforts of RCTs. It is also an important instrument in gathering data which cannot be gleaned from RCTs: data on long-term effects, on patients who do not wish to be randomized, patients with strong preferences and belief systems; in short, on typical users of CAM. Outcomes research needs RCTs in order to strengthen and qualify its results. It is not a short cut attempting to influence members of the public and purchasers but part of the landscape of evidence needed to evaluate CAM. As such, sponsors, reviewers and the scientific community at large should be urged to be more open-minded about unconventional methods for CAM research, as these are particularly needed in the evaluation of chronic illness.

REFERENCES

Abel U, Koch A 1998 The mythology of randomization. In: Abel U, Koch A (eds) Nonrandomized comparative clinical studies. Symposon Publishing, Düsseldorf, pp 27–40

Antonuccio DO, Danton WG, DeNelsky GY, Greenberg RP, Gordon JS 1999 Raising questions about antidepressants. Psychotherapy and Psychosomatics 68: 3–14

Arnkoff DB, Victor BJ, Glass CR 1993 Empirical research on factors in psychotherapeutic change. In: Stricker G, Gold JR (eds) Comprehensive handbook of psychotherapy integration. Plenum, New York, pp 27–42

Black N 1996 Why we need observational studies to evaluate the effectiveness of health care. British Medical Journal 312: 1215–1218

Black N 1998 Why we need observational studies to evaluate the effectiveness of health care. In: Abel U, Koch A (eds) Nonrandomized comparative clinical studies. Symposion Publishing, Düsseldorf, pp 15–25

Chen H, Rossi PH 1981 The multi-goal, theory-driven approach to evaluation: a model linking basic and applied social science. Evaluation Studies Review Annual 6: 38–54

Chen HT, Rossi PH 1983 Evaluating with sense. The theory-driven approach. Evaluation Review 7: 283–302

Conferences on Therapy 1946 The use of placebos in therapy. New York Journal of Medicine 46: 1718–1727

Conferences on Therapy 1954 How to evaluate a new drug. American Journal of Medicine 17: 722–727

Cook TD, Campbell DT 1979 Quasi-experimentation design and analysis issues for field settings. Rand McNally, Chicago

Cook TD, Wittmann WW 1998 Lessons learned about evaluation in the United States and some possible implications for Europe. European Journal of Psychological Assessment 14: 97–115

CPMP Working Party on Efficacy of Medicinal Products 1995 Biostatistical methodology in clinical trials in applications for marketing authorizations for medicinal products. Note for guidance III/3630/92-EN. Statistics in Medicine 14: 1659–1682

Curran D, Fayers PM, Molenberghs G et al 1998 Analysis of incomplete quality of life data in clinical trials. In: Staquet MJ, Hays RD, Fayers PM (eds) Quality of life assessment in clinical trials. Methods and practice. Oxford University Press, Oxford, pp 249–280

Dawes RM 1994 House of cards: psychology and psychotherapy built on myth. Free Press, New York

Dickersin K, Min YI 1993 Publication bias: the problem that won't go away. Annals of the New York Academy of Sciences 703: 135–148

Dickersin K, Chan SS, Chalmers TC, Sacks HS, Smith HJ 1987 Publication bias and clinical trials. Controlled Clinical Trials 8: 343–353

Dowson DI, Lewith GT, Machin D 1985 The effects of acupuncture versus placebo in the treatment of headache. Pain 21: 35–42

Engel GL 1981 The need for a new medical model: a challenge for biomedicine. In: Capla AL, Engelhardt T, McCartney J (eds) Concepts of health and disease. Addison-Wesley, Reading, MA

Engel GL 1982 The biopsychosocial model and medical education. New England Journal of Medicine 306: 802–805

Ernst E 1995 Complementary medicine: common misconceptions. Journal of the Royal Society of Medicine 88: 244–247

Ernst E 1997 Integrating complementary medicine? Journal of the Royal Society of Health 117: 285–286

Ernst E 1998a Studien ohne eine Kontrollgruppe können auf unterschiedliche Art interpretiert werden! Naturamed 13(4): 7

Ernst E 1998b Are highly dilute homoeopathic remedies placebos? Perfusion 11: 291–292

Ernst E, De Smet PAGM, Shaw D, Murray V 1998 Traditional remedies and the 'test of time'. European Journal of Clinical Pharmacology 54: 99–100

Eysenck HJ 1952 The effects of psychotherapy: an evaluation. Journal of Consulting Psychology 16: 319–324

Feinstein A 1980 Should placebo-controlled trials be abolished? European Journal of Clinical Pharmacology 17: 1–4

Feinstein AR 1989 Epidemiologic analyses of causation: the unlearned scientific lessons of randomized trials. Journal of Epidemiology 42: 481–489

Feinstein 1998 Prodems of randomized trials. In: Abel U, Koch A (eds) Nonrandomized comparative clinical studies. Symposion Publishing, Düsseldorf, pp 1–13

Fischer AR, Jome LRM, Atkinson DR 1998 Reconceptualizing multicultural counseling: universal healing conditions in a culturally specific context. Counseling Psychologist 26: 525–588

Frank JD 1989 Non-specific aspects of treatment: the view of a psychotherapist. In: Shepherd M, Sartorius N (eds) Non-specific aspects of treatment. Huber, Berne, pp 95–114

Furnham A 1994 Explaining health and illness: lay perceptions on current and future health, the causes of illness, and the nature of recovery. Social Science and Medicine 39: 715–725

Furnham A, Forey J 1994 The attitudes, behaviors and beliefs of patients of conventional vs. complementary (alternative) medicine. Journal of Clinical Psychology 50(3): 458–469

Furnham A, Kirkcaldy B 1996 The health beliefs and behaviours of orthodox and complementary medicine clients. British Journal of Clinical Psychology 35: 49–61

Furnham A, Vincent C, Wood R 1995 The health beliefs and behaviors of three groups of complementary medicine and a general practice group of patients. Journal of Alternative and Complementary Medicine 1: 347–359

Garfield SL, Bergin AE (eds) 1986 Handbook of psychotherapy and behavior change. Wiley, New York

Gatchel RJ, Maddrey AM 1998 Clinical outcome research in complementary and alternative medicine: an overview of experimental design and analysis. Alternative Therapies in Health and Medicine 4: 36–42

Grawe K, Donati R, Bernauer F 1994 Psychotherapie in Wandel. Von der Konfession zur Profession. Hogrefe, Göttingen

Grünbaum A 1985 Explication and implications of the placebo concept. In: White L, Tursky B, Schwartz GE (eds) Placebo – theory, research, mechanisms. Guilford Press, New York

Grünbaum A 1989 The placebo concept in medicine and psychiatry. In: Shepherd M, Sartorius N (eds) Non-specific aspects of treatment. Huber, Stuttgart

Güthlin C, Walach H, Heinrich S et al 1998 Outcomeforschung in der Komplementärmedizin: Ein Evaluationskonzept und erste Ergebnisse. In: Bullinger M, Morfeld M, Ravens-Sieberer U, Koch U (eds) Medizinische Psychologie in einem sich wandelnden Gesundheitssystem: Identität, Integration & Interdisziplinarität (12. Kongress der Deutschen Gesellschaft für Medizinische Psychologie). Pabst Science Publishers, Lengerich

Horvath P 1988 Placebos and common factors in two decades of psychotherapeutic research. Psychological Bulletin 104: 214–225

Kaptchuk TJ 1998 Intentional ignorance: a history of blind assessment and placebo controls in medicine. Bulletin of the History of Medicine 72: 389–433

Kiene H 1993 Kritik der klinischen Doppelblindstudie. MMV Medizinverlag, München

Kirsch I 1978 The placebo effect and the cognitive-behavioral revolution. Cognitive Therapy and Research 2: 255–264

Kleijnen J, De Craen AJM, Van Everdingen J, Krol L 1994 Placebo effect in double-blind clinical trials: a review of interactions with medications. Lancet 344: 1347–1349

Lee A, Done ML 1999 The use of nonpharmacologic techniques to prevent postoperative nausea and vomiting: a meta-analysis. Anaesthesiology and Analgesia 88: 1362–1369

Lewith GT, Machin D 1981 A method of assessing the clinical effects of acupuncture. Acupuncture and Electrotherapeutic Research 6: 265–276

Lewith GT, Vincent C 1996 On the evaluation of the clinical effects of acupuncture: a problem reassessed and a framework for future research. Journal of Alternative and Complementary Medicine 2: 79–90

Linde K, Jonas WB 1999 Evaluating complementary and alternative medicine: the balance of rigor and relevance. In: Jonas WB, Levin JS (eds) Essentials of complementary and alternative medicine. Lippincott Williams and Wilkins, Philadelphia

Linde K, Clausius N, Ramirez G, Melchart D, Eitel F, Hedges LV, Jonas WB 1997 Are the clinical effects of homoeopathy placebo effects? A meta-analysis of placebo controlled trials. Lancet 350: 834–843

Lowes T, Springer W 1997 Nachlese zur Münchener homöopathischen Kopfschmerzstudie. Allgemeine Homöopathische Zeitung 242: 224–230

Lydick E, Yawn BP 1998 Clinical interpretation of health-related quality of life data. In: Staquet MJ, Hays RD, Fayers PM (eds) Quality of life assessment in clinical trials. Methods and practice. Oxford University Press, Oxford

Melchart D, Linde K, Liao JZ, Hager S, Weidenhammer W 1997 Systematic clinical auditing in complementary medicine: rationale, concept, and a pilot study. Alternative Therapies in Health and Medicine 3: 33–39

Melchart D, Walther E, Linde K, Brandmaier R, Lersch C 1998 Echinacea root extracts for the prevention of upper respiratory tract infections. A double-blind, placebo-controlled randomized trial. Archives of Family Medicine 7: 541–545

Moerman DE 1983 General medical effectiveness and human biology: placebo effects in the treatment of ulcer disease. Medical Anthropology Quarterly 14: 3–16

Moerman DE, Jonas WB, Bush PJ et al 1996 Placebo effects and research in alternative and conventional medicine. Chinese Journal of Integrated Traditional and Western Medicine 2: 141–148

Raskin I, Maklan C 1991 Medical treatment effectiveness research. Evaluation and the Health Profession 14: 161–186

Reilly D, Taylor MA 1985 Potent placebo or potency? British Homoeopathic Journal 74: 65–75

Reilly D, Taylor MA, McSharry C, Aitchinson T 1986 Is homoeopathy a placebo response? Controlled trial of homoeopathic potency with pollen in hayfever as a model. Lancet 18: 881–886

Reilly D, Taylor MA, Beattie NGM, Campbell JH, McSharry C 1994 Is evidence for homoeopathy reproducible? Lancet 344: 1601–1606

Rosenbaum PR, Rubin DB 1983 The central role of the propensity score in observational studies for causal effects. Biometrika 70: 41–55

Rosenzweig S 1936 Some implicit common factors in diverse methods in psychotherapy. American Journal of Orthopsychiatry 6: 412–415

Rossi PH, Freeman HE 1982 Evaluation. A systematic approach, 2nd edn. Sage, Beverly Hills

Rubin DB 1998 Estimation from nonrandomized treatment comparisons using subclassification on propensity scores. In: Abel U, Koch A (eds) Nonrandomized comparative clinical studies. Symposium Publishing, Düsseldorf, pp 85–100

Schuck JR, Chappell LT, Kindness G 1997 Causal modeling and alternative medicine. Alternative Therapies in Health and Medicine 3: 40–47

Seligman M 1995 The effectiveness of psychotherapy. American Psychologist 50: 965–974

Standish LJ, Calabrese C, Reeves C, Polissar N, Bain S, O'Donnell T 1997 A scientific plan for the evaluation of alternative medicine in the treatment of HIV/AIDS. Alternative Therapies in Health and Medicine 3: 58–67

Strupp HH, Hadley SW 1979 Specific vs. nonspecific factors in psychotherapy. Archives of General Psychiatry 36: 1125–1136

Uexküll TV 1995 Biosemiotic research and not further molecular analysis is necessary to describe pathways between cells, personalities, and social systems. Advances. Journal of Mind-Body Health 11: 24–27

Uexküll TV, Wesiack W 1988 Theorie der Humanmedizin. Grundlagen ärztlichen Denkens and Handelns. Urban and Schwarzenberg, München

United States General Accounting Office 1992 Cross design synthesis. A new strategy for medical effectiveness research. Report No B244808. US GAO, Washington DC

Vincent C, Furnham A 1996 Why do patients turn to complementary medicine? An empirical study. British Journal of Clinical Psychology 35: 37–48

Walach H 1996 Verblindung in klinischen Homöopathie-Studien? In: Hornung J (ed) Forschungsmethoden in der Komplementärmedizin. Über die Notwendigkeit einer methodologischen Erneuerung. Schattauer, Stuttgart

Walach H 1999 Magic of signs: a nonlocal interpretation of homoeopathy. Journal of Scientific Exploration 13: 291–315

Walach H, Brednich A, Heinrich S, Esser P 1996 Das Erprobungsverfahren der Innungskrankenkassen zu Homöopathie und Akupunktur. Evaluationskonzept und erste Erfahrungen. Forschende Komplementärmedizin 3: 12–20

Walach H, Gaus W, Haeusler W et al 1997a Classical homoeopathic treatment of chronic headaches. A double-blind, randomized, placebo-controlled study. Cephalalgia 17: 119–126

Walach H, Schüller S, Heinrich S, Esser P 1997b The test phase of the Innungskrankenkassen on acupuncture and homoeopathy (abstract). Forschende Komplementärmedizin 4: 121

Walach H, Güthlin C, Heinrich S, Esser P 1998 Effects of acupuncture and homeopathy: a prospective documentation. Intermediate results. Alternative Therapies in Health and Medicine 4: 105

Wiesendanger H, Werthmüller L, Reuter K, Walach H 2001 Chronically ill patients treated by spiritual healing improve in quality of life: results of a randomised waiting-list controlled study. Journal of Alternative and Complementary Medicine 7: 45–51

Wampold BE, Mondin GW, Moody M, Ahn H 1997a The flat earth as a metaphor for the evidence for uniform efficacy of bona fide psychotherapies: reply to Crits-Christoph (1997) and Howard et al. (1997). Psychological Bulletin 122: 226–230

Wampold BE, Mondin GW, Moody M, Stich F, Benson K, Ahn H 1997b A meta-analysis of outcome studies comparing bonafide psychotherapies: empirically, 'All must have prizes'. Psychological Bulletin 122: 203–215

Weeks J 1997 Operational issues in incorporating complementary and alternative therapies and providers in benefit plans and managed care organizations. Agency for Health Care Policy and Research, Bethesda, MD

Weinberger J 1993 Common factors in psychotherapy. In: Stricker G, Gold JR (eds) Comprehensive handbook of psychotherapy integration. Plenum, New York

Weinberger J 1995 Common factors aren't so common: the common factors dilemma. Clinical Psychology: Science and Practice 2: 45–69

Wilkins W 1985 Placebo controls and concepts in chemotherapy and psychotherapy research. In: White L, Tursky B, Schwartz GE (eds) Placebo – theory, research, mechanisms. Guilford Press, New York

Wittmann W 1985 Evaluationsforschung. Aufgaben, Probleme und Anwendungen. Springer, Berlin

Wittmann W 1988 Multivariate reliability theory: principles of symmetry and successful validation strategies. In: Nesselroade JR, Cattell RB (eds) Handbook of multivariate experimental psychology, 2nd edn. Plenum Press, New York

3

Inspiration and perspiration: what every researcher needs to know before they start

Andrew J Vickers

INTRODUCTION

Art, we are often told, is 10% inspiration and 90% perspiration. The moment of brilliance on stage or on the art gallery wall is the result of thousands of hours of learning, planning, rehearsal and laborious attention to fine detail.

A similar adage for science might be: '10% statistics, 90% logistics'. As a clinical researcher, I spend less time devising protocols, analysing results and writing papers than I do organizing staff, checking work that I have delegated, sorting out financial administration and programming databases.

Research is a *practical* business and unless you get the practicalities right, your research will fail, no matter how brilliant its design or conception. Unfortunately, few methodology books will tell you this. This chapter will review some of the practical aspects of research. My aim is to give some simple advice and guidelines based on my own personal experience as a researcher.

QUESTIONS

Defining the question

Research is a tool for answering questions. Unless you know what your question is, you will be unable to design your research. A good proportion of those who ask me for advice on research find it hard to frame a simple question to illustrate their research interest, even after repeated prompting. For example, one researcher told me that his question was 'to demonstrate the effectiveness of herbal medicine for cystitis' and another 'to investigate massage for cancer patients'. These are clearly not questions.

I have three general guidelines for defining a research question.

Questions should be in four parts

Many questions in health research can be formulated in four parts.

- An intervention
- A comparison
- An outcome measure
- A population

Each of these four parts can be seen in this question for a clinical trial: 'What are the effects of acupuncture compared to no acupuncture on headache, health status, days off sick and resource use in patients with chronic headache in primary care?'.

The four-part question can be applied to many other types of research, including prognosis (e.g. 'What proportion of coronary heart disease patients who develop heart failure will die compared to those who do not develop heart failure?') and diagnosis ('What is the reproducibility of IgG/IgE testing for food intolerance in patients with chronic disease'?). In the last case, the 'intervention' is IgG/IgE testing and the 'comparison' is a second test.

Not all forms of research involve a comparison and in these cases the four-part question becomes the three-part question. Examples include case series ('What is the average reduction in pain scores [outcome measure] in pain clinic patients [population] undertaking an integrated package of care [intervention]?') or surveys ('What proportion of UK adults [population] have seen a practitioner [outcome measure] of complementary medicine [intervention]?'). Some research questions, particularly qualitative studies, are difficult to put into the three- or four-part format; nonetheless, the format remains a useful rule of thumb.

Questions should be focused

A colleague of mine was once asked to advise a researcher who wanted to know 'What forms of discourse were used by doctors in discussing cancer with their patients, what did patients think of this and what were the effects on outcome of the different styles of discourse?'. A vague question of this sort will often produce a vague answer and, accordingly, research which benefits no-one. Your question must be focused. A quick test of focus: give an imaginary answer to your question; the shorter the answer, the more focused your question. A possible exception to this is qualitative research, the results of which can sometimes be difficult to summarize.

Questions should be explicit

A quick test of explicitness: a research question is explicit if it immediately suggests a research design.

One question at a time

Research, like a 'journey of a thousand miles', goes one step at a time. Questions such as 'Does homeopathy work?' or 'What are the effects of patient expectations on outcome?' will not be resolved by a single research study. The researcher needs to break down large, global questions into manageable stages, a series of questions each associated with a single study.

Build on existing research

Science is a cumulative enterprise. A review of the background can help you define a study topic, identify appropriate research designs and avoid the mistakes of previous workers. Locate as many studies as possible on both the therapy and the condition under investigation and look up other examples of the type of research that you would like to conduct (e.g. have a look at some classic surveys, if you want to conduct a survey). In-depth reading of the research literature is one of the most important preparatory steps for a prospective researcher.

Keep things simple

Given that research will almost inevitably turn out much more complicated than you could possibly imagine, it is a good idea to keep things simple at the start Studies involving multiple endpoints, complex designs or large numbers of participants should be avoided by all but the most experienced researchers.

One 'red flag' to watch out for: if anyone comes to you while you are planning your research and says 'Wouldn't it be nice to know . . . ', panic! Of course it would be 'interesting to know' all sorts of things; the point is that you cannot answer all of them in your research. This seems a particular problem in questionnaire surveys, where the temptation is always to add just one more question. The problem is that the longer a questionnaire, the less likely you are to get good-quality data from your respondents.

The importance of keeping things simple is inadequately recognized at present in the complementary medicine research community. For example, a first-time researcher was recently told by a funding committee to change a simple comparison of Alexander technique with no extra treatment to a complex three-way trial of Alexander technique, contact with the Alexander teacher but no teaching and no contact. This was on the grounds that 'it would be interesting to know' which components of Alexander technique were of value: was it the actual teaching itself or just the time and touch of the teacher? This more than doubled the cost of the trial and because the funding committee was unwilling to provide the extra money, the trial is currently on hold. My own view is that the initial two-arm trial should have been funded with further research questions addressed subsequently.

PROTOCOLS
What is a study protocol?

A study protocol is a precise description of all methodologically pertinent features of a study. The point of a protocol is that it should provide a complete guide to all aspects of trial management and analysis. It should be extremely detailed and explicit: a protocol I recently wrote, for instance, was nearly 8000 words long. As an illustration, here is a short section, chosen pretty much at random which describes the rules for data entry if data are ambiguous.

- *Chronicity*: rounded to nearest year; if a range is given, the highest number will be taken.
- *Age*: rounded to nearest year on date of recruitment.
- *Severity*: if two tick boxes marked, take the higher.

Many protocols are inadequately detailed, particularly the plan for statistical analysis. Examples I have seen recently include: 'We expect to measure the proportion experiencing pain relief of at least 35–50%' and 'The main outcome measure will be forced expiratory volume'. Compare this to 'The primary outcome measure will be the change in mean daily headache score between baseline and the 1-year follow-up'. This is an absolutely explicit guide: you do not have to guess whether to choose 35% or 50% as a cut-off nor guess at which follow-up point forced expiratory volume should be assessed.

Checklists

A good way to make sure that you have incorporated all appropriate detail in your protocol is to use a methodological checklist. An example of a checklist, in this case for clinical trials, is given in Box 3.1. One useful trick is to go through the checklist a second time, this time asking 'who?' rather than 'what?' (e.g. 'What measurements will be taken before treatment?' becomes 'Who will take measurements on participants before treatment?').

Getting the basics right

There has been a good deal of discussion about the importance of adapting research methodologies to the 'special needs' of complementary medicine research. Though I do believe that this is important, I also believe the foundations of any research study have to be absolutely sound. Research with basic methodological flaws is as good as worthless, no matter how 'appropriate' it might seem for complementary medicine. If you are undertaking a survey, make sure you get a high response rate. If you conduct a randomized trial, make sure you randomize properly. If you analyse any numerical data, make sure that you have a good statistician on hand. You should have a thorough understanding of the criteria used to assess methodological rigor for the type of research you wish to undertake well before you start.

PEOPLE
Collaboration

A wide range of skills is needed for research

Research requires specialist skills and knowledge. More often than not, you will need skills or knowledge that you do not have. Here are some of the areas of skill or knowledge used in a trial I am currently running.

- Searching bibliographic databases: to find relevant background material
- Clinical trial design: to write the protocol
- Acupuncture: to advise on the acupuncture content of the protocol
- General practice: to understand the perspective of the doctors in the trial

---

Box 3.1   Methodological checklist for clinical trials

- From where will patients be recruited?
- How many patients will be recruited? Has statistical power been calculated?
- What are the criteria for including patients?
- What are the criteria for excluding patients?
- How will ethical approval for the study be obtained?
- How will informed consent be obtained?
- What control group will be used?
- How will patients be assigned to treatment and control groups?
- For a randomized trial: What method will be used to generate the randomization schedule? What method will be used to conceal allocation until subject entered into the trial? What method will be used to ensure that treatment allocation cannot be changed after subject entered into trial?
- What measurements will be taken before treatment?
- What other information will be taken before treatment?
- What is the treatment to be given to patients in each group?
- Will treatment be standardized or might it vary?
- How many treatments can be given over what length of time?
- Who will give the treatment? Are they sufficiently trained and qualified?
- How will the quality of any medicines used be ensured?
- Is there evidence that the treatment used will be effective in the patients?
- Will patients be blinded to their treatment allocation? If so, how?
- How will blinding be checked?
- Will statistical analysis be conducted blind?
- Will the researcher assessing outcome be blinded to patient treatment allocation? If so, how?
- What outcome measures will be used?
- When will the outcome measurement be made?
- What is the primary outcome measure?
- How will you monitor flow of participants through the trial: number eligible; number randomized; number receiving intended intervention; number not receiving intended intervention; number providing data for each outcome measure; number withdrawing for each of the following reasons: intervention thought harmful or ineffective, lost to follow-up (e.g. moved away), other; number completing trial?
- What will you do about missing or illegible data?
- What statistics will be used to present the results?

- Consumer perspective: to ensure that the trial meets consumer needs
- Statistics: to aid protocol design and analyse data
- Typing and word-processing: to put together the funding application
- Financial administration: to prepare estimates of costs for the funding application
- Database programming: to design the databases to manage trial data
- Questionnaire design: to design questionnaires
- Typesetting: to produce questionnaires
- General practice computer systems: to search for data needed for the trial

If we did not have these skills on the study team, we would not be able to undertake the trial. The most difficult thing for most first-time researchers is that they have few skills. For example, few if any of the researchers I have advised had good knowledge and experience of statistics; similarly, very few have programmed a database. How are you going to analyse your results if you are not confident with statistics? How are you going to manage the huge amounts of data which a study produces without a database? The answer is that you need to collaborate, particularly with experienced researchers.

In-depth knowledge is needed for research

I am often asked to talk at 'research days' which aim to teach complementary practitioners how to do research. I sometimes start by saying 'I am a researcher but I have become interested in [say] acupuncture. Could you quickly show me in a day or so how to do acupuncture?'. Just as it takes many years of training and practice to become a good clinician, so it takes many years to become a good researcher.

I would expect any researcher to have formal training in research design and statistics, a research-related higher degree, a track record of publishing original research in health-related, peer-reviewed journals and at least 3 years experience of original research. This, to me, seems a fairly basic requirement: as an analogy, would it be unreasonable to expect an acupuncturist to have formal training in diagnosis and treatment, an acupuncture qualification, a track record of satisfied patients and at least 3 years experience of giving treatments?

Anyone considering research should either fulfill these criteria or work with someone who does.

Study manual

A study manual describes, in detail, the practical procedures for a trial. It includes information on issues such as running the study databases, how to file and check study materials, interviewing participants and the like. Box 3.2 includes some example sections from a study manual of a trial I recently completed. To give an idea of the sort of detail you need to go into, the study manual of this relatively simple trial was nearly 5000 words long.

Management

Research requires careful management. There should be regular team meetings where problems are discussed and progress reviewed. The principal investigator needs to keep careful track of financial expenditure and recruitment. It is also necessary to monitor a trial, to check that what *should* be happening *is* happening. The following is an excerpt from a study protocol about trial monitoring.

The principal investigator will conduct an internal audit at the study centre every 3 months to ensure: confidentiality and integrity of databases; effectiveness of database back-up systems; confidentiality and integrity of paper records; reconciliation of enquiries with enquiry outcome; number of treatments received by each patient; data entry procedures; minimization algorithm and numbers allocated to each group; comparison of paper records and electronic records. Each month, the principal investigator will review the progress of recruitment by recording number of letters sent, number of enquiries received, number of calls made, number of patients entered, number of migraine patients randomized, number of patients without migraine randomized.

Box 3.2   Example of contents of a study manual

Preparing for interviews

1. Add data from 'subjects agreeing to interview form' to the database. As data for each subject is added, tick by the subject's name. Double-check that the data on screen match the data on the form and then write the date added and your initials on each sheet. File in the 'Proving Recruitment Pre-Interview' folder

2. On Friday of every week, run the macro 'information letters needed' on the database (the green icon). This finds recruits who have not been sent confirmation of their interview date and prints out a cover letter and audit sheet of letters sent, changes trial status field to 'information letters sent [date]'. Send these letters on hospital headed notepaper with a patient information sheet (blue) and how to get to the hospital. File audit sheet in 'Proving Recruitment Folder' stapled to appropriate 'subjects agreeing to interview' form.

3. On Friday of each week, run macro 'print out study appointment sheets' (the blue icon). This prints out the appointment details and contact details for each volunteer scheduled to attend a recruitment interview in the next week. Give these to the study nurse.

4. On Friday of every week, run the macro 'reminder calls to make' (the red icon). This prints out a list of forthcoming appointments with subject names and numbers.

5. **Every day**, check whether there are any reminder calls to make. The day before each recruitment interview, call relevant subjects and say:

'My name is . . . and I am calling from the Proving trial. You may remember that you have an appointment tomorrow at . . . am/pm. This is partly a reminder call and partly a chance to check to see if you have any questions or difficulties.'

If the subject is unable to come or wants to come at a different time, write a note to the study nurse specifying the person's name and the time of the appointment. Do NOT make changes to the database (do this when you get the study appointment sheets back).

The dry run

I always undertake a 'dry run' of a study to test all procedures before involving any patients. I get the study team to go through the trial day by day ('Okay, it is now Monday November 13 2000') with imaginary participants ('Joe Blow has now completed treatment') and imaginary events ('Jo Schmo has telephoned to say that she has decided not to take part'). We add appropriate data to the study databases, print off letters and forms, fill in questionnaires and role-play interviews.

One particularly important aspect of the dry run is to play devil's advocate. We imagine situations such as: what do you do if a patient withdraws after baseline but before randomization? What if a patient telephones to say that he will be on holiday during follow-up? What happens if a patient forgets to send back a questionnaire? We then see what, if any, problems this causes in our procedures.

DATA
Databases

Research involves managing large amounts of data. This applies not only to results and outcomes but details of participants' names and addresses, the stage they are at in the study, their GP's name and so on. It is absolutely essential to manage this data with a computer database. You need a good computer, good software (I personally recommend Filemaker Pro) and someone experienced in database design.

One of the best things about databases is that they can be used to maintain study quality. For example, you can program a database to prompt you to send out follow-up questionnaires at the right time or print out the telephone numbers of participants who are late returning data. You can also program it to check your data for you (see 'Data checking' below).

A word of warning, however: it is all too easy to end up with a database with hundreds of fields, dozens of macros and scores of layouts many of which you have forgotten what they do and why you added them. When you are working on a database you should document your design in what is known as a 'codebook'. This contains the name of a field, macro or layout and a description of its function. For example: 'Field name: date q2 late. Type of field: calculation date field. Description: created by calculation from the field "date q2 sent" plus 16 days. Contains the date on which questionnaire 2 should be received by the office. Used in the macro "find all late questionnaires" '.

Don't take too much data

Researchers often design studies without sufficient consideration of how they will analyse the information once it has been collected. An easy trap is to ask too many questions and take too much data. For example, an eight-item questionnaire completed daily for 10 weeks by 30 subjects will generate 16 800 data points. Who will type in all this information? How will it be analyzed?

Randomization

If you wish to conduct a randomized trial, do make sure that you get randomization right. One of the most important but least understood functions of randomization is to prevent trialists being able to influence treatment assignment. To achieve this, it is important that treatment allocation is concealed. 'Concealment of allocation' means that the researchers should not be able to guess the group to which a patient will be randomized before they are entered into the trial. If allocation is not concealed, it is possible that researchers may interfere with the randomization process, consciously or otherwise. For example, a surgeon who knew that the next patient to be entered into the trial was to be randomized to surgery may try to avoid recruiting a patient thought to have a poor prognosis. A typical example of unconcealed allocation is when a statistician produces a randomized list using a sophisticated computer program and this is then posted in the research office for all to see.

Randomization should also be designed in such a way that it should be impossible to change treatment assignments once patients have been entered into the trial. This can prevent the sort of problem reported in one case, where randomization took place by removing a colored or plain marble from a black bag. The principal investigators found that the study nurses were replacing marbles and choosing again if they felt that patients needed a different treatment to the one assigned.

One common method of randomization is the 'sealed envelope' method. You take 100 pieces of card, write 'treatment group' on 50 and 'control' on the remainder, place them in 100 opaque envelopes and then shuffle. The problem with this method is that there is nothing to stop a researcher opening and resealing an envelope or opening a second envelope if the first contained the 'wrong' allocation.

The best method of randomization is to separate the person recruiting patients from the person implementing randomization. Treatment assignment itself should be determined by using a password-protected database. In one trial I am involved in, patients are recruited by a study nurse who sends a request for randomization to the study office. A research assistant then runs a macro on the study database which automatically enters the treatment allocation from a separate, encrypted randomization database. The database is programmed so that the treatment allocation cannot subsequently be changed.

Data checking

You need to check, double-check and recheck your data. A few hints and tips.

- *Sign off on data.* When a researcher completes a form, standard procedure should be to check that it is complete, accurate and legible and then date and initial or sign. The signature means: 'I have checked these data'. Similarly, when data (e.g. the name and address of a new participant) are added from a form onto a database, the data entry should be visually checked and the form dated and initialled.
- *Double-check critical steps.* Certain parts of a study are absolutely critical to its quality. For example, if a researcher slightly misspells a participant's surname on the study database, this is sloppy but not disastrous. If, however, a researcher needs to add the information that a certain participant has withdrawn from a study but calls up the wrong participant on the database, the result will be that a participant who should be in the trial is not contacted again, reducing sample size and statistical power. A typical procedure to avoid this type of error might be to add all the results of all patient interviews at one time, have the database print out a list of the data added, check the list against the interview sheets and sign and date the sheet to confirm that a check has been made.
- *Guard your code numbers.* In most studies, code numbers rather than names are used to identify participants. Given the importance of code numbers, it is surprising to find them treated in a cavalier fashion by some researchers. In a trial I was asked to advise on, the code numbers were written by hand onto the top sheet of a questionnaire. Once the questionnaires had been photocopied it was impossible to check which participant had filled out any given page 2 of the questionnaire. Moreover, some code numbers were difficult to read. Make sure that code numbers are clearly stamped on every sheet of paper and no patient's code number can be changed on the database.
- *Automated consistency checks.* It is possible to program a database to find data which are illogical. What I have done in the past is to get the study team to think of all possible inconsistencies in the data (e.g. patients recorded as having returned data but who are not yet in the trial or those who have had study appointments pending but who are recorded as having withdrawn) and then program suitable searches into the study database. These searches are then run every day to alert the study team to possible errors.

- *Data entry rules.* Provide those entering data with a complete set of rules for missing, illegible or ambiguous data. You should also provide rules for data which might be presented in different ways. In one study, for instance, we asked runners to report how long it had taken them to complete a marathon. Because I didn't give those entering data sufficient guidance, race time was variously entered as '3 hours and 15 minutes' '3.15' and '195'.
- *Double-data entry.* Any data that you will analyze and report in the published paper of your research should be entered twice, on two separate databases, with automatic checking set up between the two.
- *Make extra checks on group assignments.* In controlled trials, make extensive checks that every patient code number has been given the correct allocation (treatment or control) and that any codes you use for treatment assignments (e.g. 1 for treatment, 0 for control) are correct.
- *Check your finished paper against the original output from your statistical software.* It is not uncommon for an experienced researcher to go to extreme lengths to ensure accuracy of data during a study but then to make a typographical error when typing up the final report.

Analysis

Many statistical software packages are programmable: you can load in a set of analyses and run them on whatever data are in memory. I recommend generating a set of simulated data, programming in your analyses as specified in your study protocol, checking that the analyses do what you want them to do and then saving your work. When it comes to adding the real data from your trial, all you have to do is load up your analysis and press the 'go' button. Incidentally, if you hear anyone say 'It took me ages to analyse my results' it is probable that they were not following a predefined protocol.

Some researchers suggest that you write up the results section of your paper, including tables and graphs, *before* you have any data; for example: 'Mean pain scores (x SD y) in the treatment/control group were z points (95% confidence interval a, b) lower than those in the treatment/control group (c SD d)'. This helps to ensure that you are doing the analyses correctly and not merely 'torturing the data until it confesses'.

PATIENTS

Recruitment is generally cited as the number 1 problem experienced by researchers. A large number of studies run into difficulties because insufficient numbers of participants are recruited. Given below are a few brief hints and tips on study recruitment.

Getting participants into a study

- *Motivating gatekeepers.* Many trials rely on a 'gatekeeper', such as a patient's doctor, to refer patients to a study. An extremely common problem is that gatekeepers lose motivation and refer far fewer patients than expected. They forget to tell appropriate patients or fail to do so because of lack of time or simply decide not to because it is not a priority. It is essential to keep gatekeepers involved, to help them feel ownership of a project. Arrange regular face-to-face meetings, send a 'thank you' letter when a patient is referred and send a regular newsletter with information about the progress of the trial.

- *Keep things as simple as possible for gatekeepers.* Use clear and simple forms with tick boxes and a place for a signature at the bottom.
- *Reminding gatekeepers about the study.* Some studies have used complex reminder systems to prompt doctors to refer patients. These include computerized reminders or placing a reminder sticker on notes of patients who could be eligible for a study. Other studies have used simpler approaches, using cups, pens and posters with the trial logo (e.g. 'MI < 6 hours? Think ISIS trial').
- *Recruitment materials should be attractive and professional.* Remember that 'the medium is the message': sending poorly photocopied or badly laid out information will not help recruitment.
- *Recruitment materials should be personalized.* Participants normally prefer a personalized letter, with their name and address.
- *Recruitment materials should be simple.* In one trial I worked on, we improved recruitment rates significantly by changing the recruitment letter. We replaced a letter which gave a detailed and complex description of the trial with one which just said: 'We are doing some research and it might interest you, give us a call if you want to find out more'.
- *Use the media.* A study can be a newsworthy event ('Though arthritis patients have used herbs for thousands of years, it is not really known if they can help. Scientists at the University of London are starting to look into this question...'). Call around journalists and see if any are interested in the story. Ask them to add details of the study telephone line.

Keeping participants in a study and getting good-quality data

- *Make participants feel important.* Study materials should carefully explain why you are doing a study and why the information you will get is important. Recruitment interviews and study materials should include phrases such as 'Your responses will be very helpful to us' or 'Your responses are very important for the study'.
- *Keep in contact with participants.* Calling participants ('We just wanted to check you were getting on okay') and sending thank you letters or newsletters are good ways of keeping participants motivated, particularly in longer studies.
- A hint: in any extended study, ask participants to give you the telephone number of a close friend or relative. If you cannot get hold of the participant (e.g. they have moved) you can contact the friend or relative for new contact details.

CONCLUSION

My initial response to someone asking for advice on research is often: 'Think about whether you really want this career change'. Research has to be done properly or not at all. Research cannot be done properly on an amateur basis, without an impact on the rest of a person's professional life. So if you want to do research, bear in mind first the immediate practical implications for yourself and your work.

I believe that research is important and that it has practical benefits which improve the lives of those suffering ill health. That means that all health professionals should support the conduct of research and use the results of research in making decisions. It does not mean, however, that everyone should do research. If you are considering research, think first not about methodology but about the day-to-day practicalities of managing complex systems of data gathering and analysis.

FURTHER READING

Altman DG, Schulz KF, Moher D et al 2001 The revised CONSORT statement for reporting randomized trials: explanation and elaboration. Ann Intern Med 134(8): 663–664

Barbour RS 2001 Checklists for improving rigour in qualitative research: a case of the tail wagging the dog? BMJ 322: 1115–1117

Mother D, Schulz KF, Altman DG 2001 The CONSORT statement: revised recommendations for improving the quality of reports of parallel-group randomized trials. Ann Intern Med 134(8): 657–662

Links under 'Statistics and Research Methods' on the British Medical Journal Website http://www.bmj.comscollections/

Browse 'Statics Notes' in the British Medical Journal by typing 'Statistics Notes' in 'words in title' box at http://www.bmj.com/all.shtml

4

Possible research strategies for evaluating CAM interventions

Kate Thomas   Mike Fitter

INTRODUCTION

Our aim in this chapter is to present a framework which contains the main research questions that are currently posed in relation to CAM and the range of research designs and methods that are used to address these questions. Within the limits of what is possible within a single chapter we have attempted to be comprehensive regarding the questions and designs appropriate to a focus on evaluative clinical research. To cover the full range of topics relevant to CAM research would require a book in itself. The underlying assumption of this chapter is that CAM research is not substantively different from other health-related research, especially when it is recognized that research methods draw on diverse disciplines, including biomedical, psychological and social sciences. However, research in CAM can undoubtedly present a challenge to conventional study design. Undertaking research that meets this challenge may, in turn, help to shape the way mainstream medical research is conceived and conducted.

We have written the chapter with the CAM practitioner in mind, as well as the more experienced researcher. We wish to encourage practitioners to play an active role in research, developing their skills as practitioner-researchers. It is our belief that only in this way can a profession and the therapy it practices be fully alive and growing. No results last forever; as our culture evolves so do our health-care practices and for this the practitioner needs the essential qualities of curiosity, commitment and critical thinking.

However, not all of the research designs presented here are suitable for the practitioner-researcher, unless they happen to have considerable experience in research and access to immense resources, both financial and human. It is an unfortunate but understandable fact that many practitioners, when they become enthusiastic about research, want to do the definitive study that 'proves' that their therapy works. We need to say to such people, 'Don't!' but add that there are research designs suitable for a practitioner with few resources beyond their own time and commitment.

For many of the research designs described in the chapter, we have illustrated the principles with an example from practice. All the examples are from CAM research and, where appropriate, we have used examples from our own research practice. These examples have been chosen as good illustrations of the designs that we are describing, rather than because they are necessarily exemplary studies in their practice and reporting. Indeed, one provides a good example of the serious potential pitfalls of employing a particular design.

The chapter is organized into three sections. First, we have described a group of study designs that aim to provide definitive information about efficacy, effectiveness and safety. We have termed these 'proving studies'. Second, we have described study designs that are concerned with providing less definitive data. These are smaller studies which, while not being conclusive, will nevertheless contribute to the pool of information. Such studies also provide the groundwork for making decisions about the appropriateness of undertaking a full study. We have termed these 'exploratory studies'. Finally, we describe a group of research designs that have stronger roots in everyday practice and share the aim of improving practice through greater understanding of the clinical process and its components. Not surprisingly, we have called these 'improving studies'. They are presented in this order for clarity, rather than because of any implied hierarchy of value. Done well, all these types of evaluative research have an important contribution to make to the growing body of evidence about CAM.

We aim to clarify the terms used to describe the various types of research design. The fact that so many different terms are used so loosely only adds confusion to an already complex topic. In choosing our descriptors we have been guided by the terms currently in use in CAM research and in the larger fields of biomedical and health services research. All the designs we have presented here are in active use in health-related research. Most, if not all, are in active service in CAM research. If we were to write a new edition of this chapter in 5 years time, it is our hope that we would find ample examples of each research design applied in the CAM field with skill and elegance.

All good, i.e. carefully conducted, research is worth doing. A relevant 'small' question answered well, with limited resources, is likely to be worth more than a 'big' question answered badly due to the use of inappropriate methods or inadequate resourcing. To this end, and as a rough guide, we have placed asterisks against each research design in the tables. The classification we have adopted is as follows.

* Can be accomplished with relatively few resources beyond those available in clinical practice, though there may be a need for specialist research skills that can be acquired through training.
** Requires significant resources, often including cooperation between several practitioners. Such a study could feasibly be undertaken by a practitioner with some research experience but is likely to need some specialist advice.

*** Requires substantial resources; only likely to be feasible with a major research grant, almost certainly needs to be conceived as a multidisciplinary effort to be undertaken in partnership with researchers with a recognized track record, who are able to compete for funding against experienced university researchers.

PROVING STUDIES

- Efficacy
  Placebo-controlled randomized trial
- Comparative effectiveness
  Pragmatic randomized controlled trials
  Randomization with choice (patient preference trials)
  Cost-effectiveness studies
  Non-randomized matched cohort studies
- Evidence review
  Systematic reviews
  Meta-analysis

Research studies falling into the category of 'proving' have in common the aim of answering a variation on the question 'Does it work?'. All health-care practice needs to ask this question and there is still much care delivered for which we cannot answer this question definitively. This is due in part to the fact that 'Does it work?' is never a simple question. There are often many questions to answer; any single therapeutic intervention raises a number of separate questions relating to the intervention itself (which remedy, how much is an optimum dose, for how long should the treatment continue), the implementation of the intervention (by whom, where) and the recipients of the intervention (which patient groups, with which conditions, defined how). Even the outcome measures used can shape the question itself (objective measures, subjective measures, clinical and non-clinical). Different methods tend to work best for different questions. Research methods follow from questions, not the other way around.

Efficacy: placebo-controlled randomized trial

'Efficacious' literally means capable of, or successful in, producing an intended result. In health-care research, efficacy studies aim to provide definitive evidence ('proof') of a specific effect, to isolate and test the particular hypothesized active ingredient. These questions generally stem from the desire to find and use the most efficacious treatments or combinations of treatments.

'Is there a specific (beneficial) effect?'

The need for CAM to provide evidence of efficacy is further fuelled by the fact that it embraces many treatments for which no scientifically acceptable (or scientifically plausible) mechanism of action is currently available. In the absence of accepted mechanisms, alternative explanations for observed effects will tend to be sought. Under these circumstances, a study design which systematically attempts to exclude (or control for) all potential causal factors except the one under scrutiny will have a better chance of convincing the skeptical.

Table 4.1 Proving studies

Research domain	Some research questions	Research focus / Reasons for asking the question	Some appropriate designs and methods (* Relative resources required)	Distinctive features of method
Efficacy	Is there a specific beneficial effect? What is the active ingredient?	Individual patient care focus • The desire to use efficacious treatments • Challenge to CAM to demonstrate specific effects	Explanatory randomized controlled trial (RCT)***	• Experimental design • Compares outcomes following treatment or placebo • Standardized patient entry criteria to trial • Randomization to group • Single standardized active intervention • Practitioner and/or patient 'blinding' to treatment
Comparative effectiveness	How well does it work in practice? How does it compare to other treatments or services?	Population care focus • The need to compare two or more active treatments • The need to establish what is best treatment option (or package of care) for a given population of patients • To aid decisions about services which should be provided	Pragmatic RCT*** Randomization with choice*** Non-randomized matched cohort studies**	• Compares outcomes following two or more different treatments or services • Tests real-world practice • Uses predefined patient inclusion criteria • Allows individualized treatment • 'Open' design possible – does not assume patient and/or practitioner 'blinding' • Uses wide range of outcomes, including longer term outcomes.

Economic evaluation	Is it value for money?	Commissioning focus	Cost-effectiveness studies***	• Collects predefined cost data relating to direct treatment costs and/or social costs • Compares relative costs per unit of benefit achieved for two or more treatments • Needs to be conducted alongside effectiveness studies (pragmatic trial or matched cohort study)
		• How to spend the finite resources available for health care in order to achieve maximum benefit for the maximum number of patients		
Evidence review	What do we already know?	Service development focus	Systematic literature reviews**	• Synthesizes results from multiple trials • Uses a replicable, comprehensive and systematic search strategy to identify suitable studies • Applies quality criteria to the selection of studies included
	What does the cumulative evidence tell us?	• The need to promote the practice of evidence-based medicine	Metaanalysis techniques**	• Metaanalysis entails the statistical pooling of results from selected studies using a common outcome measure.
	What further studies are needed?	• The need to design systems of care which incorporate the best available evidence of efficacy and effectiveness		

Relative resources (time, skills and funding) required to undertake this type of research – least, moderate**, most*** (see Introduction section of chapter for full description)

Some appropriate methods for questions of efficacy

If the intended result can be demonstrated and the extraneous causal factors are excluded by the design, then the outcome observed will be due to the intervention. Such research can be seen as empirical experimentation and the best available method for its application in health-care research is the placebo-controlled explanatory randomized trial or explanatory randomized controlled trial (RCT).

Distinctive features of explanatory RCTs

Explanatory RCTs entail an experimental design conducted under near as possible 'laboratory' conditions. They have the following characteristics.

- The administration of a 'placebo' intervention to the control group, which mimics the true intervention but does not contain the active ingredient under investigation such that all possible causal elements are held constant except the one under investigation.
- Standardized entry criteria (so that it is possible to generalize the results in terms of *who* benefits).
- A single standardized active intervention (so that it is possible to explain the result in terms of the specific intervention).
- The allocation of subjects into an intervention and a 'control' or comparison group according to a random method (so that patients cannot be allocated to treatment according to prognostic or other characteristics that might influence their outcome following treatment).
- Where possible, randomization is undertaken using a concealed method so that both patients and practitioners will be ignorant of the group to which the patient will be allocated (so that expectations of positive or negative outcome cannot bias the results).

Example from practice: a placebo-controlled explanatory RCT

Placebo-controlled randomized controlled trials are most commonly undertaken for drug therapies. The pharmaceutical industry has a clear need to provide definitive evidence of efficacy and the design works well for this purpose. Rigorous explanatory trials are less common in CAM. Efficacy tends to have been addressed within many CAM traditions through observed clinical practice, rather than experimental research. One well-known exception is a trial of homeopathy undertaken in the 1980s (Box 4.1). This study was a classically designed placebo-controlled randomized trial that attempted to exclude all extraneous factors and, by ensuring that only the experimental group received the active ingredients in the tablets, was able to address the question: 'Is homeopathy a placebo response?'.

A common criticism of this study from the CAM perspective is that the treatment offered did not reflect the optimal use of homeopathy because the study design required that a single standardized treatment be used. In the 'real world', as opposed to the 'laboratory', homeopaths would not necessarily use this remedy and individualized diagnosis and treatment would be the norm. The trial was successful in its aim of testing the efficacy of a particular homeopathic preparation but it was not a trial of homeopathy as it is practiced.

Box 4.1 Is homeopathy a placebo response? (Reilly et al 1986)

Objective: To test the hypothesis that homeopathic potencies are not active.

Design: Randomized, double-blind placebo-controlled trial. Patients allocated by random numbers to intervention or control group. Randomization undertaken to ensure no differences between groups for demographic characteristics or duration of hayfever or for severity of hayfever and antihistamine use at the outset of the trial. Neither the doctors nor the patients knew which treatment patients were receiving.

Setting: Homeopathic hospital clinics in Glasgow and London.

Subjects: 144 patients with active hayfever aged over 5 years with at least 1 year history of seasonal hayfever and current symptoms. Patients identified by general practitioners and referred to one of the study hospitals over a 10-month period.

Intervention: Homeopathic preparation of 30c mixed grass pollens. One tablet taken twice daily for 2 weeks. The control group received identically packaged lactose tablets with 10% alcohol, to be taken in the same way.

Main outcome measures: Patient and doctor assessed symptom scores at 5 weeks. Pollen count, month of referral and use of antihistamines were taken into account in the analysis.

Selected reported results: 'Patients taking a homeopathic preparation showed a greater improvement in symptoms than those taking a placebo. This difference was reflected in a reduced need for antihistamines, increased in significance when adjusted for pollen count and time of season, and was confirmed by the doctors' assessments.' 'No evidence emerged to support the idea that placebo action fully explains clinical responses to homeopathic drugs.'

This illustrates an important point. If the same single remedy is not the normal way a homeopath would prescribe for all patients, then the results of this explanatory RCT cannot be used to inform practice. This problem is not unique to this study or to research in CAM (Fitter & Thomas 1997).

Comparative effectiveness

Results from placebo-controlled RCTs may also be less helpful in clinical practice where practitioners are trying to decide between two different interventions; trial results may tell them that each intervention works when compared to a placebo but not which one works better and hence which should be adopted in practice. Results from an explanatory RCT may also lack external validity (i.e. the results cannot be generalized). For example, this will be the case if strict entry criteria mean that the patient population in the study is not sufficiently similar to the patient groups encountered in normal clinical practice. This is a question of effectiveness, not efficacy, and requires the application of different research methods.

'How well does it work in practice?'

Comparative effectiveness studies aim to answer the less fundamental but more practical questions associated with health-care delivery. The question in each case is not 'Does it work?' but 'Would it be better than the other option(s) on offer?'. Effectiveness studies are concerned with the comparative performance of treatments, packages of care or services. The focus of the research is not the specific effects of a treatment but rather the measurable comparative benefits that can be seen as outcomes of the different treatments received. For example, complementary therapies may be proposed as an alternative to existing treatment, as an adjunct to usual clinical management or as one of a range of treatments or packages of care that patients or practitioners may be in a position to choose. Comparative effectiveness studies are needed to develop an appropriate evidence base to aid practical decisions relating to the use of complementary therapy in the NHS or their integration into mainstream medical care.

Some appropriate methods for assessing comparative effectiveness

Comparative benefits can only be measured if the study design incorporates a comparison group receiving a different treatment or package of care. Like the placebo-controlled explanatory trial, effectiveness studies require a comparison group that is similar in all other respects to the study group. Unlike explanatory trials, effectiveness studies do not require that all possible causal effects are held constant except the one under review. A number of research designs are appropriate to this practical, or real-world, orientation: pragmatic randomized trials, partially randomized trials, randomization with choice, non-randomized matched cohort studies and cost-effectiveness studies.

Distinctive features of the methods used in comparative effectiveness studies

Effectiveness studies share a number of important characteristics.

- They compare one treatment, package of care or service with one or more alternatives (including what might be described as current normal clinical management).
- Their subject is usually real-world practice; they evaluate care which is close to the way it is usually delivered.
- Non-standardized or individualized treatment can be incorporated into the evaluation design.
- Patient and practitioner blinding are not a requirement of the design; an 'open' design is usually assumed.
- They incorporate a wider range of possible outcomes, including longer term outcomes, whilst accepting that these might not be the direct effects of the intervention itself.

Pragmatic randomized controlled trials

Pragmatic trials incorporate some key features of an explanatory trial; the patients are randomly allocated to groups and comparisons are made between the groups in terms of the measured response to treatment. In a pragmatic trial, however, treatment conditions are deliberately kept as close as possible to how they would be delivered in day-to-day practice. In this way they can also accommodate an individualized treatment approach; a whole 'package' of individualized care can be evaluated, rather than standardizing a single active ingredient. In the event of a positive outcome, the result of these studies is not certainty about which element of the care received was responsible for the outcome but rather confidence that a similar patient population receiving a similar package of care is likely to do better than those receiving the alternative or the 'usual' package of care.

Example from practice: a pragmatic RCT

A number of pragmatic RCTs have been conducted in CAM. In 1990, Meade et al published a study of a chiropractic service for patients with back pain. This study illustrates the features of a pragmatic RCT, where the chiropractic treatment was given as closely as possible to how it would be delivered in everyday practice. In particular, the number and type of treatments were given at the discretion of the treating practitioner (Box 4.2).

This trial, with its favorable conclusions regarding chiropractic, has been influential in the debate regarding the inclusion of CAM in the NHS, as well as the applicability of conventional research methods to CAM evaluation. Many potential trial entrants identified at the chiropractic clinic declined to participate, because they were unwilling to be randomized to conventional treatment. This problem can be addressed by modifying the trial design to take into account such patient preferences for treatment.

Randomization with choice (patient preference trials)

This can be approached in two ways within a trial design. Both may be particularly appropriate to the evaluation of CAM.

Box 4.2 Low back pain of mechanical origin; randomized comparison of chiropractic and hospital outpatient treatment. (Meade et al 1990)

Objective: To compare chiropractic and hospital outpatient treatment for managing low back pain of mechanical origin.

Design: A pragmatic randomized controlled trial (N=741)

Setting: Paired private chiropractic clinics and hospital outpatient departments in 11 centers in England.

Subjects: Men and women aged 18–65 presenting at clinics or hospital departments with low back pain, having no contraindications to manipulation and no treatment in the previous month.

Intervention: Treatment at the discretion of chiropractors or hospital team. Chiropractic manipulation was offered to most patients at the clinics, up to a maximum of 10 treatments. Hospital treatment was most commonly Maitland mobilization or manipulation or both.

Main outcome measures: Differences in the change in mean score on the Oswestry Pain Disability Questionnaire at 6 weeks, 6 months, 12 months and 2 years. Secondary outcomes included straight leg lumbar flex, further treatment, pain at 1 year, use of drugs at 6 months, 1 year and 2 years, time off work, satisfaction with treatment at 6 weeks.

Selected reported results: A difference in change in mean Oswestry score was observed between the groups at 2 years of 7.16 (95% CI, 1.86 to 12.45, P<0.01). For nearly all subsidiary measures, including satisfaction with treatment, patients treated by chiropractors did better than those treated in hospital. Most differences did not reach statistical significance. 'For patients with low back pain in whom manipulation is not contraindicated, chiropractic almost certainly confers worthwhile benefit in comparison with hospital management. Introducing chiropractic into NHS practice should be considered.'

- Partially randomized trials
- Randomization to choice (patient preference trials)

In a partially randomized trial design, patients who express a preference are allocated to the treatment that they prefer and those patients who express no preference are randomized to a treatment arm. Assuming that the trial attracts sufficient numbers in each group, analysis is undertaken comparing the randomized groups independently of the analysis that compares patient outcomes for the groups that expressed a preference with those allocated to treatment. In this way, the effects of receiving a treatment of choice can be measured. However, it is not possible to combine the data to answer the more practical question of how a population of patients would fare in conditions where a treatment was offered as an option. To do this it is necessary to adopt a different design that allows the comparison of the option of a new treatment with the absence of that option.

Example from practice: a pragmatic RCT with randomization to the option of acupuncture

This type of design is relatively uncommon but may be particularly relevant to research which addresses the appropriate use of CAM treatments within the NHS, where treatments are likely to be offered as an optional management strategy, rather than recommended as the routine treatment (Thomas & Fitter 1997). An example is shown in Box 4.3.

Box 4.3 Longer-term clinical and economic benefits of offering acupuncture to patients with chronic low back pain assessed as suitable for primary care management. (Thomas et al 1999)

Objective: To test the hypothesis that a population of patients offered the option of acupuncture for low back pain of more than 4 weeks duration gain more benefit for the same or less cost than a similar population offered normal management by their GP and assess the potential benefits of having an acupuncture service available on the NHS for GPs to offer to those patients who are suitable and who wish to use it.

Design: A pragmatic randomized controlled trial of clinical and cost-effectiveness of different treatment packages for low back pain. Patients randomized to control group receiving usual care or the offer of the option of acupuncture. Analysis is by allocated group, irrespective of whether subjects choose to take up the option of acupuncture if allocated to the 'offer' group.

Setting: Primary care and acupuncture clinics in York, England.

Subjects: Patients aged between 20 and 65 presenting to GPs with a current episode of low back pain of between 4 weeks and 12 months duration (N=240 patients randomized 2 to 1 in favor of option of acupuncture).

Intervention: Traditional acupuncture provided in accord with the normal practice of the acupuncturist and the clinic, with up to 10 treatment sessions available, or usual management from their GP.

Main outcome measures: Oswestry Low Back Pain Disability Questionnaire; Present Pain Intensity Scale of the McGill Pain Questionnaire; SF-36 General Health Status Profile; EQ5. Change measured at 3 months and again at 12 months, satisfaction with care received. Direct health-care costs to the NHS.

Selected results: Study in progress.

The outcome of this study will clearly be dependent on the level of uptake of acupuncture in the study population. Clearly if no, or very few, patients choose the option of acupuncture then the potential effects will be weakened. In this case a pilot study demonstrated that the majority of patients would be interested in taking up the option of acupuncture if it were offered to them. The strength of this design lies in the fact that if the study demonstrates clinical effectiveness, it will also be able to show whether or not the offer of the option of acupuncture for this group of patients is a cost-effective use of NHS resources.

Cost-effectiveness is an important issue in pragmatic research. In the chiropractic study by Meade et al, the benefits of chiropractic were obtained at an apparently higher cost, due principally to the greater number of treatments received by this group of patients. Thus one possible interpretation of the results obtained in that study is that the relatively small benefit observed in the chiropractic group might not be enough to justify the additional costs. Without the collection of data on all relevant costs, it is not possible to reach a conclusion about this.

Cost-effectiveness studies

Addressing the problem of relative costs requires the systematic collection of detailed costing data for both groups in the study. In this way the economic costs, as well as the benefits, can be compared between the two treatments.

'Is it value for money?'

Cost-effectiveness studies provide the best evidence for decisions relating to the commissioning of services or rationing of existing health care – the need to establish the best way to spend finite resources available for health care at any given time. Cost-effectiveness studies usually run alongside pragmatic trials, collecting appropriate data relating to the costs of treatment in both arms of the trial; these costs will often include longer term NHS resource use which may have an important impact on the overall cost of treatment. This type of data may be very important if a complementary therapy is believed to reduce drug costs following treatment or reduce the number of subsequent physician contacts, referrals for investigations or even surgery. Costing data may simply be reported alongside clinical outcomes or the data can be analyzed in conjunction with clinical outcome data to produce the relative costs per unit of benefit achieved for each of the treatments or packages of care being studied. Combining the results in this way can be particularly useful if there is a debate about the most appropriate number of treatments to be allowed per patient. Using these methods, it is possible to demonstrate the cost of any extra gain obtained from additional treatments and hence get a measure of value for money.

Example from practice: cost-effectiveness study of chiropractic, physical therapy and education booklet

Cost-effectiveness studies are relatively rare in CAM. This is perhaps unsurprising as the main motivation for conducting them relates to service commissioning and complementary therapies are still not widespread in mainstream medicine. As the demand for complementary therapies grows and with it pressure to provide certain

---

Box 4.4 A comparison of physical therapy, chiropractic manipulation, and provision of an educational booklet for the treatment of patients with low back pain. (Cherkin et al 1998)

Objective: To assess the relative effectiveness and costs of three treatments for low back pain (McKenzie physical therapy, chiropractic and a patient education booklet).

Design: A pragmatic randomized controlled trial of clinical and cost-effectiveness of different treatment packages for low back pain.

Setting: USA primary care; large staff-model HMO.

Subjects: Patients aged 20–64 with 7 days persistent low back pain following a primary care visit (N=321).

Intervention: Up to nine visits at discretion of therapist for physical therapy or chiropractic or the provision of an educational booklet on low back pain management.

Main outcome measures: Roland Disability Scale, Bothersomeness of Symptoms Scale, measured at 1, 4 and 12 weeks and again at 1–2 years. Satisfaction with care received. Direct health-care costs to the HMO.

Selected results: Small non-significant benefits were found for chiropractic and physical therapy. Satisfaction with care was significantly higher in these groups. Mean total costs of care to the HMO were $437 for the physical therapy group, $429 for the chiropractic group and $153 for the booklet group.

---

therapies within the NHS, or Managed Care in the US, so the need for this type of study will grow. The study outlined in Box 4.4 typifies this type of study, taking into account the direct health-care costs (treatment and subsequent investigations, consultations, etc.) to the health maintenance organization (HMO) over an extended period, to assess the total resource consequences of chiropractic treatment.

The results of this study have been interpreted as indicating that both physical therapy and chiropractic confer small clinical benefits over the provision of a $1 educational booklet and cost considerably more to deliver. However, patient satisfaction was clearly higher in the actively treated groups. An editorial published alongside the study results commented that the challenge for chiropractic is to demonstrate that it can achieve such benefits at a cost that US health insurers are willing to pay (Shekelle 1998).

To randomize or not to randomize?

All the study designs described above necessitate the setting up of a study in which at least some patients are willing to be randomly allocated to study treatments or sometimes to a placebo. Notwithstanding the benefits of these designs, there will be times when it is not possible to randomize patients to a study group, either because it is perceived as unethical or because it is impractical. CAM may fall into this category when suitable patients are unwilling to be randomized, having already made the decision to seek alternative health care. In these cases, it may still be important to evaluate CAM treatments against existing provision. Under such circumstances, it may be possible to obtain similar information on outcomes, clinical, cost and satisfaction, for a treatment group or 'cohort' of patients and a non-randomly allocated, matched comparison group.

Non-randomized matched cohort studies

In a matched cohort study, the goal is to identify a 'control' group of patients similar in all relevant ways to the study or intervention group. 'Matching' of cases is undertaken on factors such as age and severity of disease/problem at baseline, plus any other factors thought to influence outcome. Done well, these studies can provide valuable information about the relative effectiveness of various interventions. However, the problem is, of course, that it may be hard to match for all such factors. Any unaccounted-for factors that remain differentially distributed in the compared groups may create systematic differences in the outcomes. This means that there is increased uncertainty about whether the results are due to the treatment or to the uneven distribution of the unmatched characteristics. Insofar as this problem is due to random variation, it may reduce if the groups identified are sufficiently large. However, if the differences are due to a systematic difference in the pool of patients from which the two groups are drawn, then the risk of confounding remains, no matter how large the sample is.

Example from practice: a prospective cohort study of care for breast cancer patients

This study was undertaken with a matched design, rather than as a randomized controlled trial, because the patients were all self-referrals to a charitable cancer care centre and it was thought to be unethical to randomize them under these circumstances. This study illustrates the design and the pitfalls of matched control studies. Box 4.5 summarizes the study.

Box 4.5   Survival of patients with breast cancer attending Bristol Cancer Help Centre. (Bagenal et al 1990)

Objective: To compare survival and metastasis-free survival in patients treated at the BCHC and patients in a matched control group.

Design: A prospectively matched cohort study with outcome assessed 2 years after recruitment of the first patient.

Setting: Bristol Cancer Help Centre, a specialist NHS cancer hospital and two NHS general hospitals.

Subjects: All 344 women aged under 70 with a diagnosis of breast cancer attending the BCHC for the first time. The matched control group comprised 461 women taken from all women with breast cancer attending NHS hospitals. The pool of potential controls was stratified into four groups by age and year of diagnosis. Matched cases were selected at random from the appropriate group.

Intervention: At least one visit to the BCHC, which might include special diet advice, counseling and alternative therapies. The matched controls received conventional NHS management.

Main outcome measures: Survival and metastasis-free survival 2 years after the first patient was recruited. All patients were followed up for at least 1 year.

Selected results: For patients metastasis free at entry, relapse rate in the BCHC group was significantly poorer than in the controls. Survival in relapsed cases was significantly inferior to that in the control group. The authors concluded, 'These results suggest that women with breast cancer attending BCHC fare worse than those receiving conventional treatment only'.

This study became well known because the negative conclusions regarding the impact of Bristol Cancer Help Centre (BCHC) attendance received a great deal of media attention. The authors, following a public debate about the study design, however, formally withdrew the main conclusions from the study. The appropriateness of the conclusion was challenged because the matching process was shown to be inadequate and the two groups were deemed to be different with regard to disease severity as evidenced by local recurrences of the disease prior to entry to the trial. Local recurrence is known to be a prognostic factor in breast cancer and this was not controlled for in the selection of matched cases. Local recurrence was much more common in the BCHC group, leading one commentator to speculate that it might have been this that prompted attendance at the BCHC for many women. As the two groups were different in this important respect, the results could not be interpreted as the effects of attendance at the BCHC. The authors concluded that individual matching of cases and controls taking this factor into account would avoid the problem. However, an impracticably large pool of potential controls would be needed to do this. A randomized design would clearly have removed this particular problem.

Systematic evidence review

If undertaken rigorously, reviews of existing research can provide more robust evidence than any single trial. Systematic evidence reviews are also needed to inform the practice of evidence-based service development and to design systems of care that incorporate the best available evidence of efficacy and effectiveness.

'What does the cumulative evidence show?'

Reviews of existing literature are an essential starting point for any research. With the advent of on-line databases searching, identifying and gaining access to published research findings have never been easier. Reviews are necessary to answer the fundamental questions 'What do we already know?' and 'What research do we still need to do?'.

Some appropriate methods for evidence reviews

Methods for rigorous reviews of existing literature include systematic reviews and meta-analysis (statistical pooling of data). Both should be regarded as empirical research methods as both entail a detailed protocol and explicit design, which mean that the study can be replicated and the results verified.

Distinctive features of evidence reviews

Protocols for systematic reviews and meta-analyses share a number of characteristics.

- The identification of existing studies using a replicable, comprehensive and systematic search strategy.
- The systematic application of explicit quality criteria to the selection of studies.
- The synthesis of study results.
- In addition, meta-analysis involves the statistical pooling of results from trials that have been adequately reported and have an identifiable shared outcome.

The principle behind all systematic reviews is to find and review all potentially relevant data and to systematically select the data of the highest quality for inclusion. The recent explosion of systematic reviews in conventional medicine has been fueled by the promotion of an evidence-based medicine culture. The systematic scrutiny of trials means that quality standards of design, conduct and reporting have never been more important; in both conventional medicine and CAM, many published trials are being discounted due to a failure to meet these standards. However, these standards are not unachievable in CAM research and do not necessarily require huge resources. Evidence from a number of small, well-conducted trials may be equally, if not more valuable than evidence from a single large trial. The message for CAM is that high-quality, smaller trials should be encouraged, especially where resources for larger trials are hard to obtain (Edwards et al 1997).

Meta-analysis techniques

Even where an appropriately designed study results in a statistically significant finding, it is likely that more evidence than that provided by a single trial will be needed to convince the skeptical of a real effect. Replication is a cornerstone of scientific validation. As more studies are published in a particular area of research, it becomes possible to synthesize the results and thus create greater certainty regarding the direction and size of the effects reported.

Meta-analysis or the statistical pooling of data can only be undertaken on data of high quality where sufficiently similar data items exist. Meta-analysis techniques may be particularly useful in CAM research where studies have failed to show statistically significant results (no good evidence of an effect in either direction) due to the small numbers recruited to the trial. However, for this to be possible trials need to conform to recognized quality standards relating to the avoidance of bias and confounding in the data. In CAM, a depressingly large number of reviews have concluded that there is no good statistical data to be synthesized from existing studies. 'No evidence of effect' suggests that further research is needed but in the meantime this result may have the same impact on policy formation as one that shows 'evidence of no effect'. The apparent lack of good evidence in CAM may be due to inappropriate quality criteria being applied in some cases; it is hard to provide sensible placebo treatments for many CAM therapies and yet practitioner and patient blinding are almost invariably included in the list of criteria used. However, good reviews, using appropriate quality criteria, have definitely contributed to raising the standards in reporting of research studies in recent years.

Example from practice: meta-analysis of RCTs of St John's wort for depression
An example of a meta-analysis in CAM is given in Box 4.6. In this study a systematic review and meta-analysis were conducted looking mainly at non-English language published papers. Thus for many readers the review presented new data, as well as synthesized data.

The authors of this meta-analysis argue that pooling studies may be problematic because we may be pooling data on very different preparations of St John's wort and thus risking obscuring as much as we reveal. This is a potential problem in every meta-analysis and may also be relevant to other types of CAM. For example, reviews of acupuncture may combine study results using traditional acupuncture with those using formula acupuncture or reviews of homeopathy may combine

> **Box 4.6** St John's wort for depression – an overview and meta-analysis of randomized controlled trials. (Linde et al 1996)
>
> *Objectives:* To investigate if St John's wort is more efficacious than placebo in the treatment of depression and to investigate if St John's wort is as effective and has fewer side effects than low-dose standard antidepressant drugs.
>
> *Design:* Systematic review and meta-analysis of published trials of patients with mild or moderate depression identified using computerized and manual searches.
>
> *Main outcomes:* A pooled estimate of the ratio of 'treatment responders' to 'non-responders' in the groups treated with St John's wort compared to the control groups.
>
> *Selected results:* 23 RCTs of adequate quality were identified. The number of patients in each trial ranged from 30 to 162. A total of 13 trials (830 patients) had extractable data. The overall treatment response rate with placebo was 22% compared to 55% with St John's wort. No difference was found in treatment response rate in the five trials (317 patients) comparing St John's wort to antidepressants (64% and 59%). Reported adverse events were higher in the group taking low-dose standard antidepressants (36% compared to 20%).

individualized classical homeopathy with single remedy prescribing. In these cases meta-analysis is unlikely to be appropriate.

EXPLORATORY STUDIES

- Pilot studies
- Clinical outcome studies

Not all research aims to be definitive. There are a number of reasons why it is not appropriate to use definitive study designs. Resources and practicalities may militate against large-scale studies and well-conducted smaller studies may be able to make very good use of limited amounts of practitioner time which would otherwise be lost to research endeavor. Exploratory research is always needed, firstly as a means of developing hypotheses for research, allowing curiosity-led research questions to flourish, and secondly as a practical means of testing out the feasibility of conducting a larger scale study.

Some appropriate methods for exploratory research

Exploration implies less formal design but a number of research methods lend themselves to exploratory research. Pilot studies are small-scale 'dry runs' of planned or proposed further work. They offer the opportunity to test out elements of the process of research, e.g. identifying suitable patients or gauging their willingness to be involved. They also offer the opportunity to develop and test appropriate outcome measures for use in a full study and to obtain some data on the expected treatment effects that will help to define the size of the trial needed to produce statistically significant results. While the results from previous studies can sometimes be used to inform the design of new research, all too often there are no directly relevant data relating to a particular patient group or a particular treatment or service. Pilot study data help to fill these gaps by testing the conditions for a full trial.

Table 4.2 Exploratory studies

Research domain	Some research questions	Research focus/Reasons for asking the question	Some appropriate designs and methods (*Relative resources required)	Distinctive features of methods
Exploratory research	Does this procedure appear to be safe and offer benefits? Is there sufficient evidence of benefit to justify a full trial? What are the appropriate outcome measures? Is a trial feasible?	Pretrial focus ● Developing new practice ● Supporting bids for definitive research ● Refining research design ● Testing research conditions	Clinical outcome studies* N = 1 studies* Pilot studies**	● Are generally small scale and require a relatively low level of resourcing ● Lend themselves to practitioner-based research ● Do not require changes in the delivery of care to conform to an experimental design ● May involve the repeated applications of a recognized clinical outcome measure ● Comparison groups will not usually be included in the design ● Provide indicative, not conclusive or definitive evidence

Relative resources (time, skills and funding) required to undertake this type of research – least, moderate**, most*** (see Introduction section of chapter for full description)

Pilot studies may be needed when planning a full-scale trial or if there is a need to convince an external audience, such as funders, that the investment in a large study will be appropriate and the aims achievable. In contrast, observational studies do not attempt to mimic or test the process of a larger scale trial; instead they attempt to gather outcome data to address the question of possible benefits. They can also be used to test the suitability of a particular outcome measure in terms of its acceptability to patients and its sensitivity to changes following the intervention.

In contrast, the focus in clinical outcome studies is less on the testing of conditions for a trial and more on clinical process and outcomes with the aim of providing preliminary evidence of benefit and safety. What such exploratory studies have in common is that they cannot provide any conclusive evidence of an effect that can be confidently attributed to the treatment or intervention.

Distinctive features of exploratory research

Exploratory research is best seen as the beginning of the research process and should not be regarded as providing or aiming to provide conclusive evidence. Exploratory studies share a number of characteristics.

- Generally small scale and require a relatively low level of resourcing.
- Lend themselves to practitioner-based research.
- Do not require changes in the delivery of care to conform to an experimental design.
- Comparison groups will not usually be included in the design.
- Provide indicative, not conclusive or definitive evidence.
- May provide the justification for further research.
- Inform design for further research.

Pilot studies

'Is a definitive trial appropriate?'

Positive results from smaller studies are often cited as part of the justification for a larger trial. Such studies do not need to be definitive; it is enough that they indicate the possibility of a beneficial effect. It is also the case that any full trial will entail a number of decisions which will shape the final results of the trial and its interpretation: which patients will be included and which excluded, how will patients be recruited, what form will the treatment take and how much variation will there be between practitioners, which outcome measures will be used and how big does the trial need to be? All these decisions need to be informed by careful testing of the process proposed if the trial is to succeed in its own terms. All too frequently trials are reported which have failed to recruit patients in sufficient numbers. Pilot studies do not require large numbers and are therefore usually much less resource intensive. Done well, they can provide all the information required to justify and plan a successful trial.

Example from practice: a pilot study of acupuncture for low back pain

An example of a pilot study that preceded a full trial is given in Box 4.7. This pilot study tested the conditions for a trial as well as generating data on the sensitivity of

---

Box 4.7 Acupuncture for low back pain: results of a pilot study for a randomized controlled trial. (MacPherson et al 1999a)

Objective: To pilot procedures to be used in an RCT of the longer term outcomes of acupuncture for low back pain.

Design: Feasibility study and uncontrolled clinical trial.

Setting: Primary care and acupuncture clinics in York, England.

Subjects: 20 patients with low back pain lasting 1 month or more.

Intervention: 10 sessions of individualized acupuncture from traditional acupuncturist.

Main outcome measures: Oswestry Low Back Pain Disability Questionnaire; Present Pain Intensity Scale; Effect on Daily Living Scale and SF-36 General Health Index. Change measured post-treatment and 6 months after end of treatment.

Selected reported results: Substantial and statistically significant reductions were found in all scale scores post-treatment and at 6 months. Procedures used were shown to be appropriate for a full RCT. The authors conclude that although improvements observed may have been due to the natural course of back pain, the responses justify a full RCT.

the outcome measures. It led to a successful bid for national funding to conduct a full pragmatic RCT. The evidence from the pilot study demonstrated a potentially large health benefit, a feasible mechanism for referral and an appropriate level of acceptability of the treatment process to the patients. The pilot suggested that important patient benefits could be detected with the measures used, but was not able to demonstrate whether the benefits observed were due to the acupuncture treatment itself.

Clinical outcome studies

'Does this procedure appear to be safe and offer benefits to patients'

This question is the key starting point for most clinical research. Valuable information can be obtained with relatively few resources by research methods that entail the systematic monitoring of the outcomes of normal clinical practice. The choice of outcome measure is important. It needs to be easy to administer in the context of normal clinical practice; it also needs to be able to measure appropriate aspects of the patient's condition or to assess broader aims of the treatment. Although the range has expanded in recent years, published outcome measures rarely appear to meet the needs of a specific study. It is sometimes tempting to create new outcome measures to suit particular circumstances. However, the study when reported will have greater authority if the outcome measure employed has been used previously and validated, i.e. shown to measure what it claims to measure and to be sensitive to change. A number of different measures may be employed in a single study. In making this decision, consideration should be given to the fact that the more a patient is asked to do for the purposes of the research, the less treatment will represent normal clinical practice.

The most common design used for these studies entails the application of an outcome measure at baseline that is repeated after treatment for a specified series of patients. This design tests the range of responses to treatment found in a given patient group and gives a representative picture of the average response. In some circumstances, multiple measures may be taken before and after treatment, often with a crossover design that entails periods of active treatment followed by periods of no treatment. Typically, these experimental '$N = 1$' designs are applied to a single patient and derive their name from this fact. $N = 1$ designs (also known as 'n of one trials' or 'single subject trials') enable the testing for variation in the measurement process itself and thus provide an accurate measure of the change for a single patient. They are thus a stronger design than the general clinical outcome study and can provide persuasive evidence that any specific effect found is due to the treatment.

Distinctive features of clinical outcome studies

- Adoption of a systematic approach that nevertheless permits normal treatment relatively unfettered by research design.
- Repeated application at stages in the treatment process of a recognized clinical outcome measure.
- Identification of factors related to the treatment and/or to the patient that *may* indicate a causal effect on outcome.

Example from practice: factors that influence clinical outcomes

The study outlined in Box 4.8, in addition to demonstrating factors affecting outcome, was used to introduce acupuncture practitioners to research practice and to identify the circumstances and conditions in which patients consulted.

Practitioners in the study had the benefit of being part of a group working collaboratively on the research project – initially contributing to the design, collecting data in their own practices, having the data analyzed for them by a researcher experienced in data handling and statistical testing and finally meeting together to review the results and interpret their significance. Thus the research process was both educative and supportive to practitioners with little prior research experience.

IMPROVING STUDIES

- Clinical and reflective practice
  Case studies
  Diagnostic concordance studies
  Differential diagnosis and treatment (screening tool) studies
- Service delivery
  Service evaluation
  Cooperative inquiry and action research studies

Whereas research studies falling into the category of 'proving' have a common theme of addressing variants on the question 'Does it work?', 'improving' studies

---

Box 4.8 Factors that influence outcome: an evaluation of change with acupuncture. (MacPherson & Fitter 1998)

Objective: To evaluate change following treatment by acupuncture and to identify patient and treatment-related factors that affect outcome.

Design: Multicenter 'before and after' assessment of patients presenting for acupuncture with a new complaint. The participating practitioners collected data at each site.

Setting: Seven clinics in which a traditionally trained acupuncturist practiced.

Subjects: Men and women aged 18–80 with a new complaint for which they had not seen the practitioner in the previous 12 months (N= 58).

Intervention: Treatment at the discretion of the practitioner. The usual clinical service that would be provided.

Main outcome measures: A visual assessment scale, the Delighted-Terrible Faces, assessing the current experience of the complaint and a verbal scale assessing effect of complaint on daily living and well-being. Measures administered at 1st, 4th, 7th and 10th treatment sessions if patient continued to be seen. SF-36 administered prior to first treatment as a baseline measure of severity.

Selected reported results: There was a progressive and statistically significant improvement in both measures over the course of treatments. Patients with more severe initial conditions tended to make more rapid improvement, as did patients who had had their condition for a shorter duration. Measured improvement tended to level off after seven treatments and the authors discuss whether this indicates there is an optimum number of treatments from a cost-effectiveness perspective.

share the theme of 'Can it be improved in the way it works?'. Thus these studies are likely to be undertaken by practitioners interested in developing their practice in one way or another. As such there is some similarity with the exploratory studies, carried out as a prelude to a 'definitive proving' study and described in the previous section, both 'exploratory' and 'improving' studies being of particular interest to practitioners. The former focuses on developing research practice, the latter on developing clinical practice. In contrast, research can be used to develop clinical practice without any intention to proceed to a 'proving' study, such as a full clinical trial. Nevertheless, 'improving' studies can produce valuable findings and suggest avenues for further research.

As with the 'proving' studies, there are many dimensions on which change may be assessed; in addition to the primary one of clinical effectiveness, practitioners will likely have an interest in patient satisfaction and in cost effectiveness, for example. There are two broad categories of 'improving' studies: those concerned with clinical practice – practice that comprises the diagnostic and treatment processes – and those concerned with service delivery – the organization of the services that form a system enabling and supporting clinical practice.

Clinical and reflective practice

The focus in clinical practice studies is on the clinical process, the desire of the practitioner to 'do their best' for their patients and their own need for learning and professional development.

Case studies

Research-minded practitioners can use their day-to-day work as an opportunity to observe and reflect on their own practice. If tackled in a thoughtful and systematic way, the case study is a form of research that can address a wide range of interesting questions. Although such case studies in themselves are unlikely to give any definitive answers, the inquiring practitioner can make a valuable contribution to the development of practice of their profession. In the history of medical journals there are many examples of observations first written up as an 'interesting' case study, that act as a catalyst for further research, leading to important findings in medical research. When a new therapeutic method is developed initially evidence for its effectiveness will be based on the case study. For example, Levine (1997), in a book describing a new approach to healing people who have experienced trauma, states 'Somatic Experiencing® is new and is not subject to rigorous scientific research at this time. What I have to support the validity of this approach are several hundred individual cases in which people report that the symptoms which once impaired their ability to live full and satisfied lives are gone or greatly diminished'.

'By monitoring and reflecting on practice, can I improve my practice?' A particular form of clinical study is where practitioners enhance their normal practice by monitoring the process and effects of treatment. Although such studies are not able to demonstrate that any improvement in the patients' condition is unambiguously due to the treatment, they can nevertheless be of value because they can provide answers to questions such as 'Which patients do I seem to help the most' or 'In what way can I develop my skills and my practice to be more effective?'.

Table 4.3 Improving studies

Research domain	Some research questions	Research focus/ Reasons for asking the question	Some appropriate designs and methods (* Relative resources required)	Distinctive features of methods
Reflective and clinical practice	By monitoring and reflecting on practice can I improve my practice? Is this diagnostic procedure valid and reliable? Can use of a diagnostic test result in more cost-effectively targeted services?	Clinical/patient focus • The desire to learn from practice and, as a result, to change practice • Encouraging curiosity-led research • Communicating potential benefits and risks to clinical colleagues • The challenge to show that diagnostic categories have validity • If diagnostic categories can be used to discriminate between cases for which the treatment is more / less effective it can be used as a screening tool.	Case studies, including case histories, case series and reflective practice studies* Diagnostic concordance studies** Differential diagnosis and treatment studies (screening tools)**	• Usually carried out by practitioners exploring issues about which they are curious • Using a systematic process that permits normal treatment • An experimental design that presents all relevant information to multiple assessors • Use of a statistical procedure to assess whether there is sufficient agreement • Validation of differential diagnosis applied under normal clinical conditions • Demonstration that the differential diagnosis is predictive of clinical outcome and has pragmatic value.

Service delivery		Service/organization focus		
Is this new service effective in the wider service framework within which it has been established?	• If a new service is effective it may have a 'knock-on' effect on other services, with cost-benefit implications • To secure future funding of the service by demonstrating feasibility and benefits	Service evaluation**	• Evaluation of the main effects and side effects of the new service in the wider context	
What factors are enabling or impeding effective organization and delivery of services?	• In order to assess a new model of service delivery it needs to be possible. Can its operation be made more effective?	Cooperative inquiry and action research**	• Aims to understand the organization as a 'system' of interacting parts comprising 'stakeholder' roles and perspectives • An action focus with the intention of 'making a difference' in the organization • Possible blurring (or crossing) of boundaries between researchers and practitioners	

Relative resources (time, skills and funding) required to undertake this type of research – least, moderate**, most*** (see Introduction section of chapter for full description)

Some appropriate case study designs and methods The case history or case report has a long tradition within medicine, biomedical and traditional, and is still playing a prominent role. A recent collection of case histories in acupuncture practice (MacPherson & Kaptchuk 1997) brings together cases from many of the most experienced traditional acupuncturists in the West. The book explores the effect of transferring a therapy of Oriental origin into a context in which patients have different cultural experiences and beliefs about matters such as diet, lifestyle and illness. An aim of the book is to 'uncover the various ways in which leading acupuncturists engage with these experiences and issues, and how they work with the complexities and uncertainties that are inherently part of an ongoing therapeutic relationship'.

The case series is a particular type of case study that entails the reporting of responses to treatment for a systematically chosen sequence of patients (the first 10 patients treated with a new procedure, for example). The study may, for example, entail asking patients to assess side effects and benefits following treatment or to monitor subsequent resource use.

Reflective practice studies are another type of case study. Their distinctive feature is that the practitioner engages in a systematic process of self-reflection. One such way of engaging is to begin with a 'critical incident' and then explore its antecedents and consequences. Another is to regularly review practice, focusing on emotional reactions or surprises as triggers to a reflective process. Reflective practice is a form of critical thinking that requires emotional awareness in addition to thought processes. For this reason it is sometimes referred to as 'critical being' (Barnett 1997). Carried out well, with a commitment to potentially deep personal learning, the reflective practice study can produce profound results for the practitioner as well as suggesting topics for further, more objective research.

A value of the case study approach is its potential as a mechanism for communicating clinical practice, for alerting the practitioner community to possible adverse effects and for facilitating curiosity-led research. What such studies cannot do is provide any conclusive evidence of a specific effect that can be attributed to the treatment.

Distinctive features of case study research

- Adoption of a systematic approach that nevertheless permits normal treatment in a real-world context, unfettered by research design.
- Identification of factors related to the treatment and/or to the patient that *may* indicate a causal effect on outcome.
- Understanding of a therapy in its cultural context in a way that allows the exploration of curiosity and critical thinking.

Diagnostic concordance studies

When a diagnostic procedure has evolved as part of clinical practice an obvious question to ask is whether the procedure has any 'objective validity'.

'Is this diagnostic procedure valid and reliable?'

If a diagnostic procedure is not valid and reliable it may be regarded as a feature of clinical practice but its role in differentiating between clinical conditions, and thereby having value in the process of choosing an appropriate treatment, will be called into question.

Some appropriate designs and methods for assessing diagnostic concordance

An important aspect of the validity of a test is whether a number of appropriately skilled practitioners, given the same information, would make the same diagnosis. If they do, to a sufficient degree, there is tangible evidence that the diagnostic procedure is more than a chimera – it is able to differentiate reliably. Diagnostic concordance (the assessment of consistency in diagnosis across practitioners) requires each practitioner to be given:

- all necessary information to make a diagnosis
- the same information.

These requirements raise a difficulty in the design of such studies. Often it will not be possible to ensure each practitioner gets exactly the same information. In situations where it is possible, for example a photograph or a video recording is regarded as adequate information, then the research design can use a large number of practitioners assessing a small number of cases. Where it is necessary that each practitioner gets direct access to the patient, it is likely to be practical for only two or three practitioners to see each patient (and then the sequence in which they see the patient needs to be considered as a factor). In this case, a larger number of cases will be required to reach a statistically valid conclusion. Nevertheless, despite the design challenges, such studies can provide a scientific underpinning to procedures that may appear to lack a scientific foundation.

Distinctive features of diagnostic concordance studies

- An experimental design that aims to present all relevant information required for making a diagnosis to practitioners in a consistent form.
- Clinical practice needs to be able to distinguish a diagnostic process leading to distinct diagnostic outcomes (diagnoses). This may not be the case for therapies in which diagnostic and treatment processes are fully enmeshed.
- For the test to have validity requires that qualified practitioners participating in the study accept that they have all (or sufficient) relevant clinical information to make a diagnosis. They need to agree this before the results of the test are revealed.
- A statistical procedure is used to analyze data and determine whether the level of agreement (concordance) between practitioners is (a) greater than chance and (b) sufficient for the procedure to have practical clinical value.

Examples from practice: diagnostic validity and interpractitioner consistency

In CAM research, such studies have tended to focus on therapies that appear to lack a scientific basis, for example iridology (the example presented in Box 4.9) and kinesiology, a procedure commonly used for testing for food allergies. See Garrow (1988) for an assessment of the use of kinesiology in allergy diagnosis.

Box 4.9 Looking for gall bladder disease in the patient's iris. (Knipschild 1988)

Objective: To test the validity of iridology as a diagnostic aid.

Design: Blinded case-control study of the diagnosis of gall bladder disease amongst skilled iridologists.

Setting: University hospital in the Netherlands.

Subjects: Five volunteer iridologists, of whom two were medical doctors, 39 patients awaiting gall bladder removal, 39 matched controls with no gall bladder disease. Gall bladder disease was confirmed post-surgery in all 39 cases.

Intervention: The iridologists agreed to undertake diagnosis using stereo colour slides of the right iris of all subjects. Additional information on patients was limited to age and sex.

Main outcome measures: Accuracy of diagnosis (proportion of all subjects correctly assigned to positive or negative for gall bladder disease), sensitivity of iridology diagnosis (proportion of all true positives identified correctly) and specificity of iridology diagnosis (proportion of all true negatives that were diagnosed as negative). Consistency of diagnosis between practitioners was also measured.

Selected reported results: All results for validity of diagnosis were close to those that would be expected by chance; median accuracy 51%, sensitivity 54% and specificity 52%. None of the individual practitioners reached high validity. Median interperformer consistency was 60%, only slightly higher than would be expected by chance. The author concludes, 'This study shows that iridology is not a useful diagnostic tool'.

The author of the iridology paper conducted a parallel study of doctors and practitioners who had recently published in mainstream and alternative medical journals to gauge changes in their belief in iridology as a diagnostic tool (Knipschild 1989). Two hundred practitioners were surveyed before and after the publication of these results. Participation in both surveys was low (39%), but the results obtained from responders showed the results to have had a measurable impact on beliefs; the majority of responders were uncertain before reading the report and two-thirds of these did not believe in iridology as a diagnostic aid after reading the paper. Impact on practice was not researched. The negative trial result was reported as 'disappointing' to the participating iridologists, who felt that the conclusions were too final. We can only speculate whether a positive result would have been taken as conclusive evidence and whether it would have facilitated a change in either beliefs or practice.

Differential diagnosis and treatment (screening tool) studies

'Can use of a diagnostic test result in more cost-effectively targeted services?' If there is a diagnostic test that can be shown to discriminate reliably between clinical conditions, does it have prognostic value? That is, will it make any difference to practice and clinical outcomes if it is used?

Some appropriate designs and methods for developing and assessing screening tools

To assess a potential screening tool requires two stages. The first is to validate a diagnostic procedure that can reliably discriminate between conditions (see previous section). The second is that the differential diagnosis can be shown to be predictive of different outcomes.

Distinctive features of studies that develop screening tools

- Validation of a differential diagnosis applied under normal clinical conditions.
- Demonstration that the differential diagnosis is predictive of clinical outcome.
- Pragmatic value in applying the screening tool, for example, through early detection or cost-effective use of resources.

Example from practice: assessment of a diagnostic framework as a potential screening tool

The development of a potential screening tool may take place within another larger study. For example, a pragmatic RCT of the offer of acupuncture for low back pain (Thomas et al 1999) contains within it a substudy to evaluate the reliability of the diagnostic categories of traditional Chinese medicine (Box 4.10). If the categories are shown to be reliable for use in differential diagnosis and if it turns out they can discriminate between clinical outcomes (for one diagnostic category the prognosis following treatment is good, for another it is poor) then it may be possible to adapt the diagnostic framework for application at the referral stage, thereby selecting patients where the prognosis is good and thus making more cost-effective use of the service.

A particularly interesting feature of this study is that it is evaluating diagnostic categories that have no theoretical meaning within a Western biomedical framework. Were they demonstrated to be of practical value for screening patients, the study would be an interesting example of the integration of diverse medical frameworks.

Box 4.10 Evaluating the reliability of the diagnostic categories of traditional Chinese medicine. (MacPherson et al 1999b)

Objective: To assess the reliability of the diagnostic categories of traditional Chinese medicine (TCM) and to compare clinical outcomes for each of the categories. To explore the question of why some people are more likely to benefit from acupuncture than others.

Design: Patients seen by one of five acupuncturists for an initial diagnosis. Another practitioner acts as a 'bench mark' and sees all patients. For each patient the diagnosis made by the two practitioners is compared and the statistic kappa, a measure of agreement, is calculated. If the kappa indicates sufficient agreement the clinical outcome from the course of treatment is then aggregated for each diagnostic category to determine the TCM diagnosis-specific effectiveness of treatment.

Setting: Two clinics providing traditional acupuncture as part of a pragmatic RCT evaluating the longer term effectiveness of the offer of acupuncture for low back pain.

Subjects: 120 patients aged between 20 and 65 presenting to GPs with a current episode of low back pain of between 4 weeks and 12 months duration.

Intervention: Traditional acupuncture provided in accord with the normal practice of the acupuncturist and the clinic, with up to 10 treatment sessions available.

Main outcome measures: The diagnostic categories based on TCM syndromes. Clinical outcome assessed by the Bodily Pain dimension of the SF-36, the Present Pain Intensity Scale of the McGill Pain Questionnaire and the Oswestry Low Back Pain Disability Questionnaire. Outcomes assessed at baseline, at 3 months and at 12 months.

Selected reported results: Study in progress.

Service delivery

With CAM being a growth area in health care, there are numerous examples of new services being established, both in private clinics and in the NHS (and generally in Managed Care outside the UK). Often little formal research or evaluation is carried out. However, where a study is established, often by committed practitioners working together with researchers, sometimes prompted by the service commissioner requesting formal evidence of benefit, there can be much to learn if the study is well designed and executed.

Within evaluation research there are two broad categories of research design – summative and formative evaluations. A summative evaluation is one that addresses the question 'Is this service one we want to continue funding?' and it is usually therefore asked by commissioners of health-care services, though practitioners are also likely to be interested in showing that they provide a service that is of value. It is called summative because it assumes the service has been developed to the point where it is operating optimally and now it is time to ask whether it should continue, summing up what we know about it. In contrast, formative evaluation addresses the question 'How can we improve the organization of this service?' and is usually of primary concern to those developing the service. Clearly, logic suggests that formative evaluation should precede summative evaluation, though sadly this is not always the case. In practice many evaluations have both elements within them, though usually one is the primary focus.

Service evaluation studies

'Is this new service effective in the wider service framework within which it has been established?'

This question usually indicates a summative evaluation, though frequently there will be a formative component. It will be important to use the evaluation to learn lessons about how the service could be improved, unless the intention is to close it down! The evaluation needs to provide clear evidence of effectiveness and therefore will usually adopt formal clinical and economic outcome measures.

Some appropriate designs and methods for evaluating a new service

The research designs available tend to parallel the designs for evaluating a clinical intervention. Thus, for example, it may be possible to design a pragmatic RCT to 'prove' the effectiveness of the new service. However, in many situations such a rigorous design is either not practical or too expensive. Alternatives are designs that use a matched control group and designs that have no control group but compare the results produced by the service under evaluation with data available from other sources. These include data from the same context but collected prior to establishment of the new service and data from similar services elsewhere that do not have the benefit of the new service under test. As with the clinical intervention studies, the same issues of 'rigor at the expense of realism' vs 'pragmatism at the expense of confounding factors' apply.

In order to evaluate outcomes in the wider context, the study may examine the impact of the new service on the service within which it is established. Thus there may be an assessment of the impact of a new in-house service on the number of referrals to outside agencies (see, for example, Peters et al 1994). This study design may provide important information justifying the cost of a new service by savings elsewhere.

Distinctive features of studies that evaluate new services

- Use of formal clinical and economic outcome measures. It is important that the measures to be used are agreed with stakeholders to represent the important evaluation criteria.
- Evaluation of the direct effect of the service on patients referred to it.
- Evaluation of the side (or knock-on) effects of the service on other linked services.
- Identification of lessons learned that may be useful for the further development of the service.

Example from practice: evaluation of a new hospital-based CAM service

The example chosen to illustrate this type of study (Box 4.11) was not published in a journal but is a good example of a comprehensive evaluation using a relatively

---

Box 4.11   Complementary therapy in the NHS: a service evaluation of the first year of an outpatient service in a local district general hospital. (Richardson 1995)

Objective: To provide a planned, detailed evaluation program for a new service to address the questions 'Does the service have an effect on patients?', 'What is the nature of the effect?' and 'Would the effect have occurred without intervention?'.

Design: A quasi-experimental design with non-equivalent control groups and without randomization, using waiting list as the control group. The original intention was for a simpler 'before and after' outcome study, but quickly established demand led to the creation of a waiting list enabling the stronger design to be used. The waiting-list controls are assessed at the same 'before and after' time periods as patients in the 'new service' group even though they are still awaiting entry to the service. Examination of referral patterns and patient characteristics.

Setting: A complementary therapy center established as an outpatient clinic in an NHS hospital.

Subjects: 883 patients referred by GPs to the clinic during a 9-month period.

Intervention: Offer of up to six treatment sessions of acupuncture, osteopathy or homeopathy. The GP referral form offered the opportunity to refer for one of the three therapies on offer or for a multidisciplinary opinion.

Main outcome measures: The SF-36 health survey with its eight subscales, administered at baseline (initial assessment) and at completion of treatment (at 3 months from baseline for the waiting-list controls).

Selected reported results: Patients in the treatment group did not differ significantly from the waiting-list controls on patient characteristics and on baseline measures, with one exception: the 'role – physical limitation' scale of the SF-36. This result generally supports the quasi-experimental design, though it indicates that patients with a more serious role limitation were prioritized on the waiting list. T-tests indicated significant improvements for patients receiving treatment in the new service but not for waiting-list controls. The author concluded, 'The significant improvements in health following treatment and the absence of improvements for the controls over time suggest that the health improvement demonstrated in this study would not have occurred without treatment'. Service development recommendations were made.

strong design. That is, a quasi-experimental design was adopted in which patients on the waiting list for the new service were used as a control group to compare with those that received the new service.

Although patients were not randomized to the new service or waiting list in this study, the validity of the comparison group was demonstrated by collecting data that indicated that they did not appear to differ on any important characteristics. (Note, this also originally appeared to be the case with the Bristol Cancer Help Centre study, described previously, which acts as a reminder that the design is vulnerable to having non-comparable groups). This study is of interest for another reason. At the time that the results were made available, results that demonstrated the service's effectiveness, the health authority purchasing the service was making the decision to discontinue funding of the service!

Cooperative inquiry and action research studies

'What factors are enabling or impeding effective delivery of services?'

This question focuses on a desire to improve services by better understanding the factors that contribute to effectiveness. It is therefore primarily a question that requires a formative evaluation approach. Whereas outcome measures may be important to indicate effectiveness, the focus is on understanding those systemic factors that are influencing the outcome.

Some appropriate designs and methods for improving the effectiveness of service organization and delivery

Qualitative research methods are likely to predominate in this area. The goal is service development and improvement, from the perspective of the various stakeholder groups – patients, practitioners, managers, support staff and commissioners. Appropriate methods go under a variety of labels, each sharing some common characteristics and each with its own emphasis. Historically, action research focuses on theory-led change, recognizing the cyclical nature of research revolving through ideas, to planned interventions, to evaluation, to review and further action (Hart & Bond 1995). Cooperative inquiry has a similar cycle of action and reflection and focuses on the potential for collaboration between stakeholder groups, and particularly between practitioners and researchers (Reason 1994). Service development studies may also be called formative evaluations if the focus is on evaluation against an objective. Action research is also likely to start with an action-focused goal, whereas a cooperative inquiry may be more exploratory; for example, 'What might we learn by working together in this new way?'.

Distinctive features of studies that aim to improve the organization and delivery of services

- Usually explicit recognition of different stakeholder perspectives.
- An action focus; research that will make a difference in the organization where it is being carried out.
- Primarily use of qualitative methods and measures.
- A blurring (or crossing) of the boundaries between researchers and practitioners.

• Possibly, but not essentially, a result that makes a contribution to knowledge by generalizing to other contexts or by revealing some general principles.

Example from practice: cooperative inquiry on collaboration between practitioners

Since most CAM practitioners work in private clinics and historically there has been little experience of working in collaboration with mainstream health service practitioners, when a clinic is set up with the intention of practitioners working closely together it is of considerable research interest (Box 4.12).

Reading this paper today, one is struck by how the possibilities and the experience of collaboration have increased since this seminal study was conducted and also by the continuing relevance of the issues that were identified as important when practitioners with different belief systems and assumptions about practice work in collaboration.

CONCLUSION

In this chapter our aim has been to present the main research questions that are posed and the range of research designs and methods that are used to address these questions. In particular, we have not covered research designs relating to picturing current practice, understanding the mechanisms of different therapies or the

---

Box 4.12   Towards a clinical framework for collaboration between general and complementary practitioners: discussion paper. (Reason et al 1992)

Objective: To investigate the model of cooperative clinical practice being used in a health center from the perspective of each of the clinical disciplines. To identify lessons learned and ideas for improvement of service delivery.

Design: Cooperative inquiry between practitioners and researchers, working together as co-researchers; five cycles of action and reflection over an 8-month period.

Setting: Health center in inner London with a newly established multidisciplinary clinic.

Subjects: Three general practitioners and four complementary practitioners with the Director of Clinical Research as facilitator.

Intervention: In each cycle, an action phase of two or three clinics (each practitioner made an initial assessment with each patient) followed by a reflection phase (a 3-hour facilitated meeting, tape recorded, transcribed and circulated to participants).

Main outcome measures: N/A

Selected reported results: Recognition that within the clinical team there existed several different models of multidisciplinary practice, some shared, some idiosyncratic, some explicit, some tacit. There were three areas of shared concern about multidisciplinary practice: the importance of specialist diagnosis from the perspective of each discipline; differences in emphasis and interpretation of the patient's psychosocial context; the significance of the practitioner–patient relationship. The benefits and challenges arising from the availability of multiple perspectives were identified, as were the effect of the relationship with the patient on the relationship between practitioners and vice versa. Finally, the researchers identify a core issue of the personal integration of specialized skills with an understanding of the patient's predicament and containing these within a healing relationship. This was encapsulated for the team of practitioners by the question 'Who has the juice for this patient?'.

development of new and better research tools appropriate to the study of CAM. To do so would have required a much larger treatise.

Central to our framework is the assumption that there is no absolute best research design, only ones that are appropriate to the question being asked – 'horses for courses' – and that a research strategy needs to begin with the research question and then choose an appropriate design and its associated methods. There are interdependencies between research questions; as we have indicated, within a research strategy some questions logically precede others. For example, exploratory studies lead to full clinical trials; formative evaluations lead to summative evaluations.

Questions for discussion and personal reflection

- *As a practitioner*, what aspects of your practice do you feel passionate about? What are you curious about?
- Do these thoughts suggest a research question that you would like to address? Read widely around the topic; consider doing a literature search.
- If so, what would be an appropriate research design and method? Read more about this in the Further Reading, in the rest of this book and elsewhere.
- Begin to formulate a research proposal (a research question, design and methods, an assessment of resources and support required). Is it likely to be feasible? What support will you need? Where might you get it?
- Are you still enthusiastic? If yes, go for it! If not, go back to step one.
- *As a researcher*, does any of this chapter challenge you conceptually? Do you need to reframe your understanding in any way? It may help to read some more about the ideas and values underlying CAM and CAM research.
- Are there any areas where you could add greater clarity to the framework? If yes, let us know please!

REFERENCES

Bagenal F, Easton D, Harris E, Chilvers C, McElwain T 1990 Survival of patients with breast cancer attending Bristol Cancer Help Centre. Lancet 336: 606–610
Barnett R 1997 Higher education: a critical business. SRHE / Open University Press, Buckingham
Cherkin D, Deyo R, Batties M, Street J, Barlow W 1998 A comparison of physical therapy, chiropractic manipulation, and provision of an educational booklet for the treatment of patients with low back pain. New England Journal of Medicine 339: 1021–1029
Edwards S, Lilford R, Braunholtz D, Jackson J 1997 Why 'underpowered' trials are not necessarily unethical. Lancet 350: 804–807
Fitter M, Thomas KJ 1997 Evaluating complementary health care for use in the National Health Service. 'Horses for courses' Part 1: The design challenge. Complementary Therapies in Medicine 5: 90–93
Garrow JS 1988 Kinesiology and food allergy. British Medical Journal 296: 1573–1574
Hart E, Bond M 1995 Action research for health and social care: a guide to practice. Open University Press, Buckingham
Knipschild P 1988 Looking for gall bladder disease in the patient's iris. British Medical Journal 297: 1578–1581
Knipschild P 1989 Changing belief in iridology after an empirical study. British Medical Journal 299: 491–492

Levine PA 1997 Walking the tiger: healing trauma. Berkeley, CA: North Atlantic Books

Linde K, Ramirez G, Mulrow C, Pails A, Weidenhammer W, Melchart D 1996 St John's wort for depression – an overview and meta-analysis of randomised controlled trials. British Medical Journal 313: 253–258

MacPherson H, Fitter M 1998 Factors that influence outcome: an evaluation of change with acupuncture. Acupuncture in Medicine 16: 33–39

MacPherson H, Kaptchuk T (eds) 1997 Acupuncture in practice: case history insights from the West. Churchill Livingstone, New York

MacPherson H, Fitter M, Gould A 1999a Acupuncture for low back pain: results of a pilot study for a randomised controlled trial. Complementary Therapies in Medicine 7: 83–91

MacPherson H, Thomas KJ, Thorpe L, Campbell M 1999b Evaluating the reliability of the diagnostic categories of traditional Chinese medicine. Unpublished protocol

Meade T, Dyer S, Browne W, Townsend J, Frank A 1990 Low back pain of mechanical origin; randomised comparison of chiropractic and hospital outpatient treatment. British Medical Journal 300: 1431–1437

Peters D, Davies P, Pietroni P 1994 Musculoskeletal clinic in general practice: study of one year's referrals. British Journal of General Practice 44: 25–29

Reason P (ed) 1994 Participation in human inquiry. Sage Publications, London

Reason P, Chase HD, Desser A et al 1992 Towards a clinical framework for collaboration between general and complementary practitioners: a discussion paper. Journal of the Royal Society of Medicine 85: 161–164

Reilly D, Taylor M, McSharry C, Aitchison T 1986 Is homoeopathy a placebo response? Controlled trial of homeopathic potency, with pollen in hayfever, a model Lancet i: 881–885

Richardson J 1995 Complementary therapy in the NHS: a service evaluation of the first year of an outpatient service in a local district general hospital. Health Service Research and Evaluation Unit, The Lewisham Hospital NHS Trust. Unpublished report

Shekelle PG 1998 What role for chiropractic in health care? New England Journal of Medicine 339: 1074–1075

Thomas KJ, Fitter M 1997 Evaluating complementary health care for use in the National Health Service. 'Horses for courses'. Part 2: Alternative research strategies. Complementary Therapies in Medicine 5: 94–99

Thomas KJ, Fitter M, Brazier J, MacPherson H, Campbell M, Nicholl J, Roman M 1999 Longer-term clinical and economic benefits of offering acupuncture to patients with chronic low back pain assessed as suitable for primary care management. Complementary Therapies in Medicine 7: 91–100

FURTHER READING

The following are all readable general research methods textbooks and collections of readings. They lack a specific CAM perspective but cover the full range of designs and methods used to evaluate conventional health-care interventions and services.

Black N, Brazier J, Fitzpatrick R, Reeves B (eds) 1998 Health services research methods: a guide to best practice. BMJ Books, London

Crombie IK, Davies HTO 1996 Research in healthcare. Wiley, Chichester

Jenkinson C (ed) 1997 Assessment and evaluation of health and medical care. Open University Press, Buckingham

Ovretveit J 1998 Evaluating health interventions. Open University Press, Buckingham

Robson R 1993 Real world research: a resource for social scientists and practitioner-researchers. Blackwell, Oxford

5

Evaluating complementary medicine: lessons to be learned from evaluation research

Werner W Wittmann   Harald Walach

INTRODUCTION

Evaluation research is the application of methods and knowledge of social science in order to make rational and well-informed decisions about social intervention programs (Shadish et al 1991). The term was coined during the 1960s when in the United States social programs were introduced in order to promote social welfare, education or other large-scale social intervention (Cook & Matt 1990). Since it was necessary to decide whether these programs were worth their money, research was started in order to find out about their general effects. Since then evaluation research has developed into a major branch of applied social science. It has given rise to a whole new profession and because its tasks and problems are comparable to research problems in other areas, evaluation research has had an impact on other areas of applied research.

There is a long history to evaluation research and the problems encountered are comparable to what research in complementary and alternative medicine (CAM) is faced with. Hence it seems advisable to look over the border of methodological wisdom in medical research and learn from what has been achieved and experienced in this comparable branch of research. We would therefore like to introduce the reader to some major aspects and results of reflection on methodology in evaluation research. Although research on medical interventions is in many aspects different from, say, educational or social interventions, there are also basic commonalities that imply common methodological problems. Learning from these problems and the solutions reached in evaluation research means avoiding the same pitfalls.

After a short introduction to the major phases and theories of evaluation research, we will describe a comprehensive model of evaluation, some sound methodological principles derived from it and practical consequences and applications for research.

A SHORT HISTORY AND MAJOR DEVELOPMENTS OF EVALUATION RESEARCH

The development of evaluation research can be ordered into two major phases which are connected with some of the leading theorists in this area (Cook & Matt 1990). Phase 1 (1965–75) is usually connected with the names Michael Scriven and Donald T Campbell and is normally referred to as the phase of objectivistic or experimental models of evaluation. Scriven introduced the discrimination between formative and summative evaluation (Scriven 1980). In formative evaluation, applied research can be used to improve ongoing social intervention programs by immediately feeding back results into the process of shaping the program. This can be seen as an early example of quality assurance or quality management. Summative evaluation, on the other hand, is evaluation in the strong sense of the word, namely summing up the results of an intervention. Its goal is to make a well-informed decision about the introduction of certain social or political intervention programs on the basis of valid and generalizable information.

It was mostly Donald T Campbell who brought forward the point that valid decisions can only be made by experimental research. He drew attention to the many drawbacks of non-experimental (i.e. non-randomized) studies, such as the problem of confounding, the impossibility of disentangling intervention effects from effects of self-selection on natural groups and the like. It was mainly due to his widely accepted authority that evaluation research adopted this strictly experimental, objectivistic point of view.

Evaluation of programs from this era usually consisted of large-scale experimental trials, in which subjects had been randomly assigned to either receive, say, a state benefit or not. In general the evaluation results of these large programs were inconclusive. Although the experimental design of these studies made them highly internally valid, other aspects of the research hampered external validity, thereby making many of the results useless. One line of criticism, therefore, was methodological: focusing only on the methodological necessities of research and leaving out the social context and other equally important aspects of the program to be evaluated inevitably leads to the overemphasis of internal validity at the expense of external validity and in some cases of the practicability of research in general.

The second line of criticism, mainly by Carol Weiss (1973, 1975), pointed out that producing valid information is only one part of the complex process of evaluation. Researchers should also be aware of the context and the aims the research is being produced for. Weiss discovered that the results of research very often did not have the impact on political decisions that they should have or were even completely ignored. That led her to the conclusion that political factors, interests and preconceived notions are very powerful in the process of decision making and that valid information is only one of many influential factors. Weiss thus directed the attention of researchers to the political and social context of research. She criticized the aloofness of the experimental evaluation paradigm and its blindness for the way results were being used or neglected (Suchman 1967).

After 1980 the second generation of evaluation researchers tried to synthesize these experiences into one coherent theoretical model of evaluation research. The most important names in this context are Peter Rossi and Lee Cronbach (Chen & Rossi 1981, 1983, Cronbach 1982, Rossi & Freeman 1982). Rossi pointed out that experimental research strategies are only one out of a multiplicity of possible methods. He emphasized the importance of external validity or generalizability as having at least the same importance as internal validity, the hallmark of experimental research. Rossi also pointed out that for an evaluation to be successful, it would have to follow a particular theory. This means that the evaluation method applied should conform to ideas of the system under evaluation. Theory-driven evaluation means that the theory of the programs or interventions being studied should be taken into account when applying evaluation research methodology. Therefore, Rossi suggests that, depending on the question, a naturalistic or quasi-experimental design could be used just as well as an experimental design.

The general thrust of this argument was extended by Lee Cronbach who criticized the overemphasis on internal validity over external validity. He also pointed to the practical ramifications of evaluation, i.e. the necessity to convince stakeholders of the importance of evaluation or various interest groups of the importance of the results and how the results could, in the end, be practically implemented. While the end of the discussion is not reached yet, a consensus is emerging among evaluation researchers. This consensus is best described as a multiplicity of research strategies and the application of research strategy according to evaluation tasks, evaluation context and evaluation goals. There seems to be agreement among researchers and theorists that there is no single best method but only a comparatively optimal method for a certain practical situation. This has been summarized by Cook & Wittmann (1998, p. 110):

We would be pleased to see European evaluators celebrate the diversity of relevant methods and not be side-tracked into sterile debates about one method being preferable to another for evaluation in general.

Evaluation research has learned a very important lesson: there is no such thing as a gold standard of methodology. There is only a very cumbersome process of understanding a research context properly and finding the research methodology best suited to that context. Having achieved that, there still remains the task of implementing results and arguing for or against political decisions made on the basis of these research results. Applied research in social science has taken more than a quarter of a century to arrive at a multifaceted theory of research methodology. The bottom line of this is that research methodology has to be geared towards questions and the context of research problems. There is no best option but only choices which have to be made. We will describe some important ones in the following sections.

A COMPREHENSIVE MODEL FOR EVALUATION
Reliability, validity and Cattell's data box

Any research result needs to be reliable and valid. While validity refers to whether research conclusions are correct and can be trusted, reliability is concerned with whether the operationalizations and the variables have been measured in a meaningful and stable way with as little error as possible (Wittmann 1988). Thus, reliability normally addresses questions of variables and their measurement, while validity is concerned with design in terms of prediction and explanation. Technically speaking, a reliable measurement is one in which the observed variance is nearly completely due to true variance and the error variance is approaching zero. Validity normally means that the attribution of effects to an intervention or to certain causes can be made with great confidence.

A reliable measurement has two aspects: inclusion of as many facets or parts of a variable as possible and assessing the stability of the variable in question. A reliable measurement of blood pressure, for instance, includes both aspects of blood pressure, the diastolic and systolic part, as well as knowledge about the stability of a certain reading at a particular time. A reliable measurement of quality of life, as another example, would include that all interesting aspects of quality of life have been tested in multiple variables, so that the global construct quality of life has been operationalized adequately. Again, for a measurement of quality of life to be reliable, we would want to know whether a measurement instrument like a questionnaire is measuring a rather stable or quite a varied construct. Therefore, for measurements to be reliable it is usually necessary to have multiple operationalizations, such as an array of items for measuring one construct, and ideally more timepoints in order to assess stability.

A third aspect is variability across persons. Since in evaluation research we normally want to assess the impact of an intervention on groups of persons it is necessary to include more than one person in scientific observations. Therefore, an assessment can, in general terms, be conceived of as a three-dimensional data box (Wittmann 1987). Figure 5.1 shows this graphically. One dimension of the box represents subjects, another one represents multiple variables and the third dimension represents time, i.e. stability. Every construct of interest can be conceptualized as such a box. In order for a measurement to be reliable, we need multiple representations of variables addressing a construct, multiple subjects being measured and ideally multiple time-points of measurement for assessing stability. These boxes can be combined into a five data box model (Fig. 5.2) (Wittmann 1985, 1990).

The five data box model

The first box, termed the PR box (classical predictors), contains all variables measured at baseline, before any intervention is applied. If only this box is addressed we have a typical cross-sectional design over multiple measurements or a cohort study. If only one slice of the first box is addressed we have the typical one time-point cross-sectional study. Ideally, the predictor box contains all those variables which might be interesting for predicting an outcome. While intervention research in a medical context is normally mostly concerned about effects of treatments, it is also interesting to study which subjects benefit from the treatment and which do not and to use predictor variables in order to discriminate between them in regression models, an option hardly used in traditional trials, let alone in CAM.

Box 2 is the experimental treatment box. It represents all variables which refer to treatments used in randomized experiments. Put differently, box 2 describes randomized controlled trials. Here it is necessary that the treatment being studied is well described and also well applied. That usually means the multiple application of treatment and a clear definition and description of the treatment. It usually also means that more than one person is being treated and more than one person is being used as a control. Also here, ideally, a multiple set of variables should be used to verify that the treatment in question has been implemented properly.

Box 3 is termed the 'non-experimental treatment box'. It is equivalent to box 2 except it refers to treatments which subjects have not been randomized into but have chosen

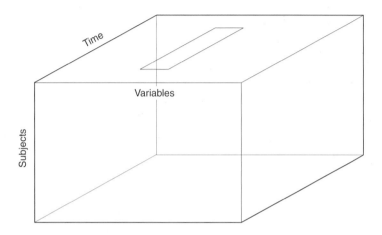

Figure 5.1 The data box (after Cattell 1957).

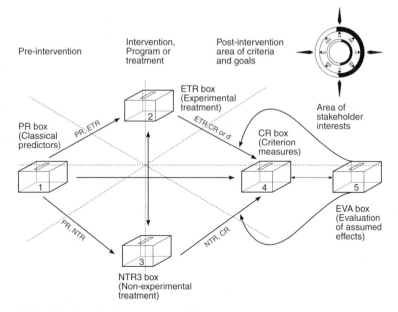

Figure 5.2 The five data box conceptualization.

naturally or as a consequence of their natural attributes, like males and females. Thus, a treatment of hypnosis, say for pain, which subjects have been attributed to randomly would be an example of treatment box 2, the experimental treatment box. Studying self-selected groups of CAM users compared to users of conventional medicine would be an example of treatment box 3, the non-experimental treatment box. Note that, ideally, box 2 and 3 are also conceptualized as boxes, that is to say that multiple variables, time points and subjects have to be evaluated.

Box 4, the criterion box, represents what is usually termed outcome variables or study targets. It contains those variables which are used for measuring effects of treatments. Also here, ideally, we would want to use a set of variables and various time-points for estimating stability, apart from the fact that all subjects who have undergone the treatment are being measured.

Treatment box 5, finally, is called the 'evaluation box'. After any type of study, the results have to be put into context and evaluated against a goal or a set of standards. Box 4 usually supplies us with information about the results which have been obtained and whether they are different from comparison standards but it does not tell us whether the differences or results obtained are in any way useful, clinically or economically relevant. This evaluation has to be made separately. And it is useful to discriminate these two processes of measuring outcome and evaluating this outcome. A good strategy of evaluating multiple outcomes is aggregating several outcomes into single or multiple criteria, which consist of higher level constructs; for example, several scales representing quality of life might be integrated into a joint score of quality of life. This integrated score might be aggregated together with other measures, like clinical or economic measures or measures of behavior change, into an overall criterion of improvement. Thus, within the evaluation box a set of strategies can be applied in order to aggregate over several domains of outcome measurement and even time. Such higher level outcome criteria may be measured either at one point in time or at several points and can accordingly be aggregated differently.

Multiple measurements to enhance reliability

Four variants of outcome criteria are to be distinguished. The first is the single act criterion, where we assess a single variable or a single item at one point of measurement. This type of outcome is known to be of low reliability. The second type aggregates an item over time and is labeled the repeated single act criterion. Hereby we strive for better reliability in terms of stability. The third type aggregates several items at a measurement point to adequately assess the breadth of a construct. Most of these scales are constructed via factor analysis. For purposes of outcome assessment, they are termed multiple act criteria. Finally, the fourth type, the repeated multiple act criterion, aggregates these multiple acts again over time to profit from higher stability and construct validity. The distinction between single and multiple act criteria goes back to Ajzen and Fishbein who demonstrated their importance in attitude research (Ajzen & Fishbein 1980). Multiple acts were much better predicted from attitudes than single acts. The types of criteria one has to use depends on the demands of the different stakeholder groups and the complexity of the implemented program, which should be tailored to the stakeholder interests.

Figure 5.2 represents several strategies. The route from box 1 over 2 to 4 is what is usually used by experimental randomized research. It has also been dubbed 'the

North-West passage' in remembrance of Donald T Campbell who worked at North-Western University, but also alluding to the near impossible North-West passage between Canada and Greenland. Although experimental studies provide us with highly internally valid information, it is very difficult to conduct such research so that the results are also externally valid and usable. Therefore, the alternative strategy of comparing natural groups, the route from box 1 over 3 to 4, has been fairly frequently used in evaluation research studies.

A novel aspect has been brought into research by adding box 5, the evaluation box (Wittmann 1990). This box maps the interests of different stakeholder groups. It is not always obvious to researchers that the results have to be put into context and evaluated against a background of political and social demand. Medical research usually incorporates the methodological postulate that outcome measures have to be clinically relevant and that surrogate measures have to be avoided. This is reflected in this model by the fact that box 5, the evaluation box, is added to the model as an explicit separate step which has to be applied to the data.

Measurement symmetry

Validity not only refers to matters of design but also to the question whether the measures and operationalizations correctly reflect or represent the constructs which have to be measured. One principle which comes into play here is that of symmetry, introduced by Brunswik (Brunswik 1956, Wittmann 1990). Its relevance for explaining success and failure in prediction and explanation is discussed in Wittmann & Süss (1999), for many research areas. Nesselroade & McArdle (1996) have extended these ideas to causal modeling.

This principle states that operationalizations have to be symmetrical in complexity and depth to the construct being measured; for example, a rather simple or unidimensional construct like momentary well-being or pain could be measured by one single visual analogue scale. However, a higher level construct like quality of life very likely has to be broken down into subcomponents like physical functioning, psychological well-being or social functioning, which in turn have to be operationalized by single statement items. Thus, an important part of validity is the question of whether complex concepts have been operationalized adequately and symmetrically to their complexity. What is essential for a fair and successful comprehensive outcome evaluation is this principle of symmetry in the level of generality between complexity of the treatment program, outcome measures and demands of stakeholders.

There are two major dangers and threats to validity here. Either a complex construct may be measured asymmetrically by a very narrow instrument or a very complex instrument, which is designed to measure a complex structure, is being used inadequately for representing a very simple construct. An example for the first problem might be the usage of one single laboratory parameter for measuring a complex disease process; an example for the second problem could be the use of a whole battery of quality-of-life items for answering the very simple question of momentary well-being. Thus, an important part of the evaluation concept depicted in Figure 5.2 is the adequacy or symmetry of variables in accord with the concept or construct being measured. It has been a principle in evaluation research for many years now that complex constructs and outcome criteria should be operationalized in multiple ways (Wittmann 1985, 1987). This also means that these constructs have to be measured on different levels or facets; for example, if a treatment is supposed to improve sleep, one would ideally want to measure not only self-reported sleep behavior or quality of sleep but also objective sleep parameters like hours slept or latency until sleep and possibly even EEG data on different sleep phases.

This measurement of outcome variables on different levels and facets ought to reflect the richness of the reality of measured constructs. Note that this view is in contrast to some prevailing methodological wisdom (Lara-Munoz & Feinstein 1999). While in traditional RCT methodology one selects a simple and very often unique outcome criterion and tries to streamline and simplify measures, the approach taken by evaluation researchers usually calls for a multiplicity of measures. This conceptual difference has to do with the testing procedure of RCTs which are conceptually derived from a falsificationist theory of science. While this is useful for answering very particular questions it is usually too narrow to study complex interventions.

Thus, traditional RCTs can be seen as a special case of the experimental strategy. They are specifically adapted to answering very simple and specific questions of efficacy but are not suited to evaluating complex interventions. RCTs with randomized treatment and control groups are traditionally analyzed with the analysis of variance (ANOVA) workhorse but they can also be analyzed with multiple regression or the general linear model (Cohen & Cohen 1983). The treatment/control group contrast mapped with a simple dummy variable, e.g. a score of 1 for the treatment and a score of 0 for the control group, uncovers the paucity of assessing a complex and multifaceted treatment package this way. The experimental treatment box thus contains only one simple dichotomy and is thus doomed to remain a real black box where the researcher has no chance to look inside. Asking for the reliability of that dummy variable and assuming that reliability is the quotient of systematic true between group variance in relation to total variance, we note that this coefficient is always one, meaning that RCTs assume the treatment dummy reliability to be one.

Good trial practice uses manipulation checks to test whether the treatment really differs from the control to ensure that the between-group variance mapped with the dummy variable is no fiction. The variability within groups is rarely investigated as differences in compliance, levels of dosage, etc. The larger the unmeasured variability within groups, the lower the reliability and the power to detect significant differences independent of sample size. Lipsey & Cordray (2000, pp. 349–354) give a whole list of these sources of within program variation as, for example, delayed, incomplete or failed program implementation, individual engagement in services, extracurricular services, aptitude by treatment interactions, among many others. Lösel & Wittmann (1989) reanalyzed a program comparing a behavioral to a Rogerian type of treatment program. The intervention intended to train prison officers to better deal and cope with prisoners. The original analysis showed no significant effects on various outcome criteria. After reclassifying the type of treatment which really was delivered, significant effects were found in terms of what would be expected of these interventions according to theory.

Experimental and quasi-experimental strategies: the conflict between internal and external validity

The disjunction of the routes from box 1 via box 2 or 3 to box 4 also reflects the partial incompatibility of internal and external validity. While internal validity refers to the question whether the conclusions drawn from intervention studies are likely to be unbiased, external validity refers to the question whether results are applicable in real life and generalizable to persons or situations likely to use or represent the intervention in real life. Very often these two types of validity are very difficult to balance in one study. The more rigidly controlled a study is and the more error variance is being reduced by using homogeneous groups and applying strict inclusion and exclusion criteria (see Chapter 9), the less likely it is to be widely generalizable. Thus, in extreme cases, studies may be highly internally valid and the conclusions unbiased but their external validity may be severely hampered and thus the information produced could be useless.

A good historical example of this problem is the history of evaluation of Antabuse, a drug used for treating alcoholics. While the original trials, all RCTs, were positive and led to the conclusion that Antabuse is an efficacious medication for alcohol abuse, the information was practically useless. Analysis of those trials from a later vantage point shows that only a very small proportion of possible subjects had agreed to be treated (Howard et al 1990). Most of them had refused to enter the trials in the first place or had dropped out again. Thus, although the treatment is efficacious, it is practically irrelevant and no longer used very widely.

Modern trial methodology tries to design trials which are both internally and externally valid by conducting large pragmatic trials with as few inclusion and exclusion criteria as possible and by using very simple and robust outcome criteria like quality-of-life measures or patient-reported well-being. This certainly improves on the problems encountered with small trials which have been designed to answer questions of causality. However, the problem still remains that those trials are only conducted with subjects who agree to be randomized and evidence is accumulating that these patients are not comparable to what is found in clinical practice (Kaptchuk 2000, Llewellyn-Thomas et al 1991, Netter et al 1986, Patten 2000, Wragg et al 2000). Moreover, there are many areas in which interventions are carried out on self-selected groups of subjects and where the question arises how effective interventions are for these self-selected persons. In other words, self-selection, like virtually any variable, can be a confounder or a predictor, depending on the outlook.

In CAM we usually have two separate strands of questions. One is that of efficacy in general and the second is that of efficacy or effectiveness and usefulness for certain subjects. While RCTs answer the question of efficacy, they do not tell us whether self-selected groups of patients profit or not from certain interventions. In order to design externally valid studies which can be applied to those patients who select certain CAM treatments for themselves, non-randomized, quasi-experimental studies of natural groups are the better choice. Non-randomized comparisons are usually much more difficult to conduct in such a way that the results are useful. This may be one reason why RCTs have conquered the scene of medical research. In order to design an internally valid quasi-experimental study (a cohort study or a case-control study), it is important to measure as many confounding variables and predictors as are known to be possibly related with outcome (Cook & Campbell 1979, Rubin 1998). Thus, the predictor box in Figure 5.2 becomes very important for quasi-experimental studies. This means that in a study of natural comparison groups it is important to know as much as possible about possible confounders. Thus, if it is known that age, income or duration of illness is in any way correlated with the outcome, it is of vital importance to assess these variables at baseline. The problem which researchers in non-experimental settings usually face is that they can never be certain of knowing all the important and relevant variables beforehand.

Thus, quasi-experimental studies are always open to criticism (Rossi & Freeman 1982). If variables are not measured at baseline we can never be sure that the intervention and not some other variable has affected measurement after intervention. Thus, the stance taken throughout this book is that no single research methodology will give us certainty. Randomized studies can give us a clear picture about efficacy and causal attributions. Quasi-experimental comparison studies and outcome studies can tell us something about practical effectiveness and generalizability of results obtained in randomized studies. Thus, Figure 5.2 reminds us of the conceptual equality of both randomized and non-randomized approaches to research. Both have their strengths and shortcomings and they balance each other's weaknesses. Two recent metaanalyses have dispelled the myth that non-randomized evidence is inferior to that obtained from RCTs (Benson & Hartz 2000, Concato et al 2000). On the contrary, it is even stronger because it is derived from real-life situations. The presupposition, of course, remains that non-randomized controlled trials have to be conducted as rigidly as RCTs and even more skills are necessary to extract the information from them.

Differential indication: predicting successes and failures

What is usually disregarded in classic intervention research is the question of differential indication. Hardly any treatment is good for everybody. In most cases, there are certain types of patients or certain groups of persons who profit more and others who profit less or are even aggravated by a treatment. Therefore, broad measurement of possible predictor variables at baseline, i.e. the predictor box 1 in Figure 5.2, is of vital importance. If the information taken at baseline is rich and comprises many areas of the treated subjects, then it is easier to find out which patients would profit from the treatment, by conducting regression analyses. Since it is impossible to measure everything, good theories are called for at this point. For instance, if a theory predicts that patients who are more severely ill or who are more motivated or believe more in the treatment will profit more, then obviously it is necessary to have a good measure of those variables at baseline. Medical research is surprisingly lacking in such measures, which might be useful for differential indication.

There is a strong a priori possibility that CAM treatments are better for certain kinds of patients including those who choose treatments, believe in them or are willing to be actively engaged. While on average, CAM treatments might be either just as effective as other treatments or even less effective than conventional treatments, nevertheless for certain patients CAM treatments might be vastly superior. In order for practitioners to advise patients whether a CAM treatment is possibly beneficial for them, they have to know which patients are likely to profit more. Thus, predictor research, either as a specific type of research or included within a conventional trial, is an important part of evaluation which is completely neglected at present.

PRACTICAL IMPLICATIONS

The picture drawn so far has some clear-cut implications.

Methodology as a flexible tool

Quite contrary to the normal opinion that there is a hierarchy of methodological approaches, the lesson to be learned from evaluation research is that there is only research methodology which is well adapted to certain problems and questions and that every research methodology is deficient in some way and has to be complemented by others. Thus, while RCTs produce very good information on efficacy, this information has to be complemented by other types of studies such as outcomes studies or cohort studies of natural groups. Methods have to be geared to questions, otherwise research produces answers to questions which have never been asked.

The principle of fair evaluation

Very often, the treatment being studied, i.e. box 2 or box 3 in Figure 5.2, is being neglected when collecting data. That is to say that the treatment is just applied and briefly described but it is not clear to the reader of the study (and often to the researcher) whether the treatment studied was really a good representation of the treatment which is applied in practice; for example, many studies of homeopathy or acupuncture have used formula acupuncture or homeopathy which is rarely applied in practice. In those cases, researchers used the mistaken concept of standardized treatments as the only ones which can be studied scientifically. Thus, the study may not even tell us a single thing about the treatment in normal practice.

The principle of fair evaluation draws our attention to the treatment boxes 2 or 3 in Figure 5.2. The treatment should be described in detail as really representative of what is done in practice. Also, its application within a study should represent normal and good practice. Otherwise, a study will always be open to criticism by practitioners who feel that their practice has not been reflected adequately by research. For example, the treatment under study could be supervised by acknowledged experts, given by an accepted practitioner in a field or given by diverse members of different branches, depending on the question asked.

The principle of rich and valid measurement

Measures should be rich, reflecting the complexity of the construct being measured, and valid. Validity here means the measures have been tested before they are used. Very often researchers make the mistake of using validated measures which have been used in other studies or reported in the literature but which are not adequate for the problem being studied. Very often, constructs which are the target of a CAM treatment have not been studied before in other research contexts and thus no measurement instrument exists. For instance, a CAM treatment might purport to affect vital energy. In order to test this it would be important to find a valid and reliable measurement instrument for vital energy. While existing scales like the Vitality Scale of the SF-36 could be used (McHorney et al 1993, Stewart et al 1988, Ware &

Sherbourne 1992), it is good research practice to try to understand the concept in question well enough in order to judge whether existing scales really do reflect the concept being studied. Thus, it might turn out that the Vitality Scale of the SF-36 measures something quite different from vital energy, as understood, for instance, by traditional Chinese medicine.

If a researcher comes to the conclusion that no existing measurement instrument would adequately reflect the construct in question, it is good practice not to use a surrogate measure but to construct a new measurement instrument or commission such a construction if knowledge of how to do this is lacking. This can mean that other studies have to be conducted in order to construct and validate such a measurement instrument before the study on the effectiveness of a CAM treatment can be carried out. For example, if the effect of homeopathic treatment on the quality of life in children with asthma is to be studied, it might well turn out that no suitable instrument for this variable exists. The researcher then has to decide whether to drop the subject or invest in the construction of such an instrument. This can be a difficult and time-consuming task.

While traditional psychometric theory usually presupposes that a complex construct is more validly and reliably measured by multiple items and questions, it can also be useful to just use some global scales. Multi-item instruments are usually more sensitive and can reflect changes and different aspects of a construct more validly. Simple single-item questions, on the other hand, are very robust indicators. It has been argued that a simple question like 'How is your quality of life?' scaled on a 5-, 7- or 10-point scale might give us all the information we need (Lara-Munoz & Feinstein 1999). This could be true if it is hypothesized that the impact of treatment is strong and can easily be seen. If this impact is hypothesized to be rather small and subtle, then more complex measurement instruments designed for sensitivity and broadness have to be employed.

Relevance of measures

A common mistake is to use irrelevant measures in order to determine the efficacy of a treatment. In medical research this problem has been known under the term 'surrogate measures' which refers to the fact that some easily measurable endpoint is used instead of one which is complex and difficult to measure.

Another aspect of this problem is the question of data sources. For instance, researchers could ask the doctor, the patient or the patient's relatives about the general state of health of a subject. Depending on the question and intervention, they might get some very different pictures. It is known that doctors' judgments and patients' estimations of their state of health are only weakly correlated and sometimes not correlated at all (Koller et al 1996). Thus, it might be necessary to include questions from both the patient and the doctor perspective. If a study is designed to find out whether a treatment is useful in reducing work absenteeism, neither doctor nor patient is a very reliable source for this information and so insurance or work registers have to be employed. On the other hand, if pain is the target of the study, it is not very useful to ask the doctor whether the patient is in pain because the doctor would have to ask the patient in the first place.

Effect size and clinical importance

Relying on statistics for decisions is a central part of the modern scientific approach. Thus, looking for significance has very often become the sole arbiter of effectiveness. Significance, however, is a concept which is dependent on the magnitude of the effect and the size of the study (Cohen 1987, 1992). Thus, theoretically, even very small and practically irrelevant effects could be made statistically significant provided the numbers in a study are large enough. On the other hand, small studies will only produce significant results if the effects are rather large. As a rule, the more fine-grained and sensitive measurement instruments are, the easier it is to show statistical significance with them. But it remains a question whether effects found in a study with a sensitive instrument are really important. Thus, rather robust measures like single-item visual analogue scales ('How are you today?') might be preferable if one wants to demonstrate a clinically relevant effect.

Researchers and readers of studies should be aware of the fact that significance is only a very formal criterion for judging a study. More interesting for patients and practitioners, as well as for purchasers, is the question of whether the effects demonstrated by a study are in any sense practically relevant. If a large study of, say, 500 patients showed just one single significant effect in a highly sensitive and somewhat artificial scale but did not show differences in other more relevant measures, then it is likely that the treatment under study is not of much practical relevance.

A way of formalizing this is the calculation of effect size measures. These are unitless measures, which standardize differences across studies. There are two families of effect size measures: those for continuous and those for dichotomous variables. Effect size measures of dichotomous variables are more common in medical research. They are known as odds ratios, rate ratios or risk ratios. Effect size measures of continuous variables are usually known as effect size d or g. While odds or rate ratios are simply ratios of improved patients in experimental and control groups, effect sizes d or g are defined as differences between groups divided by standard deviation.

Calculation of effect size is something which can easily be done on data reported in the results tables of studies. But it is necessary to calculate effect sizes in order to understand whether a study has produced a sizeable effect. It is enough to look at the size of the study, the measure being used and the level of significance, for all practical purposes. By the same token, a researcher planning an evaluation study should keep in mind that the treatment should be practically relevant and use well-known, robust and not oversensitive measures. While it might be important for efficacy trials, as used for drug-licensing processes, to show very small changes by using sensitive scales, the same is not true for trials which want to convey that a CAM treatment studied is useful in practice. For that purpose measures should be used which are meaningful to patients and can reflect clinically important change.

Results in social, scientific and political contexts

Results of research studies in CAM are never just bland facts. They are always facts for an audience, facts in favor of or against practical decisions. It is wise to have possible audiences in view right from the start of a study. Thus, if a study is meant to address purchasers or political decision makers, it is wise to consider what type of information is going to impress them; for example, while legal authorities might require a demonstration of specific effects of a CAM treatment against placebo, this might be irrelevant for purchasers or patients. While for political authorities or health-care decision makers sound scientific evidence of statistical superiority of a treatment over control might be mandatory, for purchasers it could be enough to demonstrate a certain level of practical usefulness. Thus, before designing and planning a study one should be aware of the persons to be addressed by it.

By the same token, it should be clear who the main critics of the results will be. Usually there are always groups who will try to oppose research results, no matter how sound a study is. If the audience to be addressed is the medical research community, then it is likely that they will ask questions about specific efficacy and want to see a well-controlled RCT. The other danger could be that the research results are being used by interest groups for their own purposes. Thus, the researcher who wants to be active in CAM research should always be aware of the social and political dimension of such work (Cronbach 1982, Rossi & Freeman 1982, Suchman 1967, Weiss 1973, 1975).

CONCLUSION

Instead of summarizing what has been said so far, we would like to make a simple statement as a concluding remark.

The history of evaluation research teaches us that there is no such thing as the right method, the best method or the gold standard of research. There is only good research applied to a relevant question with the appropriate consideration of measurement and socially skillful manipulation of the results. It is only the multiplicity of methods and the variety of approaches, as well as complementary skills of the researcher, which will help us solve the questions in front of us. What lies ahead is seen in the switch of the funding policy by one major funding organization, namely the National Institute of Mental Health. While in the past mainly efficacy-oriented research was commissioned, funding activities are now being directed to effectiveness research of practical real-world interventions.

The new emphasis breaks sharply with traditional treatment studies that often look at select patients in academic settings: it will study large numbers of diverse patients in real-world settings, follow them for lengthy periods of time and measure progress by the patients' functioning in school, work and other areas of life. (Foxhall 2000)

REFERENCES

Ajzen I, Fishbein M 1980 Understanding attitudes and predicting social behavior. Prentice-Hall, Englewood Cliffs, NJ

Benson K, Hartz AJ 2000 A comparison of observational studies and randomized controlled trials. New England Journal of Medicine 342: 1878–1886

Brunswik E 1956 Perception and the representative design of psychological experiments. University of California Press, Berkeley, CA

Cattell RB 1957 Personality and motivation: structure and measurement. World Books, New York

Chen H, Rossi PH 1981 The multi-goal, theory-driven approach to evaluation: a model linking basic and applied social science. Evaluation Studies Review Annual 6: 38–54

Chen H, Rossi PH 1983 Evaluating with sense. The theory-driven approach. Evaluation Review 7: 283–302

Cohen J 1987 Statistical power analysis for the behavioral sciences. Lawrence Erlbaum, Hillsdale, NJ

Cohen J 1992 Statistical power analysis. Current Directions in Psychological Science 1: 98–101

Cohen J, Cohen P 1983 Applied multiple regression/correlation analysis for the behavioral sciences. Lawrence Erlbaum, Hillsdale, NJ

Concato J, Shah N, Horwitz RI 2000 Randomized, controlled trials, observational studies, and the hierarchy of research designs. New England Journal of Medicine 342: 1887–1892

Cook TD, Campbell DT 1979 Quasi-experimentation design and analysis issues for field settings. Rand McNally, Chicago

Cook TD, Matt GE 1990 Theorien der Programmevaluation – Ein kurzer Abriß. In: Koch U, Wittmann WW (eds) Evaluationsforschung. Bewertungsgrundlage von Sozial- und Gesundheitsprogrammen. Springer, Berlin, pp 15–38

Cook TD, Wittmann WW 1998 Lessons learned about evaluation in the United States and some possible implications for Europe. European Journal of Psychological Assessment 14: 97–115

Cronbach LJ 1982 Designing evaluations of educational and social programs. Jossey Bass, San Francisco

Foxhall K 2000 Research for the real world. NIMH is pumping big money into effectiveness research to move promising treatments into practice. Monitor on Psychology 31(7). http://www.apa.org/monitor/julaugoo/research.html

Howard KI, Cox WM, Saunders SM 1990 Attrition in substance abuse comparative treatment research: the illusion of randomization. In: Onken S, Blaine JD (eds) Psychotherapy and counseling in the treatment of drug abuse. National Institute of Drug Abuse, Rockville, MD, pp 66–79

Kaptchuk TJ 2000 The double-blind randomized controlled trial: gold standard or golden calf? Journal of Clinical Epidemiology (in press)

Koller M, Kussmann J, Lorenz W et al 1996 Symptom reporting in cancer patients. The role of negative affect and experienced social stigma. Cancer 77: 983–995

Lara-Munoz C, Feinstein AR 1999 How should quality of life be measured? Journal of Investigative Medicine 47: 17–24

Lipsey MW, Cordray DS 2000 Evaluation methods for social interventions. Annual Review of Psychology 51: 345–375

Llewellyn-Thomas HA, McGreal MJ, Thiel EC, Fine S, Erlichman C 1991 Patients' willingness to enter clinical trials: measuring the association with perceived benefit and preference for decision participation. Social Science and Medicine 32: 35–42

Lösel F, Wittmann WW 1989 The relationship of treatment integrity and intensity to outcome criteria. In: Conner RF, Hendricks M (eds) International innovations in evaluation methodology. Jossey Bass, San Francisco, pp 97–108

McHorney CA, Ware JE, Raczek AE 1993 The MOS 36-item short form health survey (SF-36): II. Psychometric and clinical tests of validity in measuring physical and mental health constructs. Medical Care 31: 247–263

Nesselroade JR, McArdle JJ 1996 On the mismatching of levels of abstraction in methematical-statistical model fitting. In: Franzen MD, Reese HW (eds) Life-span developmental psychology: biological and neuropsychological mechanisms. Lawrence Erlbaum, Hillsdale, NJ: pp 23–49

Netter P, Heck S, Müller HJ 1986 What selection of patients is achieved by requesting informed consent in placebo controlled drug trials? Pharmacopsychiatry 19: 335–336

Patten SB 2000 Selection bias in studies of major depression using clinical subjects. Journal of Clinical Epidemiology 53: 351–357

Rossi PH, Freeman HE 1982 Evaluation. A systematic approach, 2nd edn. Sage, Beverly Hills, CA

Rubin DB 1998 Estimation from nonrandomized treatment comparisons using subclassification on propensity scores. In: Abel U, Koch A (eds) Nonrandomized comparative clinical studies. Symposion Publishing, Düsseldorf, pp 85–100

Scriven MS 1980 The logic of evaluation. Edge Press, Inverness, CA

Shadish Jr WR, Cook TD, Leviton LC (eds) 1991 Foundations of program evaluation. Theories of practice. Sage, Newbury Park, CA

Stewart AL, Hays RD, Ware JE 1988 The MOS short-form general health survey. Reliability and validity in a patient population. Medical Care 26: 724–736

Suchman EA 1967 Evaluation research. Russell Sage Foundation, New York

Ware JE, Sherbourne D 1992 The MOS 36-item short form health survey (SF-36) I. Conceptual framework and item selection. Medical Care 30: 473–483

Weiss CH 1973 Where politics and evaluation meet. Evaluation 1: 37–45

Weiss CH 1975 Evaluation research in political context. In: Struening EL, Guttentag M (eds) Handbook of evaluation research. Sage, Beverly Hills, pp 13–26

Wittmann W 1985 Evaluationsforschung. Aufgaben, Probleme und Anwendungen. Springer, Berlin

Wittmann WW 1987 Grundlagen erfolgreicher Forschung in der Psychologie: Multimodale Diagnostik, Multiplismus, multivariate Reliabilitäts- und Validitätstheorie. Diagnostica 33: 209–226

Wittmann WW 1988 Multivariate reliability theory: principles of symmetry and successful validation strategies. In: Nesselroade JR, Cattell RB (eds) Handbook of multivariate experimental psychology. Plenum Press, New York: pp 505–560

Wittmann WW 1990 Brunswik-Symmetrie und die Konzeption der Fünf-Datenboxen – Ein Rahmenkonzept für umfassende Evaluationsforschung. Zeitschrift für Pädagogische Psychologie 4: 241–251

Wittmann WW, Süss HM 1999 Investigating the paths between working memory, intelligence, knowledge, and complex problem solving performances via Brunswik-symmetry. In: Ackerman PL, Kyllonen PL, Roberts R (eds) Learning and individual differences. Process, trait, and content determinants. APA, Washington, DC

Wragg JA, Robinson EJ, Lilford RJ 2000 Information presentation and decision to enter clinical trials: a hypothetical trial of hormone replacement therapy. Social Science and Medicine 51: 453–462

6

Improving patient care in complementary medicine: using clinical audit

Rebecca W Rees

INTRODUCTION

The idea behind clinical audit is extremely simple – that patient care can often be improved. Audit is a framework of reflection and action aimed at making appropriate changes in practice happen. This chapter presents audit as an approach that can be applied in anyone's day-to-day practice. It briefly describes the usual components of an audit and then presents several case studies. These illustrate what audit can do and give some pointers to practitioners to help them make choices over different audit approaches. A final section puts audit in context, examining its place in current developments in health care and comparing it with the other, more frequently discussed forms of systematic enquiry.

This chapter is based upon a programme of work carried out at the Research Council for Complementary Medicine in 1998. As part of this programme, 16 complementary therapists attempted clinical audit in their own clinics or professional organizations, the first time that audit as an activity had been implemented across complementary therapy professions in the UK. This chapter depends considerably on the work of these therapists and their work needs to be acknowledged. They found audit to be achievable and useful. They highlighted issues that need to be considered by practitioners preparing for audit. Like any systematic endeavor undertaken by practitioners, audit takes time and other resources and is best done with the support of someone who has successfully done it before. This chapter should enable practitioners to see what audit involves so that they can use it to help improve patient care.

WHAT DOES AUDIT DO?

Audit is a framework that helps change in clinical practice happen. And the reality of clinical practice is that there are always aspects that could be improved: practitioners are often aware of areas of their work where they suspect they could do better; a profession's understanding of good practice develops from year to year. Audit has been developed to deal with this need for change, to help ensure that clinical practice stays responsive to the needs of patients, practitioners and society as a whole. There will be nothing new to complementary practitioners about the idea of reflection followed by action: practitioners are used to thinking about what is best for patients on a case-by-case basis. The main difference between usual practice and audit is in the degree to which this reflection and action are made systematic and explicit. The place of audit in professional practice is discussed further towards the end of this chapter. First, we will look at the components that make audit what it is and illustrate these with examples from actual complementary medicine practice.

What makes an audit?

Audit is often thought of as cyclical. In brief, it starts with looking at an aspect of care and deciding how it should be carried out. It moves on to a reality check, to see how day-to-day practice compares with these aims. At its heart is the next step – actually making changes to the way things are done and checking that these changes have made a difference.

In more detail, at the start of the cycle, practitioners draw upon their own and others' expertise to look at how they want one aspect of patient care to be. For example, a group of herbalists might look at handling answerphone messages left by clients. They would start by identifying a number of criteria for good practice. These might include returning calls within 24 hours or ensuring that outgoing answerphone messages are modified if a therapist is due to be away for more than one day.

The audit then moves on to see if what practitioners currently do actually meets this ideal. In our example, the herbalists might keep a simple record of a week's calls, with notes about how they were handled.

The most challenging part of audit follows: if change is due, practitioners then take steps to make sure it happens. If the herbalists' records show that they are not meeting the standards they have set they could then spend time discussing possible reasons why their current answerphone systems are not working and pool ideas for improving: maybe changing their outgoing answerphone messages in some way. To keep the audit's momentum going, they would then make plans to change and set a date for reassessing. They would possibly repeat the whole exercise if message taking was still not working as they'd like, as long as this area was still a priority for them.

The processes involved in audit are often summed up by an audit cycle (Fig. 6.1).

The audit cycle simply breaks down change into several explicit stages. Each stage is important in itself if valuable and lasting changes are to be made.

- *What am I trying to do?* At this stage, an area of care is selected and ideas about good practice are sought. Research may have been done that indicates that certain approaches are appropriate. Where there is no research, professionals can get together to come up with a consensus.

- *Am I doing it?* This stage is the one that requires measurement, to see how close current practice is to good practice. The techniques and tools used for measuring in audit are relatively simple.
- *Why am I not doing it?* It is often far easier to see what it is you are not doing than to work out why. And yet, knowing why aspects of your work are not getting done is usually key to working out what can be done to improve matters.
- *What can I do to make things better?* Simply wanting to improve an aspect of practice is rarely enough. A plan of action helps. Frequently, new systems need to be set up.
- *Have I made things better?* This stage is used to check whether the plan of action has (a) been carried out and (b) been effective. If the plan hasn't worked, it may be necessary to go back a stage, maybe working further with colleagues who hold the key to change taking place. If things have gone to plan, the audit cycle has been completed, at least for the time being. The cycle can be repeated if ideas about good practice develop further or if it is suspected that actual practice is again not as it should be.

The next section illustrates the purpose and possibilities of audit further, using a set of four case studies.

Learning points

* Audit is a framework that helps change in clinical practice happen.
* Audit aims to make the process of clinical reflection and action systematic and explicit.
* Audit can be summed up as a cycle that asks and then addresses the implications of the following questions in turn: What am I trying to do? Am I doing it? Why am I not doing it? What can I do to make things better? Have I made things better?

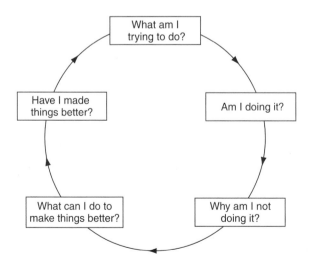

Figure 6.1 A basic audit cycle.

CASE STUDIES: CLINICAL AUDIT IN ACTION

The following case studies use fictional settings but are based around real audit projects carried out by complementary therapists as part of the Research Council for Complementary Medicine's Clinical Audit Project. They illustrate how different audits may be appropriate at different times for different practitioners. Look out for the kinds of changes that these audits helped bring about and ask whether such an approach may be suitable for you.

The case studies have also been chosen in order to start showing what audit can do and what its limitations are, something that is discussed further in the last section of this chapter. Practitioners might find it helpful to look at the audits and think over whether bringing about change really is their immediate goal or whether they are more interested in focusing in more detail on what is going on or how different approaches might affect patients. If the latter is the case, they may be more interested in undertaking survey or outcomes-focused research.

The case studies illustrate how individual practitioners can choose their own audit topics and then use the principles of audit in a relatively flexible way. When it comes to this kind of 'practitioner-driven' audit the goal of bringing about valuable change is ultimately far more important than carrying out each audit stage as outlined in a text book. Another distinct but valuable approach to audit is occasionally demanded of practitioners by therapy bodies working on behalf of the profession as a whole. This type of audit will be discussed towards the end of this chapter.

The audits described here all take slightly different routes around an audit cycle. They help illustrate a number of key audit concepts. A more theoretical approach to audit methods and further examples from outside complementary medicine can be found in a large number of easily available texts (see Further Reading). Look out for the following key concepts in each case study.

- *Defining the problem.* Why this area of care is important.
- *Purpose of the audit.* This makes the aims of the audit explicit from the start.
- *Criteria.* These are definitions of good practice. They can be generated from many sources, including research evidence, professional organizations, the Patient's Charter, peer group consensus, etc.
- *Standards.* These show how vital it is that each criterion is met. Some criteria will be more critical than others and so need a higher standard. While it is not always done, setting standards helps prioritize action.
- *Data collection.* Tried and tested techniques can investigate how well you are doing. Data may be previously recorded information. Fresh data can be collected by questionnaires or forms, both of which need careful thought in preparation if they are not to be problematic. Most audits summarize information using simple data collection sheets.
- *Analysis.* Having collected information about your practice, it is time to compare your results against the standards set at the start of the audit. This stage asks, 'Where am I meeting the standards, where not?'.
- *Discussion.* Discussion with colleagues or peers helps even if they are not directly involved with your audit project. Reassess your criteria and standards

and generate ideas about what can be done to improve things. Sometimes an audit of one area will highlight problems in another area. An audit of record keeping, for example, may suggest that more time is needed for a first consultation.

- *Managing change*. The most critical part of the audit comes when you decide what can be improved and how. If you are working in a team it is important to reach agreement about what needs to be changed and the means of doing it. It is equally important to take steps to manage the changes. Agree what will be done, by whom, by what date. Implement the changes and re-audit at an agreed date in the future.

Case study 1: recording patient information – the initial consultation

Defining the problem

The collection and recording of information during a patient's first consultation is a fundamental aspect of clinical practice. Certain information needs to be in a patient's notes for reference. Some say that if it isn't written down, it didn't happen. Nevertheless, poor standards of note taking are common across all health professions. Few complementary medicine professions have looked into this aspect of practice.

Purpose of this audit

This audit was carried out by four osteopaths working in a multi-partner clinic. They wanted to:

- see how well they collected and recorded information from patients in a first consultation
- compare practice amongst themselves
- compare this with best practice and improve where necessary.

Criteria

Practitioners are taught to collect and record specific clinical information during their undergraduate training. Often techniques are then adapted with experience. The osteopaths referred to documents produced by their professional body and decided that the following should be recorded at a first consultation.

Box 6.1   Benefits of this audit

- Vital information about each patient will be in place for future consultations.
- Notes will act as a record that certain questions have been asked.
- Colleagues will be more able to use notes, improving the continuity of patient care.
- Notes will be of more use in future audit or research projects.

- *Personal details.* Name (first and surname), address, telephone number, date of birth, gender, occupation, GP name and contact details.
- *Presenting complaint.* Site, nature, date of onset, causative factors, duration and progression, factors affecting symptoms, past history.
- *Medical history.* Current general health, medication, investigations and treatments, illness/accidents/surgery.
- *Other.* Family medical history, diagnosis, treatment plan. Records should also be signed, dated and legible.

Standards

The osteopaths decided:

- just over half of their criteria were 'critical' and needed targets of 100% (e.g. name, address, gender, site and nature of presenting complaint)
- others (e.g. GP details and medical history criteria) were considered a lower priority and were therefore set lower targets of 80% or 90% in this audit round.

Data collection

- The osteopaths in our program wanted an up-to-date picture of their practice and so sampled all new patients over the previous month ($N=36$).
- Figure 6.2 shows the simple data collection sheet developed to assess patient records.
- The criteria were defined in detail to make assessment as precise as possible.
- A '1' was entered in the appropriate box when the criterion was met fully, a '0' inserted when the criterion was not met fully (e.g. to receive a tick for the first criterion, a record should contain the patient's name in full; a record featuring only the second name would receive a '0').

Criterion	Record no.						Total %	
	1	2	3	4	5	35	36	
Name in full	1	1	1	0	1	1	1	33	92
Address including postcode	1	1	1	1	1	1	1	36	100
Telephone no.	1	1	1	1	1	1	1	36	100
Date of birth	1	1	1	1	1	1	1	36	100
Gender	1	0	1	0	0	1	0	15	4
Occupation	1	1	1	1	1	1	1	36	100
GP name, surgery and tel. no.	1	0	1	0	0	1	1	27	75
Site of complaint	1	1	1	1	1	1	1	36	100

Date	1	1	1	1	1	1	1	36	100
Legible – mark 1 if assessed readable by practice manager	0	1	1	1	0	1	1	21	58

Figure 6.2   Data collection sheet. Patient information collected at first consultation.

- Simple percentages were used to sum up how well each criterion was met over all the sample and for each osteopath.

Analysis and discussion

The group of osteopaths each received a summary of their own record keeping along with anonymous copies of their colleagues' results. As a group they found that:

- they were meeting just over half of the criteria at near to or above the desired standard
- the remainder of the criteria were being met less than 60% of the time.

They were shocked by their findings and looked again at their professional guidelines.

- Few had realized that signing and dating made notes more valuable as legal documents.
- They initially disagreed about whether it was necessary to record gender if also recording a full name but finally agreed that names alone can mislead.
- The group felt that they would be far more likely to record gender and the other patient details now that the reasoning behind their professional guidelines was clear to everybody.

Managing change

The osteopaths:

- agreed to a re-audit of their notes in 1 month and in a further 3 months time
- suggested printed case notes with prompts as a possible solution
- decided to wait for the results of the next audit round to see what effect increased awareness had on their record keeping. Most standards were met on their first re-audit but they plan to re-audit again to see if this continues.

Box 6.2 Is this audit for me?

- Case note taking is simple to assess and is a common first topic for practitioners new to audit.
- This audit will help you see where you need to record more carefully and, perhaps, where you are doing more than you need to.
- Look at the criteria described and ask yourself, 'Am I 100% certain that I am recording the patient information that I should be?'.

Case study 2: communicating with other health professionals – letter writing

Defining the problem

A growing number of complementary therapists find that they need to write letters to their patients' GPs. These might describe a course of treatment or ask for information.

Box 6.3 Benefits of this audit

- Good communication between health professionals improves continuity of care; for example, reducing the number of unnecessary tests patients receive.
- A letter-writing system can reduce workloads for both writer and reader.

Illegible, poorly structured correspondence is common in all health professions. It is possible to systematize letter writing to some extent so that it takes less time and still transfers vital information.

Purpose of audit

A peer group of four chiropractors from several different practices used this audit because they were concerned about the relevance and content of their letters to GPs.

Criteria and standards

The chiropractors consulted their professional body's guidelines and met with local GPs. They decided that 100% of patients who consent to contact with their GP should have a letter written within a month of their initial presentation. These letters should:

- have no errors in legibility or spelling (in 100% of cases)
- contain a brief history, X-ray report, summary of diagnosis, treatment type, advice given, outcome and prognosis (in at least 90% of cases – the chiropractors thought these aspects were likely to be a problem and wanted to be realistic in early audit rounds)
- be short – no longer than one side of A5/250 words (in at least 80% of cases – the chiropractors felt this criterion was a lower priority).

Data collection

- The chiropractors drew up a data collection sheet (Fig. 6.3).
- All the last 3 months' records were searched for new patients giving consent for GP contact and letters written.
- The last 20 letters for each chiropractor were examined by the clinic manager for compliance with the remaining criteria.

Analysis and discussion

Each chiropractor received their results and those of the practice as a whole. They found that, for the group:

- only 76% of letters were being sent on time
- 90% were too long

1) Number of new patients: 60
2) Marked as 'do not inform GP': 10
3) Number of 'eligible' letters [1–2]: 50
4) Number of 'eligible' letters sent within 1 month of presentation: 38
5) Proportion of 'eligible' letters that were not sent on time [(3–4)/3]: 24%

Sample of 20 consecutive letters sent since: 1/11/97
Practitioner: 02

Case no.	No. words in letter	Too many words?	Spelling errors	Legible		Outcomes of care	Prognosis
A123	160	0	1	0		1	0

A141	350	1	0	0		1	0
A142	450	1	1	1		1	1
Total		18	8	10		20	16
%		90	40	50		100	80

Figure 6.3 Summary sheet of letters written to GPs.

- except for prognosis, the clinical content of letters was sufficient over 90% of the time
- they did poorly on spelling and legibility (meeting standards in 50% or fewer cases).

Managing change

The team was heartened by their findings on the clinical content but concerned by the late and overlong letters. They decided to:

- improve their clinic system for notifying chiropractors when letters were due
- try to shorten letters and use computer spellchecks
- do a second, identical assessment of letters in another 3 months, raising their standards for the criteria about clinical content to 100%.

Three months later the chiropractors found that all but one of the criteria were met – their record on recording prognosis was still slightly below target. They agreed to continue auditing letters to ensure that their standards did not slip.

Box 6.4   Is this audit for me?

- It is relatively simple to assess the letters you already send, perhaps using your own criteria or those described here.
- Getting feedback from health professionals in your vicinity will take more planning and persistence but will improve relations if it is done well.

Case study 3: communicating with patients – individuals who discontinue treatment

Defining the problem

Patients who fail to complete a course of treatments may not get the full benefits of a therapy. There will be different reasons for not returning but misunderstandings about what treatment involves are common. Effective communication, both before and during a first consultation, increases attendance at further treatment. Many therapists do not know how many of their patients fail to complete treatment or why this might be. It is often possible to improve communication.

Purpose of audit

This audit was done by an osteopath who worked in a GP practice. He was concerned that several patients had recently not completed their planned courses of treatments. He suspected that they might not have known what to expect and had been disappointed. His audit aimed to:

- identify the numbers of patients discontinuing treatment
- find out patient perceptions about why they discontinue
- identify mismatches between patient expectations of treatment and reality and take steps to address these.

Criteria

The osteopath wanted to ensure that 100% of his patients:

- received diagnostic information at their first consultation
- felt that they had had treatment explained to them
- felt that they had been told about the expected number of treatments.

Data collection – stage 1

The osteopath:

- wanted a longer term picture so looked at all patients seen in the previous 3 months
- identified patients who had failed to rebook appointments using the clinic's appointments register and patient notes

---

Box 6.5   Benefits of this audit

- It is essential to find out how much non-attendance is a problem to a clinic before you take any steps to change clinic procedures. The perceived problem may not be too great after all.
- Feedback from patients is always enlightening, as long as good questions are asked. Patients who have not completed treatment are an ideal group to question about possible shortcomings.

- drew up a summary sheet that listed each patient who did not attend for the expected number of treatments.

Analysis and discussion – stage 1

- Out of 480 patients, 53 had not completed their expected number of treatments.
- The osteopath presented these findings to colleagues, including the practice manager and receptionist. The group decided that this was a high enough number for concern and talked about the kind of information patients might need.
- The GPs gave some feedback to the osteopath from their discussions with patients.
- The group drew up several questions to ask discontinuing patients. The questions asked about information requirements both before and during treatments.

Data collection – stage 2

- The osteopath drew up a draft questionnaire. This was tested on five discontinuing patients identified in stage 1. Figure 6.4 shows some questions from the final version.
- The questionnaire was posted to the remaining discontinuing patients.

Analysis and discussion – stage 2

When the questionnaires were back all the responses were typed onto a single, large summary sheet for quick reference. The osteopath asked himself:

- how do questionnaire responses compare with my criteria and standards?
- are there any surprises in my results? If so, what is surprising?
- does the questionnaire indicate particular problems with my service? If so, what can be done?

Feedback on the osteopath's skills in explaining treatment was encouraging but patients often reported that they did not feel that their condition had been explained. While the osteopath often remembered a discussion there was rarely mention of it in the notes. Patients reported practical reasons for discontinuing that were not related to treatment; 50% said that they would like better information before treatment.

The osteopath looked again at his criteria for good communication. Patients may forget about aspects of their treatment and it will often be better to record discussion of diagnosis in the notes and audit this; 100% patient satisfaction is extremely rare.

Managing change

- The case note form was modified to prompt and record discussion about diagnosis and treatment. An audit of case notes is planned.

Your osteopathy treatment

We are looking at how we can improve the services we provide at the clinic. We would be very grateful for your cooperation in completing this questionnaire. The questionnaire should only take a few minutes of your time. Please note that all information you provide will be kept **strictly confidential** and cannot affect any future treatment in any way.

If you have any questions about this survey please do not hesitate to contact me at the clinic by telephoning 0181 333 2222 in between 2 and 4pm. Thank you for your help.   Signed..............

Please complete the following questions (please continue over the page if you need more space)

1 For which complaint(s) were you referred to the osteopath?

2 Before your first consultation with the osteopath, did you feel you knew what osteopathy treatment would involve?

                                    Yes [ ] No [ ]

Please state how you knew if you ticked 'yes'

3 Did you feel the osteopath listened well to you when you told him of your complaint?

                                    Yes [ ] No [ ]

4 Did he explain what he thought was wrong with you?

                                    Yes [ ] No [ ]

5 Was there anything unexpected about the treatment?

                                    Yes [ ] No [ ]

If you ticked 'yes', please state what was unexpected.

----

12 Your answer to this next question is particularly valuable.

We note that you did not complete your course of treatment. Please state why:

Thank you for taking the time to complete this questionnaire. Please return in the stamped addressed envelope provided.

Figure 6.4 Part of the questionnaire sent out to discontinuing patients.

- A second questionnaire to a further 20 patients found that they still wanted more information.
- The clinic manager has drawn up a leaflet to give to patients on referral. Another questionnaire to discontinuing patients is planned to obtain feedback on the leaflet's contents. It is likely that lower targets for satisfaction will be set.

Box 6.6   Is this audit for me?

- The first stage of this audit mainly uses records of patient appointments and attendance. You will also need patient notes. This stage should be relatively quick to complete.
- The second stage uses questionnaires and is more challenging. You will need help from someone with expertise in designing questionnaires so they are easy to understand and provide the information you want. Handling mailouts and the new data they produce can be quite time consuming. Advice on sampling will help to keep the workload manageable.

Case study 4: communicating with patients – discussing progress during consultations

Defining the problem

Many therapists practice without systematically assessing their patients' progress. This can be a problem because we all have selective memories, tending to remember events that have gone particularly well or particularly badly. It is difficult to see things as a whole, both within the course of an individual's treatment and in the context of the totality of practice. Patients benefit if they feel that health professionals understand their experience of ill health.

Purpose of audit

A practitioner of traditional Chinese medicine (TCM) used this audit to ensure he was looking critically at the progress of people attending an AIDS/HIV clinic. The practitioner also hoped to highlight areas where treatment may not have been working as well as hoped.

Criteria

The practitioner wanted to add completion of a short questionnaire to his usual consultation procedures. The questionnaire he chose, MYMOP2 (Measure Yourself Medical Outcome Profile 2), is one of a number of instruments developed recently to measure individual patient experiences of a course of treatment. MYMOP2 forms produce initial measures of:

- a primary and secondary symptom to provide the initial clinical focus
- an activity that is restricted by the symptoms
- the patient's overall feeling of well-being
- the patient's attitude to medication use.

Box 6.7   Benefits of this audit

An audit of the discussion of patient progress can:
- help practitioners ensure they keep track of their patients' experience of treatment
- maintain a clinical focus on areas needing treatment
- indicate areas of care that might require research.

Follow-up MYMOP2 forms allow patients to continue scoring their initial symptoms and activity restrictions, to introduce new symptoms and to describe any changes in medication use. The scores translate into a visually effective graph for use within the consultation.

A recent study of an earlier version of MYMOP involving NHS general practitioners and complementary therapists (Paterson 1996) showed that the questionnaire was practical to administer within a consultation. The practitioners reported increased awareness of patients' priorities.

The practitioner in this audit decided that he wanted:

- a focused discussion of treatment progress with all clients who continued with him beyond a third treatment
- to complete MYMOP2 forms for at least four treatments with all these clients if they were agreeable to this.

Data collection

Clients who had completed at least three sessions of treatment were identified from the clinic's register each week for a month and added to a list kept in the register. A set of four MYMOP2 forms was put in the notes to remind the practitioner to invite clients to fill one in at their next consultation. The completed forms were held in the notes and added to if necessary. At the end of 2 months the practitioner looked at the register list and the completed MYMOP forms.

Analysis, discussion and managing change

Eighteen of the TCM practitioner's clients saw him for three or more consultations. MYMOP2 had been used with all of these clients. All had given consent.

The TCM practitioner's patients reported that his use of MYMOP2 made them feel 'properly listened to'. He was able to present the graphs to colleagues and show that all but one of his patient's MYMOP2 main presenting symptom scores had increased, indicating improvement, or remained stable. He found that some symptoms were more commonly presented than others. These included fatigue, mental and emotional problems and ear, nose and throat disorders.

Box 6.8 Is this audit for me?

- This audit can improve communication between you, your patients and clinical colleagues.
- Other patient-generated forms may also be of value. Practitioners who want to use MYMOP2 should obtain a user's pack, complete with instructions (see Paterson 1996).
- This audit does not show whether a therapy is effective. It takes a useful procedure (MYMOP2 completion) and helps make sure it is used.
- The practitioner in this example found his audit did not identify areas needing change. It encouraged him to investigate published research in areas that did not seem to be responding to treatment.

He reported that the collection of this data gave him increased confidence about his treatment approach but left him with more questions than answers. He did not plan changes to practice.

Learning points

* There is no one, correct, way to carry out audit. Audits can take very different forms and still produce valuable changes in patient care.
* While the basic principles of audit are relatively simple, practitioners will benefit from seeking help with designing and implementing their audit projects.

AUDIT IN CONTEXT

This last section describes audit's role in professional, evidence-informed practice. The need to do audit is a fact of life in orthodox clinical practice and is fast becoming an important aspect of complementary therapy practice. Anyone thinking of undertaking audit needs to be clear as to what it can achieve and how it complements and builds upon research activity.

A commitment to audit is now a requirement for professional clinical practice in the UK. The Department of Health's Chief Medical and Nursing Officers have stated, 'Clinical Audit should be a routine practice for all health care professionals' (Department of Health 1994). Under the NHS framework of clinical governance, GPs and other purchasers of health care have responsibility for the quality of the care they provide (Department of Health 1998). They will therefore need to work with professionals who understand the principles of audit and are prepared to take part in audit projects.

Professional bodies in complementary medicine are now developing or considering audit training or formal audit programs for their members. The chiropractic and osteopathy professions, for example, have, along with general practitioners, been involved in a centrally organized 'Sentinel' audit of treatment for acute back pain. With this approach, individual practitioners are presented with a single audit topic, chosen as important for the profession as a whole, and with an off-the-shelf set of materials to help them collect and report data. The whole exercise is conducted confidentially, in such a way that no individual practitioner is identified but each can see how their practice compares with professionally defined standards and large group averages. While audit on this scale can help a profession focus on an important clinical topic and is a useful adjunct to individually driven audit, it is less able to make use of individual practitioners' enthusiasm and knowledge about their own situation.

There has been confusion in the past as to what clinical audit can do and what it requires. Box 6.9 summarizes some of the common concerns about audit and presents some initial responses. The following points may also help avoid misunderstanding and ensure that audit is an effective approach for complementary therapists and patients.

Can clinical audit help me find out if I am effective?

One of the golden rules of audit is that it should address things that are under the control of clinicians. This is why most successful audits look at processes or struc-

---

Box 6.9 Common concerns about audit – and some responses

- 'Audit is about being assessed "from above".' Audit can be self-directed by individual practitioners or coordinated by a professional body. It should always be confidential.
- 'It's not me – it's the others!' But audit raises standards throughout a profession.
- 'We already do it.' Most practitioners do look subjectively at their own work, but this can be misleading. Audit provides a more objective basis on which to make decisions.
- 'What's in it for me?' This often goes unsaid. It is important to acknowledge motivation.
- 'Not enough time' / 'I'm not being paid for it.' These are both questions of priority. Other professions report that audit has repaid the effort spent.
- 'I don't want to standardize' / 'What I do is an art.' But all artists use techniques.
- 'Outcomes research is more important.' Outcomes research helps with audit but is not a prerequisite. We need audit to improve the quality of what we do. Outcomes research helps us find out what we should be doing.

---

tures that are known to result in effective care. The outcomes for patients, complementary or otherwise, are influenced by many factors. To find out which factors are important, we need outcomes research, not audit. Outcomes research depends on the investment of a considerable amount of time in selecting research methods that will answer very specific research questions, with the endpoint being a qualified answer to that research question, e.g. in specified conditions, compared with approach x, approach y results in reduced side effects. The aim of clinical audit, in contrast, is direct, positive effects on patient care within a short timescale.

In particular, outcomes monitoring is often confused with audit. Monitoring of outcomes is a helpful way of looking at care and highlighting areas that need attention or could be usefully researched. It does not, however, explicitly aim to identify barriers and opportunities to good practice and then work on these and is therefore unlikely to lead to audit's main goal: improved care in the short term.

While the research base in complementary therapies is growing, there is still very little research that can actually guide clinical decision making. As has been shown elsewhere in this book, the complementary medicine research base provides some evidence that certain interventions may be of use for some patients. It will rarely support a specific intervention in a given clinical situation. As a result, audit criteria are unlikely to be informed by controlled complementary medicine research in the near future.

This should not impede audit, however. Conventional health professions have found that research evidence for interventions is useful if it is present, but is not essential. Audit criteria can be based upon local or national consensus about professional practice. Localized expertise – about a clinic's patients or communication systems, for example – can be used. National therapy bodies can issue guidance that can then be used to assess and improve practice. The important thing is to start audits by answering the question 'What am I trying to do?' in a reasoned way.

It is also worth asking, 'Is audit itself effective?'. This very question was addressed in a recent systematic review conducted as part of the Cochrane Collaboration's work to collate and critically appraise the evidence for different approaches to health care

(Thomson O'Brien et al 2000). This study found 37 randomized trials examining the effects of audit and feedback on the practice of health professionals and patient outcomes. The review's authors concluded that these approaches 'can sometimes be effective in improving the practice of health care professionals, in particular for prescribing and diagnostic test ordering', adding that, when effective, effects 'appear to be small to moderate but potentially worthwhile'.

Do I have the skills and technology?

Audit is easily as challenging as the other forms of systematic enquiry described in this book; however, it requires organizational and people skills far more than it does technical skills. It is rare, for example, for measurement in audit to involve anything other than simple percentages and totals. Likewise, audit shouldn't be equated with information technology. The simplest audits can be done with paper, pens and a calculator. Similarly, a helpful librarian is usually worth more than access to the Internet. The relative technological simplicity of audit may be one of the things that makes it attractive to practitioners interested in taking a systematic approach to patient care.

Learning points

* Audit is an activity expected of UK health professionals.
* Audit cannot be used to find out whether a particular approach to care is effective.
* Research evidence for interventions is useful to define practice standards if it is present, but is not essential. Audit criteria can also be based upon local or national consensus about professional practice.
* Audit is a challenging form of systematic enquiry that requires organizational and people skills far more than it does technical skills

CONCLUSION

This chapter has presented a brief introduction to clinical audit, focusing on examples of how audit can work within complementary medicine. Audit has been presented as a means of bringing about valuable change to practice that can be used in some form by any practitioner. The value of audit's explicit approach to developing practice is increasingly recognized in a wide range of health-care professions. Early reports from complementary therapists suggest that it is a valuable and do-able approach for complementary medicine. As complementary therapy practice develops and more audit is done, further lessons need to be learned and shared. Work in other health-care professions has made it clear that audit succeeds the most when the impetus and enthusiasm for it come from practitioners.

Acknowledgments

This chapter is based upon the work of 16 complementary practitioners and staff at the Research Council for Complementary Medicine in 1998. The content of this chapter, however, is the responsibility of the author alone.

Questions for discussion and personal reflection

- Which areas in my day-to-day practice could do with some improving? What could I do to find out about other practitioners' ideas about good practice in these areas?
- What aspects of my practice am I likely to be able to change and which are likely to be less amenable to change in the short term?
- Which changes in practice could make the most difference to patient care?
- How might my professional body be able to support me in audit activity?
- Where can I get help locally for any audit I do?
- Are there other people (other practitioners, practice managers, patients) who could usefully be involved in an audit of my practice?
- Am I clear about the different aims of audit and outcomes research?

REFERENCES

Department of Health 1994 Clinical audit: meeting and improving standards in healthcare. Department of Health, London
Department of Health 1998 A first class service: quality in the new NHS. Department of Health, London
Paterson C 1996 Measuring outcomes in primary care: a patient generated measure, MYMOP, compared with the SF-36 health survey. British Medical Journal 312: 1016–1020. Users' pack available from the author.
Thomson O'Brien MA, Oxman AD, Davis DA, Haynes RB, Freemantle N, Harvey EL 2000 Audit and feedback: effects on professional practice and health care outcomes. Cochrane Database Systematic Review 2000; 2: CD000259. The Cochrane Database is available on CD-ROM at most medical libraries.

FURTHER READING

British Journal of Clinical Governance (Quarterly, peer-reviewed journal, edited by staff at the University of Leicester's Clinical Governance Research and Development Unit. Describes itself as 'addressing the topics of clinical governance, evidence-based practice, guidelines, audit, risk management, user involvement and health outcomes'. It is aimed at clinical and non-clinical professionals from a wide variety of disciplines in primary and secondary care with an interest in improving the quality of health-care services)

Fraser RC, Baker R 1997 The clinical audit program in England: achievements and challenges. Audit Trends 5: 131–136
Fraser RC, Lakhani MK, Baker RH 1998 Evidence-based audit in general practice. Butterworth Heinemann, Oxford. (An introduction to the subject, with further examples.)

INFORMATION SOURCES

National Institute for Clinical Excellence
90 Long Acre
Covent Garden
London WC2E 9RZ
Tel: 0207 849 3444
Fax: 0207 849 3127
Email: nice@nice.nhs.uk
Web:http://www.nice.org.uk

Set up as a Special Health Authority on 1st April 1999 to provide the NHS (patients, health professionals and the public) in England and Wales with authoritative, robust and reliable guidance on current 'best practice'. Provides guidance on audit methods and criteria for high-quality clinical audit. Works in all sectors and with all professions.

Clinical Governance Research and Development Unit
Department of General Practice and Primary Health Care
University of Leicester
email: gcrdu@le.ac.uk
Web:http://www.le.ac.uk/gpaudit/index.html

Information service. Produces off-the-shelf audit protocols containing full instructions and evidence-based review criteria. Can direct practitioners to their nearest Medical Audit Advisory Group (MAAG/PCAG).

Primary Care Audit Groups/Medical Audit Advisory Groups
Nationwide. For local details, contact the Clinical Governance Research and Development Unit (above). Run by NHS health authorities. Can provide advice to local clinicians on planning and running an audit.

7

The placebo effect in complementary medicine

Irving Kirsch

INTRODUCTION

Everyone knows about the placebo effect but no-one seems to like it very much. Instead of investigating and using it, researchers and clinicians try to control and avoid it. This is certainly true of conventional medicine, in which there are only a few studies devoted to assessing and understanding placebo effects, against the thousands in which placebos are used as controls. Researchers in complementary medicine may be more open to examining the placebo effect, rather than just controlling for it, and this provides both a challenge and an opportunity.

There is something paradoxical in the use of placebo as a control and its neglect as an important component of treatment. The placebo effect is the only psychological variable that must be controlled before new medications can be approved by the United States Federal Drug Administration (FDA). In fact, it is the only control condition of any kind that must be bettered before a new drug can be approved. Implicitly, this means that the placebo effect must be important because if it were not important, there would be no need to control it. But if it is so very important, then why treat it only as a nuisance variable? Would it not be more reasonable to reconceptualize it as a legitimate part of treatment?

If there are placebo effects in conventional medicine, there must also be placebo effects in complementary medicine. Whatever else the herbs, needles and manipulations are doing, they are producing expectations of improvement and expectancy is the foundation of the placebo effect. In this chapter, I review a few of the many effects that placebos have been found to produce in conventional medicine. These are the effects that complementary treatments must be demonstrated to improve upon, if the claim for effects specifically due to their physical characteristics are to be substantiated. More important, these are effects that complementary medicine can lay claim do, if it does not repeat the mistake of dismissing the placebo effect as a mere nuisance variable.

DEPRESSION

Hopelessness is at the core of depression. Hopelessness is also an expectation. It is an expectancy that an intolerable situation will not improve. This being the case, one would expect depression to be very reactive to the placebo effect. Placebos instill an expectancy for improvement and this addresses a core issue of depression.

Kirsch & Sapirstein (1999) reported a metaanalysis of antidepressant medication, in which both the drug effect and the placebo effect were evaluated. They found that the effect size (D) for pretreatment to posttreatment changes in depression in patients given antidepressant drugs was 1.55 standard deviations. This is a very large effect and it indicates that administration of an antidepressant medication results in substantial clinical improvement. However, the effect size for response to placebo was 1.16SD. This indicates that 75% of the effect of antidepressant medication can be duplicated by administration of an inert placebo. In contrast, analysis of the course of untreated depression over the same time period indicated an effect size of only 0.37SD. Taken together, these effect sizes suggest that about 25% of the response to antidepressant medication may be a true drug effect, another 25% may be due to the natural history of the condition and 50% is an expectancy effect.

Despite the magnitude of the placebo effect, the data in the Kirsch & Sapirstein (1999) metaanalyses indicate a reasonably sizeable advantage for the active drug over placebo. However, there is reason to believe that much of this difference may be due to expectancy, rather than to the pharmacological properties of the drugs. Kirsch & Sapirstein reported that the correlation between response to medication and response to placebos across studies was $r = 0.90$. In an effort to track down the reason for this substantial correlation, they subdivided the set of studies by type of medication (e.g. trycyclics, SSRIs, MAOIs, etc.). They found that the pretreatment to posttreatment effect size was fairly consistent across drug type. More remarkable, the proportion of the effect size duplicated by placebo was virtually identical across medication type (range = 74–76%). The biggest surprise, however, came when they examined the effect size for a subset of studies in which the active drugs (amylobarbitone, lithium, liothyronine and adinazolam) were not antidepressants. The effect of these drugs on depression ($D = 1.69$) was as great as that of the antidepressants, and again an inactive placebo duplicated 76% of this effect.

It seems unlikely that amylobarbitone, lithium, liothyronine and adinazolam are in fact antidepressants, with pharmacological effects as great as trycyclics, SSRIs, MAOIs and the others. Instead, it is possible that all of these drugs function as active placebos. An active placebo is an active medication that does not have specific activity for the condition being treated. Greenberg & Fisher (1989) summarized data indicating that the effect of antidepressant medication is smaller when it is compared to an active placebo than when it is compared to an inert placebo. The reason for this difference seems to be related to the side effects produced by the drug. Because the active drugs produce more side effects than the inert placebo, most participants in studies of antidepressant medication are able to deduce whether they have been assigned to the drug condition or the placebo condition (Blashki et al 1971). This may produce an enhanced placebo effect in drug conditions and a diminished placebo effect in placebo groups. Thus, the apparent drug effect of antidepressants may in fact be a placebo effect, magnified by differences in experienced side effect and the patient's subsequent recognition of the condition to which he or she has been assigned. Support for this interpretation of the data is provided by a metaanalysis of fluoxetine (Prozac), in which a correlation of 0.85 was reported between the therapeutic effect of the drug and the percentage of patients reporting side effects (Greenberg et al 1994).

The Kirsch & Sapirstein (1999) metaanalysis was limited to studies of the acute effects of antidepressant drugs and placebos (the mean duration of the studies was 5 weeks). Walach & Maidhof (1999) extended these findings to their long-term effects (6 months to 3 years). In the most stringent analysis of their data (reported in Kirsch 1998), confined to studies in which drop-outs were analyzed as treatment failures, the results were virtually identical to those reported in the Kirsch & Sapirstein (1999) metaanalysis. They indicated that 73% of the long-term improvement among patients treated with antidepressant was duplicated in patients treated by placebo and the correlation between the proportion of patients responding to antidepressant and proportion of patients responding to placebo was $r = 0.93$. In addition, another metaanalysis conducted on a different set of studies (Joffe et al 1996) revealed pre-post drug and placebo effect sizes very similar to those reported by Kirsch & Sapirstein (1999). The close correspondence in the results of these three independently conducted metaanalyses, despite little or no overlap in the studies included for analysis (there were two studies that were included in both the Joffe et al metaanalysis and the Kirsch & Sapirstein metaanalysis), indicate that the data they reported are very reliable.

A methodological feature of the Walach & Maidhof (1999) metaanalysis provides further information on the relative advantage of active medication compared to inert placebo. Instead of using standardized mean improvement scores, as had been done in the other metaanalyses, Walach & Maidhof (1999) based their calculations on the number of patients showing long-term clinically significant improvement in the drug condition and the number showing long-term clinically significant improvement in the placebo condition. With drop-outs categorized as treatment failures, 63% of the patients in drug groups improved, compared to 46% of patients in placebo groups – a difference of 17% (Kirsch 1998). Thus, only one in six patients showed long-term clinical improvement following medication but would not have done so following placebo.

PAIN

Placebos are best known for their ability to reduce pain. Compared to untreated controls, subjects given placebo analgesia report less pain at similar levels of stimulation, tolerate more intense levels of stimulation and have a higher threshold for reporting that a stimulus is painful (Baker & Kirsch 1993, Camatte et al 1969, Gelfand et al 1963, Liberman 1964).

Not all placebos are equally effective in reducing pain. Placebo morphine is considerably more effective than placebo Darvon, which in turn is more effective than placebo aspirin (Evans 1974). In each case, the placebo is about half as effective as the pharmacologically active drug. Similarly, placebos produce more pain relief when given after a more potent drug than they do when given after a less potent drug (Kantor et al 1966). Thus, the effectiveness of a placebo pain reliever varies as a function of its believed effectiveness.

Early estimates suggested that about one-third of all patients are benefited by placebos (Beecher 1955) but procedures that enhance the credibility of a placebo also enhance its effectiveness. For example, Traut & Passarelli (1957) reported an improvement rate of 50% following the administration of placebo tablets to patients suffering from rheumatoid arthritis. Those showing no improvement were then given placebo injections. Sixty-four percent of them reported improvement, half of whom complained that the effects wore off after 3 days and were therefore given injections twice a week. Thus there was an overall improvement rate of 82% from either the tablet or the injection. Patients reported greater relief when the placebo was injected near the affected part of the body and continued placebo treatment was reported to be effective for as long as 30 months.

Backman et al (1960) reported similar results for placebo treatment of pain produced by peptic ulcers and other gastroduodenal disorders. Instead of administering one or two pills, the patients in this study were instructed to take six tablets, four times a day, over a 2-week period. Symptom improvement was reported for 92% of the patients.

Is there less pain or does it just hurt less?

There is some question as to whether placebos actually reduce the intensity of sensation that is produced by a painful stimulus or whether they alter the way in which the sensation is experienced. Some writers have argued that the sensation itself is not altered but that it is experienced as less painful. Placebo administration is seen as producing the reaction 'my pain is the same, but it doesn't hurt me now' (Beecher 1956, p. 111; also see Barber 1959).

This explanation has considerable intuitive appeal. There are a number of situations in which the same sensation elicits markedly different reactions in different people. For example, spicy foods contain irritants that produce a sensation of burning heat, a feeling that small children avoid. As they grow older, however, some youngsters begin to like the effect and develop a craving for spicy food. Similarly, some people experience cold as painful, whereas others learn to experience the same sensation as bracing and refreshing.

It is sometimes assumed that active pain medications are unlike placebos in that they decrease the sensation of pain as well as affecting the person's reaction to that sensation. However, Beecher (1956, 1957) has suggested that morphine and other analgesics operate in much the same way as placebos: 'Narcotics really alter pain perception very little but do produce a bemused state, comparable to distraction' (Beecher 1957, p. 152). From this perspective, placebos and active analgesics operate via similar mechanisms. According to Beecher, placebos reduce the anxiety associated with clinical pain, thereby making the pain more tolerable. In addition to reducing anxiety, active medications generate an altered state of consciousness that distracts the person from attending to the pain. But neither active nor placebo medication affects the sensation itself.

Beecher's hypothesis was based in part on the erroneous belief that the effects of placebos – and of opiates as well – were limited to clinical pain. He argued that because subjects in an experimental situation had no reason to be anxious about the meaning of their pain (e.g. it was clearly not an indication of serious disease), there was no pain-related anxiety to reduce; hence the failure of placebos and general anesthetics to relieve experimental pain. In fact, numerous early studies appeared to show that neither placebos nor opiates had any effect on experimentally induced pain. However, the failure of these studies to find an effect was at least partly due to the absence of no-treatment control groups in experimental designs. Subsequent studies indicated that repeated administration of experimental pain stimuli can produce increases in pain, which can mask the pain-relieving effects of treatment. Studies that include no-treatment control groups show reliable placebo effects on both clinical and experimental pain (Baker & Kirsch 1993, Camatte et al 1969, Gelfand et al 1963, Liberman 1964).

General anesthetics as 'active' placebos

The results of two studies suggest that Beecher may have been right in hypothesizing that placebo and pharmacological pain reduction are due to similar mechanisms (Dworkin et al 1983, 1984). However, these studies also suggest that Beecher's theory of pain reduction needs to be modified. They indicate that the altered states of consciousness produced by active drugs do not automatically reduce pain. Instead, the pain-relieving effects of some active drugs may be entirely due to expectancy. Rather than reducing pain, altered states of consciousness may act to confirm people's expectations for reduced pain. These studies also suggest that whether induced by placebos or by active drugs, expectancies can affect the sensation of pain as well as a person's reaction to that sensation.

Nitrous oxide (N_2O) is an analgesic gas that is frequently used in dentistry. As is true of other general anesthetics, nitrous oxide produces global alterations in consciousness (the 'bemused state' to which Beecher referred). However, Dworkin et al (1983) demonstrated that, depending on people's expectations, this bemused state can either decrease or *increase* sensitivity to painful stimulation. In that study, one group of subjects was given a rationale that described the common use of nitrous oxide as a pain reliever in dentistry. A second group was told that the altered state of consciousness produced by nitrous oxide can increase sensitivity to physical sensations, creating 'a kind of exquisite awareness of what's going on in the body' (p.1075). The authors reported that whereas nitrous oxide decreased pain in the first group, it led to increased pain in the second.

The effect of this expectancy manipulation was not limited to reports of pain. Besides assessing pain threshold and tolerance, Dworkin et al (1983) measured the effects of nitrous oxide on their subjects' absolute sensation threshold, a measure of sensitivity to non-painful stimulation. Their results on this measure were similar to those reported for pain. With expectations for pain relief, subjects were less sensitive to non-painful levels of stimulation with nitrous oxide. Conversely, nitrous oxide increased sensitivity to stimulation when subjects were led to believe that this would be its effect.

Placebos are generally inert substances, but 'active' or 'impure' placebos have also been suggested (Blumenthal et al 1974). Active placebos are substances that produce pharmacological effects but not for the condition being treated or investigated. They may mimic the side effects of other drugs, for example, thereby being more likely to convince recipients that they are receiving effective medication. The data reported by Dworkin et al (1983) suggest that general anesthetics can function as 'active' placebos and that their pain-relieving effects may, in some cases, be entirely due to expectancy. The superiority of these drugs to inactive placebos may be due to the convincing character of their side effects. The bemused state acts to confirm the potency of the drug, thereby confirming subjects' expectations of decreased pain. To my knowledge, no drug that produces an altered state of consciousness has been shown to not have analgesic effects. Furthermore, the degree of pain relief brought about by these drugs appears to be proportional to the intensity of the altered states of consciousness that they elicit.

In a follow-up to their earlier study, Dworkin et al (1984) tested the hypothesis that the mood-altering effect of active medication enhances expectancy by confirming that the drug is working as intended. In this study, the analgesic effects of nitrous oxide were tested with and without information intended to highlight the connection between pain reduction and the mood alterations and other side effects produced by the drug. Subjects in the 'high' information condition (the pun appears to have been unintended) were told that:

... nitrous oxide works as a sedative or tranquilizer. It lowers the brain's level of consciousness about anxiety and pain, making people feel good. Actually, the first signs that nitrous oxide is changing how your brain is processing information comes from changes you can readily experience with the lowest dosages of nitrous oxide – your toes, maybe your hands, may begin tingling and a kind of warm glow may come over you, a feeling of relaxation of muscle tension. These signs from your body, which some compare with drinking a good glass of wine or even smoking marijuana, indicate that the nitrous oxide has reached physiologically active levels. The drug is now working. (p. 343)

As predicted, this information increased the effectiveness of nitrous oxide as a pain reliever. Furthermore, as in their earlier study, this effect was obtained for absolute sensitivity to sensation as well as for pain threshold.

Taken together, these two studies suggest that active analgesic medication may function via the same mechanism as placebos; that is, by altering pain expectancies. The pharmacologically active components of these drugs enhance their effectiveness by strengthening the expectancy for pain reduction. These studies also show that the effects of expectancy are not limited to people's classification of sensations as painful or non-painful. Instead, expectancies can affect absolute sensitivity to sensation.

Additional evidence that placebos can affect the sensation of pain, rather than just the reaction to that sensation, is provided by data indicating that expectancies can generate pain, as well as alleviate it. For example, headaches are a frequently reported side effect of lumbar puncture, a clinical procedure used to administer anesthetics or to extract spinal fluid for diagnostic purposes. Daniels & Sallie (1981) performed lumbar punctures on two groups of subjects, only one of which was warned of the possibility of headaches. Approximately half of the subjects who were forewarned subsequently reported headaches, as compared to only one of the control subjects, suggesting that this commonly reported consequence of lumbar puncture is a placebo effect.

Finally, the sensory component and the emotional component of the pain response have been assessed separately in more recent studies of placebo analgesia (Montgomery & Kirsch 1996, Price et al 1999). The results of these studies indicate that the intensity of pain and its unpleasantness are very highly correlated. They also reveal that placebos have as great an effect on pain intensity as they do on the unpleasantness associated with the pain.

SKIN CONDITIONS

Because depression and pain are psychological responses, placebo effects on them are not particularly surprising. However, placebos have been reported to produce some rather startling effects on skin conditions and these are very surprising indeed.

The most impressive of these reports involves the suggestion-related production and inhibition of contact dermatitis (Ikemi & Nakagawa 1962). Contact dermatitis is a skin condition produced by chemical substances to which people have become sensitized. In the study reported by Ikemi & Nakagawa, 13 students were touched on one arm with leaves from a harmless tree but were told that the leaves were from a lacquer or wax tree (Japanese trees that produce effects similar to poison ivy and to which the boys had reported being hypersensitive). On the other arm, the subjects were touched with poisonous leaves which they were led to believe were from a harmless tree. All 13 subjects displayed a skin reaction to the harmless leaves (the placebo) but only two reacted to the poisonous leaves. Five of the students were hypnotized before being touched with the leaves but the results were virtually identical for hypnotized and non-hypnotized subjects.

In 1927, Bloch (cited in Allington 1952) followed 179 patients whose warts had been treated with an elaborate placebo procedure. The warts were painted with various colored dyes and exposed to an impressive electrical machine which was then turned on. After treatment, the patients were instructed not to touch the warts until the color had faded completely, at which time, they were assured, the warts would be cured. Bloch reported success rates of 44–88% depending on the type of wart, with most of the warts disappearing within 1 month. Although there was no control group in this study, the results can be compared with data from other studies indicating a rate of spontaneous remission of about 25% over a 6-month period (Allington 1952).

Four years after Bloch's data were reported, Memmesheimer & Eisenlohr (cited in Allington 1952) observed changes in warts among 70 patients to whom placebo treatment was provided and another 70 patients in a no-treatment control condition. Their treatment was not as impressive as that used by Bloch (only a few of their patients were exposed to the electrical apparatus) and their results were not as impressive. After 6 months, only 17 of the treated patients were cured of their warts, as compared to 20 of the untreated patients. However, the treated patients were cured more rapidly: 11 within 1 month (as compared to only two in the untreated group) and 14 within 3 months (as compared to five in the untreated group).

Johnston & Stenstrom (1986) compared the effects of hypnosis, placebo and no treatment on warts. Within 6 weeks, 50% of the hypnosis subjects had lost warts, compared to 25% of placebo subjects and 11% of untreated controls. The difference between the hypnosis and the untreated groups was statistically significant but the proportion of subjects losing warts in the placebo group did not differ significantly from that found in either of the other conditions. Similar results were reported by Spanos et al (1988). In that study, 34% of the hypnosis subjects lost warts, compared to 9% in the placebo condition but only 2% in the no-treatment control condition. These data suggest that hypnosis may have specific benefits for skin conditions, beyond those produced by the placebo effect. However, the fact that success in the hypnosis group was unrelated to subjects' hypnotizability levels suggests that these results were not due to hypnosis per se. In some situations, hypnosis can be a more credible expectancy manipulation than medical placebos and this may be responsible for its greater efficacy in reducing warts.

CONCLUSION

Depression, pain and skin conditions are but a few of the conditions that can be affected by placebos. Placebos have also been found to produce changes in phobic anxiety, bronchoconstriction in asthmatics, heart rate, blood pressure, sexual arousal, alcohol craving and consumption among alcoholics, skin temperature and gastric function (reviewed in Kirsch 1997, 1999). These powerful effects can make it difficult to find a significant effect for an active medication and the placebo effect has been the bane of medical researchers (see, for example, Enserink 1999).

The field of complementary medicine has a choice to make regarding the placebo effect and this choice may have a profound effect on its future. It may choose to emulate conventional medicine and treat the placebo as an alien factor, an outside influence to be shunned and controlled. Alternatively, it might embrace the placebo effect that conventional medicine has thrown away. There may be more than placebo effects to alternative treatments but expectancy effects might also be regarded as an important positive factor in their effectiveness.

REFERENCES

Allington HV 1952 Review of the psychotherapy of warts. AMA Archives of Dermatology and Syphilology 66: 316–326
Backman H, Kalliola H, Ostling G 1960 Placebo effect in peptic ulcer and other gastroduodenal disorders. Gastroenterologia 94: 11–20
Baker SL, Kirsch I 1993 Hypnotic and placebo analgesia: order effects and the placebo label. Contemporary Hypnosis 10: 117–126
Barber TX 1959 Toward a theory of pain: relief of chronic pain by prefrontal leucotomy, opiates, placebos, and hypnosis. Psychological Bulletin 56: 430–460
Beecher HK 1955 The powerful placebo. Journal of the American Medical Association 159: 1602–1606
Beecher HK 1956 The subjective response and reaction to sensation: the reaction phase as the effective site for drug action. American Journal of Medicine 20: 107–113
Beecher HK 1957 The measurement of pain: prototype for the quantitative study of subjective responses. Pharmacological Review 9: 59–209
Blashki TG, Mowbray R, Davies B 1971 Controlled trial of amytriptyline in general practice. British Medical Journal 1: 133–138
Blumenthal DS, Burke R, Shapiro K 1974 The validity of 'identical matching placebos'. Archives of General Psychiatry 31: 214–215
Camatte R, Gerolami A, Sarles H 1969 Comparative study of the action of different treatments and placebos on pain crises of gastro-duodenal ulcers. Clinical Terapeutica 49: 411–419
Daniels AM, Sallie R 1981 Headache, lumbar puncture, and expectation. Lancet 1 (8227): 1003.
Dworkin SF, Chen ACN, LeResche L, Clark DW 1983 Cognitive reversal of expected nitrous oxide analgesia for acute pain. Anesthesia and Analgesia 62: 1073–1077
Dworkin SF, Chen ACN, Schubert MM, Clark DW 1984 Cognitive modification of pain: information in combination with N_2O. Pain 19: 339–351
Enserink M 1999 Can placebo be the cure? Science 284: 238–240

Evans FJ 1974 The placebo response in pain reduction. In: Bonica JJ (ed) Advances in Neurology, Vol. 4. Pain. Raven, New York: pp. 289–296

Gelfand S, Ullmann LP, Krasner L 1963 The placebo response: an experimental approach. Journal of Nervous and Mental Disease 136: 379–387

Greenberg RP, Fisher S 1989 Examining antidepressant effectiveness: findings, ambiguities, and some vexing puzzles. In: Fisher S, Greenberg RP (eds) The limits of biological treatments for psychological distress: comparisons with psychotherapy and placebo. Lawrence Erlbaum, Hillsdale, NJ, pp. 1–37

Greenberg RP, Bornstein RF, Zborowski MJ, Fisher S, Greenberg MD 1994 A meta-analysis of fluoxetine outcome in the treatment of depression. Journal of Nervous and Mental Disease 182: 547–551

Ikemi Y, Nakagawa S 1962 A psychosomatic study of contagious dermatitis. Kyoshu Journal of Medical Science 13: 335–350

Joffe R, Sokolov S, Streiner D 1996 Antidepressant treatment of depression: a metaanalysis. Canadian Journal of Psychiatry 41: 613–616

Johnson J, Stenstrom R 1986 Hypnotic suggestion and placebo in the treatment of warts. Paper presented at the meeting of the American Psychological Association, Washington, DC

Kantor TG, Sunshine A, Laska E, Meisner M, Hopper M 1966 Oral analgesic studies: pentazocine, hydrochloride, codeine, aspirin, and placebo and their influence on response to placebo. Clinical Pharmacology and Therapeutics 7: 447–454

Kirsch I 1997 Specifying nonspecifics: psychological mechanisms of placebo effects. In: Harrington A (ed) The placebo effect: an interdisciplinary exploration. Harvard University Press, Cambridge, MA, pp. 166–186

Kirsch I 1998 Reducing noise and hearing placebo more clearly. Prevention and Treatment, Article 0007. Available on the World Wide Web: http://journals.apa.org/prevention/volume1/pre0010007a.html

Kirsch I 1999 How expectancies shape experience. American Psychological Association, Washington, DC

Kirsch I, Sapirstein G 1999 Listening to Prozac but hearing placebo: a meta-analysis of antidepressant medication. In: Kirsch I (ed) How expectancies shape experience. American Psychological Association, Washington, DC, pp. 303–320

Liberman R 1964 An experimental study of the placebo response under three different situations of pain. Journal of Psychiatric Research 2: 233–246

Montgomery G, Kirsch I 1996 Mechanisms of placebo pain reduction: an empirical investigation. Psychological Science 7: 174–176

Price DD, Milling MS, Kirsch I, Duff A, Montgomery G, Nicholls SS 1999 An analysis of factors that contribute to the magnitude of placebo analgesia. Pain 83: 147–156

Spanos NP, Stenstrom RJ, Johnston JC 1988 Hypnosis, placebo, and suggestion in the treatment of warts. Psychosomatic Medicine 50: 245–260

Traut EF, Passarelli EW 1957 Placebos in the treatment of rheumatoid arthritis and other rheumatic conditions. Annals of the Rheumatic Diseases 16: 18–22

Walach H, Maidhof C 1999 Is the placebo effect dependent on time? A meta-analysis. In: Kirsch I (ed) How expectancies shape experience. American Psychological Association, Washington DC, pp. 321–332

8

Conducting multicenter and large trials in complementary and alternative medicine

Richard Grimm

INTRODUCTION

The gold standard for evaluating medical treatments is the clinical trial. A clinical trial is defined by Friedman et al as a 'prospective study comparing the effect and evaluation of an intervention(s) against a control in human subjects'. It is necessary for the trial control or comparison group(s) to be evaluated concurrently against the intervention(s). Clinical trials are a relatively new methodology compared to other means of assessing medical treatments. Even as recently as the 1960s, clinical trials were done only occasionally and those that were done usually focused on infectious diseases by evaluating vaccines and antibiotics. The field has progressed dramatically and at the beginning of the 21st century, NIH and industry are conducting tens of thousands of trials. Trials are so visible now that the term 'clinical trial' has become part of the vernacular. Why have trials proliferated to such a degree over this relatively short period of time?

The primary reason is that clinical trials are the only study design for evaluating treatments that can establish a causal connection between treatment and outcome. Observational and case control studies can determine that an association exists, but they cannot prove that one is the cause of the other. In all studies except clinical trials, there is always the problem of 'chicken versus egg'.

Confounding is also a major problem in observational and case controlled studies because biases of practitioners can easily affect the outcomes. Bias can selectively direct patients with different severity of disease to different types of treatment. For example, in a data set evaluating treatments for carpal tunnel syndrome, subjects with more severe disease would tend to be directed toward surgery, while those with less severe disease would be more likely to be treated with medical therapy.

Efforts are made in observational and case controlled studies to adjust for inequalities in confounding using matching and statistical techniques, but such efforts are limited in their effectiveness. This is true because of limitations in data collected, problems selecting the best control group and unknown factors not measured which can and usually do confound the results. Confounding is not a problem in clinical trials because subjects are assigned to treatments randomly; therefore, biases of practitioners cannot come into play.

ALTERNATIVE MEDICINE: THE CONCEPT

In recent years, there has been increased interest in and use of non-traditional treatments for acute and chronic diseases. Treatments that are often lumped together as complementary and alternative medicine (CAM) include chiropractic manipulation, acupuncture and acupressure, herbal therapy, massage therapy, naturopathic medicine and various relaxation and meditation techniques.

Often mainstream allopathic physicians have suspected CAM practitioners of using methods which are neither scientific nor effective compared to conventional medical interventions. Similarly, CAM practitioners often have strong feelings and negative biases toward allopathic treatments. There are numerous reasons, some epistemological, some sociological, for this state of mutual distrust but using clinical trials to evaluate CAM treatments can go a long way toward alleviating it.

Part of the problem seems to lie in our commonly agreed definition of CAM itself. Complementary and alternative treatment is defined as any disease-related treatment that is not part of the allopathic approach. This view of alternative medicine is not satisfactory because it merely defines CAM by what it is not, without giving us any clear indication of what it is. Moreover, by this definition, what is included in CAM would have to change continually because more and more CAM treatments are being included in traditional medical practices. This is true of both acupuncture and chiropractic, for example. Does this mean that acupuncture and chiropractic should no longer be seen as CAM modalities?

Since the customary distinction between allopathic medicine and CAM is so unclear, perhaps it is more useful to view both as treatments which lend themselves to testing for benefit or harm using scientifically rigorous methods, especially clinical trials. In the evaluation of allopathic treatments, the usual outcome has been that most are found to be ineffective, some are found to be harmful and some are found to be safe and effective and therefore worthy of prescribing to patients. The same will likely be true when CAM treatments are evaluated in clinical trials.

MAIN FACTORS TO CONSIDER WHEN USING CLINICAL TRIALS

There are several considerations that need to be carefully thought out before undertaking a clinical trial.

- What is the question or hypothesis being tested?
- Is it ethical to test this hypothesis?

- What are the primary outcomes?
- Can the outcomes be measured accurately?
- Can potential bias be minimized or eliminated?
- Does the study have sufficient statistical power to answer the question?

Each of these areas will be discussed in detail.

Stating the question

In all clinical trials, it is critically important to stipulate up front the primary and secondary questions or hypotheses to be tested. If this is not done explicitly, the investigators may find at the end of the study that the design selected could not possibly answer the most important questions. Once the questions have been clearly stated, the design will follow.

It is also crucial to stipulate the primary outcomes or endpoints of the main hypotheses. For example, an outcome in an osteoporotic fracture trial might range from hospitalized fracture to dual photon-determined bone density. The occurrence of the primary outcome in the control group of the trial will be the main factor determining sample size and power. Even a large study with few of the prestipulated outcomes in the control group will have little or no ability or power to answer the question.

Ethics

Ethical considerations are important in every stage of clinical trials. As we have said, the first phase is the development of the study concept, which then leads to the formation of the primary hypotheses. At this time, it is necessary to consider whether the test treatment(s) or intervention(s) to be studied have the potential to cause harm. This determination can be based on a thorough review of the previous human and animal studies. (With drugs under the FDA approval process, this is usually accomplished in Phase 2 and Phase 3 clinical trials.)

For example, early studies of the effect of changing blood cholesterol on incidence of cardiovascular disease considered giving foods high in saturated fat to the intervention group compared to a low-fat and cholesterol diet for the control. It would have been much easier to achieve the desired difference in blood cholesterol between treatment and control groups by recommending higher fat foods to the treatment group. Instead, a diet low in fat and cholesterol was recommended to one group and usual diet to the others. This approach was necessary because of ethical considerations. In situations where standard therapy has already been demonstrated to be effective and the condition to be studied involves high risk to the patient, standard treatment is required for both the control and treatment groups. Then an additional treatment can be added for the intervention group and placebo added for the control, thus providing useful scientific data for the trial without causing undue risk to the participants. Although data regarding the comparison of treatment versus no treatment will not be yielded, the trial thus designed addresses the useful purpose of comparing the additive effect of the test treatment with standard care.

Ethical concerns are also present during the study recruitment phase. When qualifying a participant, it may be necessary for current treatments to be withdrawn. Sometimes there is a lead-in period required before randomization can be done. The investigators must be certain that by choosing to be a part of a clinical trial, the participant is not exposed to unreasonable risk.

Ethics are a major concern during the maintenance phase of clinical trials as well. Frequently issues concerning unblinding or establishing 'escape criteria' arise. When ongoing analysis reveals that the studied intervention is clearly harming the patient, patients must be withdrawn from study treatment and converted to standard care. The same is true if the studied treatment is found to have such a significant benefit over standard care that it is no longer ethical to withhold the studied treatment from the control group merely for the sake of gathering more data.

Large multicenter studies usually have an oversight group called the Data Safety and Monitoring Board (DSMB). The DSMB consists of investigators of the study group who periodically examine unblinded outcome data for evidence of harm or benefit, either of which might necessitate stopping the study for ethical reasons. Ethical concerns in the analysis phase require the unbiased release of results to the scientific as well as the lay community. Also each participant must be fully informed of the relevance of the study results to their personal health care. All these issues are dealt with through the proper application of informed consent.

Bias

In clinical trials, every effort must be made to eliminate, if possible, or minimize sources of bias. The introduction of bias is one of the biggest obstacles for conducting a successful clinical trial. Since clinical trials of CAM treatments are relatively new, elimination of bias will be particularly important. Frequently, inequalities of study groups at baseline with regard to important measures influence or confound the outcome of the trial. In order to achieve true randomization, the treatment assignment must be *unpredictable*. Using randomization with a large study population (approximately $N > 300$), one can be virtually certain of distributing the large majority of factors equally at baseline across study groups, even those that are not measured in the protocol. Table 8.1 shows baseline characteristics of two study groups in a clinical trial evaluating the influence of chiropractic manipulation compared to diet on blood pressure.

Table 8.1 Distribution of baseline characteristics by study group

	Control (N = 69) ± s.d.	Treatment (N = 71) ± s.d.	Between group P
Age (years)	47.6 ± 6.6	47.5 ± 7.2	0.95
% black	8.8	8.5	0.94
% male	46.4	42.3	0.62
Alcohol (drinks/wk)	3.1 ± 4.0	3.4 ± 4.8	0.75
Weight (lbs)	200 ± 44	187 ± 36	0.06
Systolic BP (mmHg)	136.5 ± 10.9	134.8 ± 9.4	0.32
Diastolic BP (mmHg)	88.8 ± 3.3	88.8 ± 3.7	0.95

Bias is a primary concern when it comes to determining the main outcome (endpoint) of a trial. Any bias becomes obvious when the study is unblinded and the investigators are informed of the treatment assignments, but bias can also be a problem at the outset when observers are determining the study endpoint. For example, when using two observers for measuring blood pressure when pressure is the primary outcome, one observer may systematically read higher values of pressure compared to the other observer.

These differences in observation may be accounted for by differences in acuity of hearing and eyesight as well as by type and thoroughness of training of the observers.

Generally in clinical trials both the staff and the participants should attend clinic visits at the same time of day for every visit. In a two-group parallel study, it is important to balance the observer measures between study groups. If this is not done, the difference in blood pressure revealed at study's end may be due to the measurement process itself.

Another way to ensure randomization and minimize bias is to make sure that observers do roughly the same number of measures on each study group over time. If one observer sees a higher proportion of patients from one study group compared to the other, bias would necessarily occur if there were differences in measurement technique. Ideally, the schedule of visits should be balanced so that each observer sees the same proportion of each treatment group.

This form of bias can also be addressed by using rigorously trained and certified personnel or by using only one observer for both groups; however, these solutions are not practical in most settings. The specific observer for each key measure in a study should be coded on the forms and observer comparisons, means and standard deviations of key measures should be monitored over the course of the trial.

An alternative to random assignment to treatment in a clinical trial might be to enroll patients systematically on an alternating first-come basis. Though easier to manage logistically, this approach should never be selected because it introduces predictability into the process.

For example, some years ago there was a study comparing two antibiotics, penicillin and lincomycin, for patients admitted to the hospital with lobar pneumococcal pneumonia. Residents covering the emergency room were instructed that patients admitted with this diagnosis on Monday, Wednesday and Friday were to be given penicillin; patients admitted on Tuesday, Wednesday and Saturday were to be given lincomycin. (Sunday was a day off.) The final result of the study was that there was a slight difference in favor of lincomycin over penicillin, with the primary endpoint being total days in the hospital. This was a surprising result since the house staff universally believed penicillin was the best drug. However, close inspection of the process of entry into the study revealed a major selection bias. When moderate to severe pneumonia patients presented to the emergency room on a lincomycin day, they were frequently excluded from the study so that they could be admitted to the hospital and treated with penicillin. Alternatively, these patients might be given oral outpatient penicillin medication and advised to come back the next day (a penicillin day). On the other hand, patients presenting on penicillin days were readily enrolled in the study regardless of disease severity. The result was that the more severe cases were systematically assigned to the penicillin group and severity is obviously related to stay in the hospital. This assignment method invalidated the study results. Randomization would have eliminated this source of bias.

If concerns about ensuring the right balance of participants in each study group arise, the problem can be addressed by a technique called 'blocking'. For example, groups of two, four and six participants would be randomly assigned within each block. The sequence of the blocks would also be randomized. This procedure portions out the number of participants desired in each study group.

Power

Statistical power is probably the most crucial concept to understand when designing clinical trials. It is also a poorly understood concept, even for many clinical investigators now active in the field. Statistical power is determined by the rate of occurrence of the primary outcome in the control group; the higher the control event rates, the greater the power. Power is also related to the expected effect of the intervention to be studied. This seems odd to the new investigator; if you already know the effect of the treatment, why are you doing the study? The answer is that you need to estimate the treatment effect in order to determine what treatment difference would be clinically meaningful. The rate of events in the control group as well as the estimated treatment effect are usually estimated using data from previous studies.

Statistical power is also determined by determining the chances for errors in the result. There are two types of errors: Type I and Type II. Type I errors occur when a positive effect is observed erroneously. Conventionally, in determining sample sizes, the level of probability acceptable for Type I has been set at 5% or an 'alpha' of 0.05. What this means is that if the probability or 'P value' is <0.05, the result is 'statistically significant'. In other words, one would expect to observe this particular positive result by chance in only one of 20 identical studies if such studies were carried out; a P of <0.01 would be less than 1 in 100. The concept of Type II errors is commonly less well understood. A Type II error occurs if, in a particular study, no difference is found between study groups but in fact a true difference exists. In that instance, we must determine the probability or the confidence that there is truly no difference between the study groups. Type II errors are related to the rate of events in the control group. The conventional level used in estimating sample sizes for a Type II or 'beta error' is often 0.9; if no difference is observed between groups in the trial outcome, there is a 90% chance that the studied treatment really makes no difference. Thus statistical power is determined by the chance of not making a Type II error 1, or 1-beta.

At the present time, estimating statistical power for CAM studies is particularly difficult. Often there are few, if any, previous studies available upon which to base estimates. Also, CAM studies are usually limited in sample size due to lack of sufficient resources for larger studies. Studies using smaller sample sizes tend to lack statistical power; therefore, if no treatment difference is observed, as is frequently the case, there is no confidence that the result is truly negative. Because CAM treatments are so widely used by the public, a valid negative study would be almost as valuable as a positive study. However, with little power, a negative study is not useful except for making general estimates of treatment effect and event rates for a larger definitive trial. In most instances, the results of trials should be reported as the observed group differences along with the 95% confidence limits around the observed difference point estimate. This allows a more enlightened interpretation of the results because it incorporates the concept of the study's power.

Another difficulty for CAM studies is that controls must frequently be standard treatment rather than placebo. With many diseases, it is not ethical to withhold an established treatment that is known to be effective.

CAM studies are also difficult to blind. For example, how could a treatment such as acupuncture or chiropractic manipulation be delivered without the patient knowing whether they were receiving it or not? Since many CAM treatments do not involve taking pills, it is very difficult to devise placebo controls for CAM interventions. Investigators have recently worked at developing sham 'placebo' controls; for example, acupressure has been used as a placebo with acupuncture and massage has been compared to chiropractic manipulation. Herbal treatments do allow for placebo control. For example, a large placebo-controlled trial of St John's wort for treating depression is currently being conducted by the NIH's National Center for Alternative and Complementary Medicine.

Blinding

Reducing observer bias and subject reporting bias are among the most important considerations when conducting a well-designed trial. If there is any possibility for bias to manifest in a trial, it usually will. Like water, bias takes the path of least resistance. Observer and participant bias are especially of concern when carrying out trials in the area of CAM because there are often strong opinions and beliefs concerning the benefit (or lack of benefit) among investigators and/or participants before the trial is initiated. Blinding (also termed masking) is usually the most effective method for reducing or eliminating such bias.

Blinding means that the treatment and control assignments are concealed. Single blinding occurs when either the investigator or participants are blinded. In other words, one of these groups is aware of the treatment assignment and the other is not. Single-blind procedures are especially useful in drug studies when subjects may need to take placebo before receiving their random treatment assignment or during washout periods such as are used in parallel crossover design studies.

Double blinding is commonly used and is the most desirable form of blinding because it reduces sources of bias from both the investigator and the participants. Double-blind studies are often placebo controlled. Double blinding can also be used in studies comparing multiple active treatments. For example, in CAM research, double-blind procedures are often used to evaluate herbal treatments and dietary supplements and the control is usually placebo.

Double blinding is often impossible or very difficult to achieve when evaluating procedures such as chiropractic manipulation or acupuncture. When these studies elect to use a sham procedure as control, they are usually single blinded since the investigator is aware of the study group. Single-blind, sham or even open study designs can be acceptable as long as the primary endpoint is objective (e.g. blood pressure) and the observers collecting the endpoint data are a third party not aware of the treatment group. Some treatments are impossible to blind because the treatment causes side effects such as the moderate to severe flushing which occurs in trials of nicotinic acid. When selecting the control for a clinical trial, the goal is to choose one that eliminates or reduces as much as possible the potential of introducing bias from all possible sources.

BIOMEDICAL RESEARCH PARADIGMS

The traditional approach to biomedical research in the US is viewed as a logical progression of stating a hypothesis, usually from work in molecular and basic science (Fig. 8.1). This hypothesis is then refined using animal models for the condition under study. Once the hypothesis is confirmed in these models, the effort focuses on humans. These studies lead to Phase 2 and 3 trials, which establish safety and efficacy of the treatment for human subjects. The next step may be larger clinical trials, which examine the potential benefit for managing the condition of concern (e.g. blood pressure lowering for preventing stroke). At this point, large demonstration projects may be carried out to explore successful application in the community. An example is screening mammography in the community for preventing breast cancer.

THE ROLE OF MULTICENTER TRIALS IN CAM RESEARCH

In multicenter trials, more than one independent center collaborates to answer a scientific question following an identical protocol. Multicenter trials are necessary to address questions that are too difficult or impossible to examine in a single center study. Multicenter trials have the advantage of being able to recruit a larger sample size than one center can; often large sample size are required to answer the question in a reasonable amount of time. Multicenter trials are also useful when a degree of diversity with regard to such factors as ethnicity, geographic distribution, socioeconomic status, etc. is required. The primary disadvantage of multicenter trials is that they are usually much more expensive and complicated than singlecenter trials. In the new field of CAM research, multicenter trials are also difficult because only a few CAM-oriented centers that have experience in conducting multicenter trials exist.

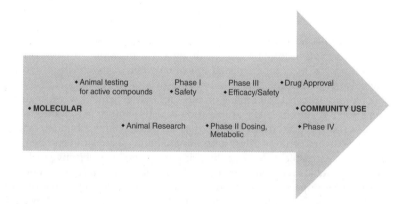

Figure 8.1 Traditional research paradigm.

Center selection

The primary consideration in selecting clinical centers is their ability to recruit and follow the study participants. This ability is related to the prevalence of the condition under study, which is in turn determined by the size and nature of the recruitment area. Centers in multicenter trials are frequently located in larger metropolitan areas because of their greater access to larger, more diverse study populations.

Another consideration when selecting study centers is the experience and special expertise of available investigators. It is important to avoid centers where the investigators and staff might have a conflict of interest and may be unduly biased in favor or against the intervention under study. If any investigators have a financial interest in the study, they should declare their interests and divest themselves of them or exclude themselves from participating in the study.

It has been crucial to exclude conflicts of interest in clinical trials of conventional treatments; the same will be true in the clinical studies of CAM. In all clinical trials, conflict of interest should be reassessed annually and updated over the course of the trial.

Role of the coordinating center

Multicenter trials also differ from single-center trials in that they have a central data-coordinating center that operates independently of the clinical centers. The central coordinating center (CTC) has broad responsibilities that include developing the study protocol and designing the randomization scheme, including block sizes and stratification. The CTC is also responsible for form development as well as training clinical center staff in data entry and special measurements or procedures. During recruitment, the CTC monitors the adequacy of randomization on baseline characteristics and once the interventions are initiated and participants followed, the CTC ensures quality control of the data collected. Data editing, analysis and central protection of the blinding process are also the responsibility of the coordinating center.

The CTC must arrange and conduct site visits to each participating clinical center. A site visit is conducted by a group made up of CTC personnel, principal investigator(s) from collaborating centers, coordinators from other clinical centers and project office representatives if the trial is funded by the NIH. The purpose of the site visit is to ensure uniformity and standardization of methods among all the participating centers. During the maintenance phase of the trial, visits are usually conducted at least annually and even more frequently in some trials. Monitoring standardization will be especially important in CAM studies until a substantial number of them develop track records and reputations comparable to those of the more established clinical trials centers.

STAGES OF A CLINICAL TRIAL

Carrying a clinical trial to a successful conclusion is a complex and arduous endeavor that must take place over a considerable period of time. For many investigators, this process is highly rewarding because the results of the trial are directly applicable to the real world of patients and practitioners in the community.

Conceptualization

All clinical trials begin as a concept in someone's mind. Ideally, the concept is formulated as a question or hypothesis. Hypotheses are generated from sources which include concerns for evaluating current practices, personal experience of the investigators and questions that are generated from the results of recently completed trials.

Even in studies with convincing outcomes, several new hypotheses can emerge. Trials frequently find results that are contradictory to conventional medical wisdom. The contradiction can prompt us to examine the problem using new paradigms and models to frame new questions. Thus large definitive trial results stimulate further investigation across the spectrum of scientific research areas from epidemiological to basic science.

Grant writing and the Institutional Review Board (IRB)

Once the hypothesis is well formulated and feasibility and ethical concerns are addressed, usually the next task is to prepare a formal grant proposal. This proposal will differ greatly in length and detail depending on the source of the potential funding. Grant writing is a scholarly activity that involves a thorough review of the topic under study, selection of study designs and establishing the variability, reliability, validity and feasibility of key measures. Once these concerns are addressed, sample size is determined using the desired power and expected treatment effects. Proposing a realistic sample size with adequate power to test the hypotheses is probably the most important component in maximizing the chances that the grant will be approved and funded and ultimately that the study will be successful.

At the same time the grant is submitted, an application must be filed with the Institutional Review Board (IRB) of the grantee's institution (university, hospital, clinic, etc.). In multicenter studies, each site submits an application to the IRB of its own institution. Very large trials with hundreds of clinical centers may also have a central IRB to expedite the process and to accommodate any centers that are not formally affiliated with an IRB. A committee reviews the IRB proposal with a view toward evaluating safety and consent procedures for the study participants. For NIH proposals involving human subjects, IRB approval must be obtained prior to funding the trial.

Protocol development and the manual of operations

It is usually necessary in large trials to build in an adequate planning phase at the beginning of the funding period. A primary task during this phase is to agree upon and write the study protocol. The protocol includes a summary of the justification of the trial, a priori statements of study hypotheses and detailed descriptions of study methods and standardization of measures. Clinic visit schedules with flow charts and time estimates for each type of visit, form development, training, certification of procedures and quality controls are also contained in the protocol as well as a description of the primary analyses which are planned and a description of the data and safety monitoring procedures. The protocol is usually a relatively compact document, designed as a quick reference for anyone interested in the overall design of the study.

The protocol is usually reviewed by an outside group (protocol review committee, DSMB, etc.) for ethics, internal consistency and omissions. Then the protocol provides the matrix for developing the manual of operations (MOP). This document covers the same areas as the protocol but with much more detail and supporting information.

Conducting the trial

Once the protocol has been completed and approved by the protocol committee and the IRB, the next phase is the actual conduct of the trial. This phase involves training of staff, recruitment of study subjects, maintaining adherence to the protocol and close out.

Training of clinic staff is especially important in a multicenter trial. Training involves standardization of procedures for filling out study forms, taking measurements and data entry. Training frequently takes place in a central location involving clinic staff from each clinical center and the CTC. A certification procedure is often used for special study interviews or measurements (e.g. 24-hour dietary recalls of food intake). Since many multicenter trials are conducted over several years, recertification at set intervals is required. In addition, staff turnover should be anticipated and a process of training and certifying new staff established.

Recruitment is sometimes given inadequate attention when preparing the grant proposal. In fact, recruitment is often the most difficult aspect of the trial. It is a common mistake to overestimate the number of eligible participants in the recruitment pool and to underestimate the recruitment yield (number of participants that must be screened to yield one randomization). Often, large multicenter trials must extend the recruitment period and add additional resources to complete enrollment of patients into the study.

Recruitment methods include:

- print and electronic media, including both feature stories and advertising
- mass brochure mailings to enriched and unenriched mailing lists
- referrals
- field screenings.

In large trials, advertising and mailings usually yield the largest number of randomized participants. Field screening is rarely successful because it is too labor intensive and expensive. Also participants recruited through field screening tend to be less motivated to join the study as well as less likely to attend subsequent eligibility visits. Professional referrals are inexpensive (except when chart reviews are necessary), but professional referrals are rarely successful unless the referral doctor is an integral member of the study team.

From the investigator's perspective, the maintenance phase can be less interesting than the conceptualization and design phases. Maintenance involves the hard work of continuing to follow the participants, collecting data and maintaining adherence to treatment assignments. Lost to follow-up and non-adherence can be devastating to the trial's power. A team approach for individual case management with problem participants has been helpful in avoiding these pitfalls.

The end of the study should include a final visit, which is called the close out visit. The purpose of this visit is to share the results of the study with the participants and to ensure a smooth transition back to regular care, whether it be allopathic, CAM or some combination of the two. At this point in blinded studies, the participants and the staff are invited to guess their group assignment (control or active treatment) so that the study's ability to maintain the blind can be determined. Even if the integrity of the blind is less than expected, the study results are still valid and knowing exactly the degree to which the blind succeeded will aid greatly when analyzing the data.

Data analysis

Analyses at the end of the trial involve comparing the outcomes in the unblinded study groups, both treatments and control. These analyses are focused on the primary and secondary questions and endpoints. It is extremely important to have data on as many randomized participants as possible and to include even those participants who were study drop-outs. Completeness of follow-up is critical because the result analyses are carried out according to the principle of intention to treat. 'Intention to treat' means that all participants are included in the analysis regardless of adherence to treatment or drop-out status. Data on intervention results and endpoints for drop-outs are imputed. A frequently used conservative method of imputation is to substitute the baseline values for the result, which assumes no change with intervention.

Efforts should be made to ensure as many participants as possible, including drop-outs, attend the final visit because the final visit values are used to assess the effects of the intervention. Intention-to-treat analysis is important because experience from past trials has shown that study drop-outs and non-adherers tend to be quite different from adherers. The alternative of on-treatment analysis is very seductive to the clinical mindset. However, using on-treatment analysis voids the validity of randomization and introduces an unacceptable degree of bias to the study.

In multicenter trials, the investigators must come to a consensus about the meaning of the results as well as the conclusions and implication of the trial's outcomes. At this point, it is important to share the results with the rest of the scientific community through presentations at the appropriate professional meetings and journal publications. This phase of the study can continue for a long time, even years, because large studies tend to reveal so much information that must be shared with the community.

Crossover designs

In crossover studies, participants are randomized initially to treatment or control. Then, after a period of time, the groups' interventions are crossed over or interchanged so that treatment becomes control and control becomes treatment. The same follow-up period is used in each study period.

Crossover studies have appeal because study participants act as their own controls, thus taking advantage of the fact that within-subject variability of essential study measures is much smaller than between-subject variability. In other words, on repeat measurement, people are much more likely to be like themselves than they will be like someone else. With this reduced variability, a crossover study can be done with a much smaller sample size than the standard parallel study. A general guideline which can be used is that the sample size in a crossover study can be reduced to one fourth of the parallel estimate; for example, the estimated sample size is N of 200 in a parallel study design could be reduced to an N of 50 using the crossover design without any significant loss of power.

In spite of this obvious advantage, crossover studies are much less common than parallel design studies. This is due to possibility of residual or lag effect of the treatment that can persist into the next study period. When this happens, the contrast of treatment versus control is contaminated.

This problem can be circumvented if the duration of the post-treatment effect is known. If not, residual effects can be eliminated by introducing a no-treatment ('washout') period between the two treatment periods.

Crossover study designs may be particularly suited to CAM studies. Their reduction in sample size with maintenance of power means more definitive studies can be carried out with the same (usually limited) resources. It is important to carry out as many CAM studies as quickly as possible, because clinical trials of CAM methodologies are a relatively new endeavor which has raised a multitude of unanswered questions. Millions of Americans are already using these treatments with little prior scientific assessment of their efficacy and safety. The crossover study allows for a faster assessment of any harm they may already be doing and increases the likelihood that the ones that prove to be safe and beneficial can be made available to a larger population of patients. In CAM crossover studies, the lag effect is not as large a problem as previously studied treatments because in order to have a residual effect persisting into the second period, there must be an effect in the first period. In addition, there are less serious concerns in CAM for having relatively long washout periods since there is often no prior evidence of treatment benefit or harm.

Large simple trials: the potential

CAM research can benefit greatly by doing large clinical trials. In the traditional FDA approach to approving new drugs, agents are developed at the molecular level either by screening or designing biologic compounds (Fig. 8.2) These are usually evaluated for activity by testing on thousands of lab mice or other animal subjects. Only a small percent of those tested are found to have biologic activity and the more promising ones go on to further animal testing. Fewer still go through the phase 1–4 clinical research sequence in humans and are finally approved for general use and prescribed in the community. This process often takes 10 years or more and costs hundreds of millions of dollars.

The opposite is true for CAM botanicals and 'food additives' which have gone through little or no previous testing and are already being used frequently by millions of people.

Figure 8.2 illustrates an alternative to the time-consuming and costly FDA approach, which could be used relatively quickly and cheaply for evaluating the

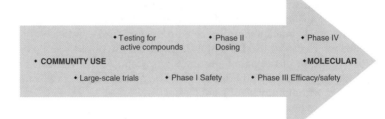

Figure 8.2 CAM research paradigm.

safety and efficacy of CAM compounds and treatments. The alternative strategy would be to do large, simple and relatively short duration trials. Since these agents are already consumed by millions of people and can be bought over the counter by anyone, the ethical barriers to studying their use in human subjects are far less formidable than when evaluating new drugs whose effects are less well known.

Large trials, placebo controlled, can be very useful for CAM evaluations. For example, a botanical commonly used for depression could be evaluated quickly against placebo by using an outcome such as a brief, self-administered depression inventory in hundreds or even thousands of participants without raising concern about exposing study participants to unreasonable risk. A huge trial can tolerate much higher drop-out and non-adherence rates while still preserving power to definitively answer the question. The maintenance phase of these trials would be much less time consuming and costly than in traditional clinical trials.

Those agents that prove safe and efficacious could then be studied in smaller, more contained trials to establish dosing range. Metabolic and animal studies could then be carried out to investigate mechanisms of action. Thus the sequence of metabolic and animal studies preceding human trials which has been necessary in allopathic medicine could be reversed in CAM research, thus enabling a much faster and less expensive scientific examination of their methodologies than previously thought possible.

In the past, the main obstacle to carrying out clinical trials has been cost. Using conventional methods, the costs of a trial are directly related to numbers of participants studied and the duration of the trial. Large trials done conventionally cost per participant year in the thousands of dollars. These studies have been so costly largely because of the necessity of maintaining a large clinic staff at one or more research facilities to collect patient data.

Using currently available technology, these barriers to CAM research can be potentially overcome. Participants could be enlisted, informed and randomized and data could be self-entered using interactive automated techniques via telephone or Internet. The active agent or placebo could be mailed to the participants and follow-up data could be collected interactively using the same media as in the recruitment phase of the trial. Since no clinics and few staff would be needed, per participant costs would be much lower than has previously been true for clinical trials and the much larger sample size would allow questions to be answered more quickly than has traditionally been the case.

Such data collection technology has been used successfully in survey and small trial research. There are feasibility and validity questions that need to be addressed. Nevertheless, the use of large simple trials may be particularly suited to CAM research on botanicals and food additives. In addition, the development of a whole new paradigm for conducting clinical trials could be of great benefit for the study of allopathic medicines as well.

9

The importance of patient selection

Fred Wiegant   Willem Kramers   Roeland van Wijk

INTRODUCTION

Interest in various forms of complementary medicine is growing among professional and lay people. As a result, there is increasing interest in performing well-designed clinical trials to study the efficacy of complementary therapies. Useful suggestions and an overview of the different aspects to be faced in preparing research protocols can be found in this volume as well as in other recent publications (Kron et al 1998, Levin et al 1997).

In medicine, claims of therapeutic efficacy will only be taken seriously when the clinical trial has been performed in a methodologically sound manner. For instance, the trial must:

- compare the effect of treatment with the effect of no treatment (or with other treatments)
- ensure that people who receive treatment are not specifically selected into either one of the groups that participate in the experimental trial (randomization)
- control for the placebo effect (depending on the research question)
- identify a clearly diagnosed illness (in order to study the effect in a homogeneous group of patients)
- use effect measures which are precise, valid, reliable and meaningful.

In general, clinical trials with randomization and blinding provide the strongest evidence for a relationship between intervention and effect. The most common version of a clinical trial that satisfies these rules is the double-blind placebo-controlled trial, where neither the patient nor the person prescribing the treatment knows who is receiving the actual treatment.

Clinical research on individualized homeopathy, acupuncture or naturopathy poses particular problems. Competence and experience are growing but are still in a developing state. Over the past decade a number of problems in the setting up of clinical studies have been discussed when conventional methodological criteria were applied to study complementary medicine therapies (such as crossover, randomization, double blind, etc.) (Heron 1986, Jingfeng 1987, Leibrich 1990, Lynoë 1989, Patel 1987, Walach 1998). However, in our opinion, one of the most prominent methodological problems has not yet received sufficient attention: namely the selection of patients.

In this chapter the problems associated with the selection of a homogeneous group of patients, which is to be included in a clinical trial, are discussed. Most often, the inclusion criteria for patients enrolled in clinical studies are based on their Western conventional diagnosis (e.g. arthritis, cancers, ulcers). Since complementary health-care systems have considerably different diagnostic systems, patients with the same conventional Western diagnosis can be subdivided into different diagnostic subgroups from the complementary medicine viewpoint. It is often on the basis of these subgroups that the specific complementary treatment plan is determined. This implies that patients with a similar conventional diagnosis will probably not benefit from the application of the same complementary treatment. Only when a group of patients is homogeneous from the viewpoints of conventional medicine and complementary medicine can a well-designed study on the efficacy of complementary medicine be performed.

SELECTION OF PATIENTS

In order to select patients for inclusion in a clinical trial, it is of crucial importance to give as complete a description of the disease or the patients' symptom pattern as possible. The group of patients should be as homogeneous as possible; that is to say, all patients included in a clinical trial should express a comparable set of symptoms. Homogeneity is important to reduce error variance and to increase internal validity of the study. Clear selection criteria are required to obtain a homogeneous group of patients. Only then can the same treatment be given to all patients in a group. When the selection criteria are incomplete, this will result in the formation of an inhomogeneous group of patients. Applying a standard treatment to an inhomogeneous group of patients holds the risk that some patients will be treated in a non-optimal way and therefore might not react to treatment. In that case no significant effect of treatment will be found.

In conventional medicine, the ICD-10 (International Classification of Diseases, 10th edition) or the DSM-IV criteria (Diagnostic and Statistical Manual of Mental Disorders, 4th edition) provide optimal assurance of obtaining homogeneous groups of patients. Following these criteria, specialists in different countries will obtain groups of patients showing the same characteristics. In essence, such standardized criteria are still lacking in complementary medicine.

The problem of inhomogeneous groups of patients is mainly encountered in those trials in which attention has only been paid to conventional diagnostic criteria and not (or not sufficient) to the diagnostic criteria used in the complementary therapy under study.

Homogeneity of groups: two different points of view

The problem of homogeneity is illustrated in Figure 9.1, where patients with COPD (chronic obstructive pulmonary disease) are taken as a rather uniform group. Out of this group a further classification of patients can be made such as those with asthma, bronchitis or emphysema. This further classification is based on specific sets of criteria used in conventional medicine. The general practitioner will consider these as homogeneous subgroups.

However, from the point of view of a homeopath or an acupuncturist, the group of patients with COPD or asthma is far from homogeneous. The complementary therapist is not only interested in the specific symptoms that are thought by conventional practitioners to be of crucial importance for the diagnosis of COPD or asthma. Other factors and additional diagnostic criteria are used, including symptoms at the physiological level (including alterations in the color of the skin, tongue or iris, the number of painful spots, alterations in the pulse characteristics) and symptoms that are psychosocial (emotional, cognitive, sometimes even the content

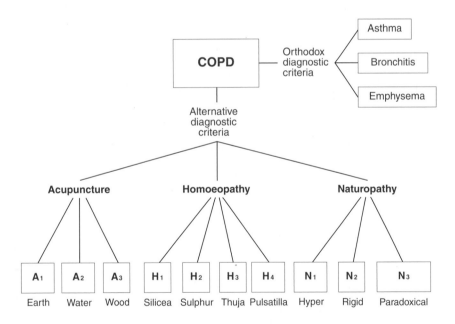

Figure 9.1 Homogeneity of patients from the conventional as well as the complementary medical point of view. Out of a group of patients with COPD, three more or less homogeneous subgroups can be formed, based on conventional criteria. However, from the viewpoint of the complementary therapist (acupuncture, homeopathy or naturopathy), these subgroups are far from homogeneous. Based on their specific diagnostic criteria, a different categorization of subgroups takes place. The other way around, a subgroup that is homogeneous on complementary medical grounds is not necessarily so on orthodox grounds (see text). An adequate selection of patients should therefore take place before they participate in a trial to study the efficacy of a complementary therapy.

of dreams) and energetic in nature. Based on an overall individual symptom pattern, a different categorization of homogeneous groups will take place.

For instance, the acupuncturist will pay attention to characteristics that can be detected by pulse and/or tongue diagnosis as well as the patient's overall appearance and specific reactions to changes in the internal and external environment. These characteristics indicate functional interactions between organ systems, flow of energy through the meridians, etc. In this way patients can be classified according to specific syndromes, as yin- or yang-deficient, in terms of the main perverse energetic influence that is present (e.g. heat, damp or wind).

In homeopathy, the principle of similars is used as a therapeutic guideline, meaning that certain compounds that induce specific symptoms in healthy volunteers ('remedy picture') are used as a remedy in patients expressing these same symptoms. Thus, in individualized homeopathy, the choice of a remedy is based on the match of the particular set of symptoms observed in the patient with the set of symptoms that is defined as the 'remedy picture'. Therefore, in addition to conventional diagnostic symptoms, symptoms and behaviors are analysed at different levels of the patient. The higher the resemblance between the symptom pattern of a patient and the symptoms characteristic for a specific remedy, the more certain the homeopath will be in prescribing this specific remedy. In homeopathy, a distinction can be made between several (constitutional) types that are more or less homogeneous (e.g. Phosphor, Sulphur, Silica types).

In naturopathy, important aspects in diagnosis involve the examination of body fluids, the level of toxicity in tissues and the condition of the detoxifying organs (liver, intestines, kidneys and skin). Furthermore, the 'detoxifying' condition on the mental level (e.g. emotional expressions and type of main psychological defence mechanism used) can be of importance to classify patients in categories. In addition, the condition of the 'basic bioregulatory system' (soft connective tissue including autonomic nervous system and immune system) is of importance in naturopathy. This system is thought to play a crucial role in the normal functioning and regulation of the organism (Pischinger 1975). Therefore the therapist will use diagnostic methods aimed at identification of the activity of these regulatory processes. In addition, naturopaths may stress the importance of the type of reaction a patient shows to stimuli and discriminate on this basis between normal reaction pattern, hyperreactive pattern, rigid reaction pattern or paradoxical reaction. A treatment protocol will be chosen based on the type of reaction pattern as well as on the degree of toxicity observed in the various organ systems of the patient.

Although in different fields of complementary medicine different categories can be identified, these categories have not yet reached a worldwide status of acceptance as, for instance, the ICD-10 or DSM-IV criteria in conventional medicine. For instance, not all homeopaths agree on the same limited set of important symptoms required to identify patients that would benefit from specific remedies. Different schools in homeopathy favor different (origin of) symptoms (physical, psychological/emotional, behavioral, dreams, etc.) as being of importance as criteria for remedy selection. Lack of consensus makes worldwide comparison of complementary medicine trials problematic.

CATEGORIES OF RESEARCH TRIALS IN COMPLEMENTARY MEDICINE

With respect to the formation of groups of patients, research trials can be categorized based on two characteristics. First, whether the patients are selected by conventional and/or complementary criteria and second, whether or not the procedure of selection is well described and controllable.

With respect to the first characteristic, three groups can be discerned depending on whether the above-mentioned selection criteria are used to obtain a homogeneous group of patients (from the point of view of conventional medicine and/or from the point of view of complementary medicine).

- *Category 1*. In the first category, only conventional medical selection criteria are used. No diagnosis is taken by a complementary therapist, which implies a standard complementary treatment for all participating patients. An individualized treatment based on guidelines used within the specific therapeutic system under study (e.g. homeopathy or traditional acupuncture) has not taken place.
- *Category 2*. In the second category, the selection of patients is based on conventional diagnostic criteria, followed by a second selection step which is dictated by the diagnostic criteria of the complementary therapy under study. Thus, a group of patients is included in the trial which can be called homogeneous from both points of view, conventional as well as complementary. In this category, attention is paid to the theory as well as to the specific way of working of the complementary therapy under study, leading to the application of an optimal individual treatment.
- *Category 3*. In the third category, selection of patients is based on the selection criteria from complementary medicine only.

The above-mentioned categorization of research trials is based on whether patients are selected from the perspective of conventional or complementary diagnostic criteria. In addition, a second aspect of the selection procedure should be considered: controllability. The question is whether other practitioners are able to control the decisions of the complementary therapist that have led to the selection of a specific remedy or therapeutic procedure for an individual patient. In conventional medicine the rationale for the application of the remedy or therapy is usually that the selected patient with a specific diagnosis shows all symptoms described in the ICD-10 or DSM-IV handbooks. Since such criteria are lacking in complementary medicine, controllability is more difficult. Therefore, the question is whether the conviction of the complementary therapist that the right remedy or treatment protocol has been applied to the individual patient has been quantified. Or whether any consensus has been reached between various colleagues that the right remedy has been prescribed to individual patients. Although different gradations exist in meeting this aspect of controllability, for reasons of clarity two approaches are discerned.

- The 'black box' approach in which no further justification is given by the complementary therapist for the choice of a certain remedy or treatment protocol. In many ways this approach is a great disadvantage since other therapists are unable to control the details or rationale of treatment.

- The 'open box' approach in which the complementary therapist gives (extensive) indication or justification of the remedy or treatment protocol applied to the selected group of patients. Ideally this approach may lead to ICD-like criteria for complementary medicine.

In the following, some examples are given of the above-mentioned three categories as well as of the 'black box' and 'open box' approaches.

Patient selection based on diagnostic criteria from conventional medicine only

Examples of trials belonging to this category are the studies of Reilly et al (1986) and Fung et al (1986). Reilly et al (1986) studied the effect of a homeopathic high-potency preparation in patients with hayfever. There were 144 patients in the trial; 74 were given a homeopathic preparation of mixed grass pollen in a C30 potency (i.e. a potentized dilution of 10^{-60}) and 70 were given a placebo. Both groups were well matched and rigorous controls were used throughout the study. After 5 weeks a statistically significant improvement ($P=0.02$) was observed in the group of patients treated with a homeopathic potency in comparison with the placebo group. This paper is considered as a landmark in homeopathic research, since it took into account all required methodological criteria. It obtained the highest score with respect to methodology in the metaanalysis of Kleijnen et al (1991). Moreover, it showed a positive effect of a homeopathically prepared remedy over placebo. Despite this result, homeopaths might have doubts, arguing that the protocol did not allow for the necessary freedom and individuality of homeopathic prescription. Only hayfever symptomatology was taken into account and not the overall symptom pattern of the individual patients. In their view, prescription of the same homeopathic remedy for all patients with hayfever is unlikely. A diagnosis from the point of view of classical homeopathy would lead to the prescription of different remedies. Therefore a group of patients with hayfever might be sufficiently homogeneous from the viewpoint of conventional medicine but from the viewpoint of classical homeopathy, this may not be the case.

The same rationale can also be used in the field of (traditional) acupuncture. The aim of Fung et al (1986) was to study whether real acupuncture provides a better protection against exercise-induced asthma than sham acupuncture. Twenty minutes before exercise, patients were treated on three asthma-related standard acupuncture points whereas the control group was treated on three unrelated acupuncture points in the neighboring dermatome. They found that real acupuncture does provide a better protection against exercise-induced asthma than sham acupuncture. Despite this result, the classically orientated acupuncturist might object that no account has been taken of the symptom pattern or specific syndrome of the individual patients. According to their view this selected group will not be homogeneous and therefore it is unlikely that the same acupuncture points should be stimulated in all patients. Furthermore, by restricting needling sites to specific loci, limiting the number of treatment sessions and not using traditional diagnostic practices, these kinds of clinical trials are reduced to testing the insertion of needles at particular points. In this way, acupuncture in not investigated as an individualized treatment modality but as a 'needling technique' (Aldridge & Pietroni 1987).

With respect to the controllability of the selection procedure, most clinical trials in which the selection of patients is based on conventional diagnostic criteria use ICD criteria. Therefore the 'black box' approach to obtaining a group of patients is usually not encountered, simply because a conventional medicine study in which clear selection criteria are not provided is usually rejected by the ethics committee. Alternatively, it will be rejected by referees of a peer-reviewed journal to which the results of the clinical trial are submitted.

In complementary studies such rigorous ICD-like criteria to define disease entities or symptom patterns do not yet exist. That is to say, the professional standards of conventional medicine have not yet been reached. Nevertheless, in many complementary medicine studies the complementary medical therapist has provided criteria to select the optimal treatment protocol for the individual patient, as will be described in the next section.

Patient selection based on diagnostic criteria from conventional and complementary medicine

In this category of clinical trials, the therapist is given the opportunity to apply an optimal treatment to each individual patient. Selection of patients takes place in two steps, the first step being based on criteria from conventional medicine, the second on the criteria of the complementary therapy under study. There are a number of ways in which this individualization has been achieved in clinical studies. In the case of homeopathy this could mean that:

- only those patients are included who meet the criteria of one specific remedy. In this respect, Fisher et al (1989) only included rheumatoid arthritis that fitted the remedy picture of Rhus tox
- only those patients are included who fit the remedy picture of one of a number of preselected remedies. An example is the study of Kainz et al (1996) who included patients with warts on the hands and selected the best fitting remedy picture out of a predefined set of 10 constitutional remedies. Also Lökken et al (1995), studying the pain after oral surgery, selected the best fitting remedy picture from six predefined remedies in D30
- all patients are included and for each patient their individual similimum is selected without any predefined restriction. For instance, De Lange-de Klerk et al (1994) prescribed constitutional and acute individual remedies as necessary in children with recurrent upper respiratory tract infections.

A subdivision of this category of clinical trials, in which two consecutive selection or characterization steps have been performed, will be illustrated by describing studies in which either the black box approach or the open box approach has been followed.

Black box approach using poorly defined selection criteria

In these clinical trials, the precise way in which a diagnosis is taken or the rationale for a specific alternative therapy is not registered nor justified. The whole treatment remains within a so-called 'black box'. The only relevant information in this type of study concerns the change in condition of patients before and after treatment. Examples of clinical trials that belong to this category are the studies of Brigo (1987) and Jobst et al (1986).

Brigo (1987) demonstrated the superiority of individualized homeopathy over placebo in migraine. A group of 60 patients was randomized to a placebo and a verum group. The homepath was allowed to prescribe one or two remedies out of a preselected set of eight homeopathic remedies in C30 potency. In comparison with the placebo group, the verum group showed a dramatic and extremely significant reduction in frequency (number/month) and duration as well as in severity of migraine attacks. Interestingly, this is one of the few studies that has been repeated by three different groups (Straumsheim et al 1997, Walach et al 1997, Whitmarsh et al 1997). None of these groups could reproduce the observations of Brigo (1987). They reported that there was no evidence for a significant effect of individualized homeopathy over placebo in migraine.

The aim of Jobst et al (1986) was to study whether traditional acupuncture influences the perception of breathlessness in patients with COPD (chronic obstructive pulmonary disease). A treatment with either real acupuncture on individually selected acupuncture points or placebo acupuncture on non-acupuncture points was given for 3 weeks. After that period, a significant improvement in the acupuncture group was found with respect to the subjective perception of breathlessness.

The advantage of these studies is that instead of a standard treatment protocol, an optimal treatment is given according to the rules of the complementary therapy under study. In these studies, the efficacy of a therapy is evaluated as a system of medical practice. However, the disadvantage of clinical trials in this category is the lack of controllability. The diagnosis and the way in which a therapy is applied from the point of view of the complementary therapist remain unknown (i.e. hidden in the black box).

Three arguments can be formulated against the use of the black box approach.

- Particularly in those trials where no effect is measured, other therapists might claim that this negative trial outcome is caused by a faulty complementary diagnosis leading to a failure to detect the characteristic symptom pattern and therefore an incorrect choice of remedies or acupuncture points to be treated. In these circumstances the quality of the therapist is at issue.
- Fisher (1990) points out the possibility that in these so-called 'one disease/any remedy' types of studies, some remedies are effective whereas others may not be. One is, of course, unable to track down which remedy has been (in)effective when a black box approach is used.
- Finally, Canter (1987) emphasized that the task of research is not only to study the efficacy of a certain intervention but also to understand the strengths and weakness of the various approaches in complementary medicine to the promotion of human well-being. To develop that understanding, research should be aimed at examining the logic upon which the different complementary practices operate and study more closely the conditions under which successes and failures occur. Therefore registration of those actions which take place during the process of diagnosis and therapy is essential for the further development of research in this field.

In a number of clinical trials an attempt has been made to 'overcome' the shortcomings mentioned above. In the remainder of this section we will focus on homeopathic trials. However, the general idea is also applicable to other fields in complementary medicine.

Open box approach using well-defined complementary medicine selection criteria

Having selected the patients who meet the conventional diagnosis, a further characterization occurs in order to individualize the complementary therapy. In contrast to the black box approach, this characterization is well defined and controllable or at least an attempt has been made to do so.

In the case of homeopathy, this means that some indication must be given that the correct similimum has been selected for the individual patient. The question is how we can be sure that the correct remedy is prescribed, i.e. the remedy showing the largest overlap between the symptoms of the patient and the characteristic symptoms of the so-called 'remedy picture'. A number of options exist.

- The selected patients are distinguished by having good or bad prescribing symptoms (Fisher 1986; Gibson et al 1980).
- The therapist expresses his degree of confidence in having prescribed the most optimal remedy for the individual patient (Jacobs et al 1997).
- The therapist is allowed to use a number of sessions, if required, to reach the most optimal remedy. In this respect, Kuzeff (1998) used up to four sessions.
- A team of homeopaths must agree on the remedy (Walach et al 1997).

All these strategies increase the controllability or confidence that the optimal treatment protocol or the correct remedy has been prescribed to the individual patient. Since this will be an important aspect in the next decade to increase the quality of clinical trials in complementary medicine, it is relevant to focus on some of the above-mentioned strategies.

Good or bad prescribing symptoms An interesting example is the fibrositis study reported by Fisher (1986). In a randomized double-blind trial, 24 fibrositis patients were selected who showed the characteristic symptomatology of one out of three homeopathic remedies (Arnica, Bryonia or Rhus tox). Moreover, an indication was given for the number of good prescribing symptoms. A three-point scale was used: no symptoms characteristic of the remedy prescribed (0), one or two characteristic symptoms (1), three or more characteristic symptoms (2). In other words, an attempt was made to establish a 'goodness of fit' between the symptom pattern of a patient and the characteristic symptoms of a remedy picture. This represents the certainty by which the homeopath prescribes the correct remedy as well as a first quantification to indicate the correctness of the similimum.

The three subgroups of fibrositis patients received either a placebo or the indicated remedy. Several variables were measured, such as sleeping problems and pain score on visual analogue scales, number of painful spots and use of analgesics. Statistical analysis was performed in two ways.

- Comparison of control group with all patients treated homeopathically (irrespective of which remedy was given). In this analysis no significant difference was found with respect to sleeping and pain scores.

- A second analysis was done including only those patients with good prescribing symptoms. Interestingly, in this second analysis, a significant improvement was found for the homeopathically treated group versus placebo. Fisher (1986) concluded that improvement is correlated with strong prescribing symptoms, irrespective of which remedy was prescribed.

This last result stresses the crucial importance of the proper selection of a homeopathic remedy, since it seems that the effect of a remedy can only be detected optimally when its prescription is based on a strong resemblance between remedy picture and the specific symptom pattern of the patient. In essence, this result supports the validity of the principle of similars.

Gibson et al (1980) reached a similar conclusion in their study of patients with rheumatoid arthritis. Forty-six patients (receiving a conventional first-line anti-inflammatory treatment) were divided in two matched groups. One group received a placebo, whereas the patients in the other group received a homeopathic remedy that was prescribed according to the individual symptom patterns. With respect to the result, a significant improvement was found in subjective pain, articular index stiffness and grip strength in those patients receiving an individually selected homeopathic remedy. In addition, the authors also characterized their patients as having strong or poor prescribing symptoms.

The strong prescribing group included patients with three or more homeopathic characteristic features. Any patient who showed less than three of these homeopathic characteristics, or who was uncertain in his reactions, was classified as having poor prescribing symptoms. The patients were then assigned to two groups (a therapy group and a placebo group), so that as far as possible there were equal numbers of strong and poor prescribing patients in each group. The results show that patients in the homeopathic group with good prescribing symptoms showed a larger improvement (although not significant in this study) than the group with poor prescribing symptoms. For example, the mean improvement in limbering up time was 52 minutes for strong prescribers and nearly 30 minutes for poor prescribers, whereas in the placebo group limbering up improvement was only 7.9 minutes.

Degree of confidence In this respect, the studies of Jacobs et al (1994, 1997) are of interest. Children who suffered from diarrhoea were rehydrated and also received individualized homeopathy or placebo. In a placebo-controlled trial the superiority of individualized homeopathy over placebo was shown in children in Nicaragua (Jacobs et al 1994). These researchers repeated their experiment in Nepal in which they observed a positive trend just missing significance (Jacobs et al 1997). Interestingly, when they restricted their analysis to cases where homeopaths were confident about the chosen similimum a significant difference was observed in favor of the homeopathic treated group. As was previously observed in the analysis of Fisher (1986), this stresses the importance of incorporating a confidence score or a 'patient–remedy score' as defined recently by Kramers (1998). This score indicates a quantitative expression of the correctness of the similimum.

Patient selection based on diagnostic criteria from complementary medicine only

The third category represents clinical trials using homogeneous groups of patients that were selected on complementary criteria only. In the field of homeopathy, the study of Kuzeff (1998) is an example of including any conventional diagnosis of consecutive patients presenting in his practice. All patients who gave consent were included in a placebo-controlled trial studying the effect of individualized homeopathy. Kuzeff (1998) only included patients when an appropriate similimum was identified. When after four sessions a remedy still could not be selected with complete confidence, the patients were not included in the trial. The study looked at whether homeopathy causes a greater improvement in feelings of well-being than placebo and whether it changes immune function. Kuzeff concluded that homeopathy significantly improved feelings of well-being.

Is this a black box or an open box approach? Due to the fact that up to four sessions were possible until the correct remedy was found, a strong attempt has been made to be confident about the correct similimum. If after four sessions this confidence was not reached, the patients were not included. Therefore we classify this study as an open box approach.

A further example of this category would be a group of patients suffering from any type of disease but who resemble the remedy picture of a specific compound, e.g. Bryonia. In this trial across conventional diagnoses, the typical Bryonia symptoms could be followed in a placebo-controlled randomized trial in the same way as a trial that evaluates the change in symptoms of, for instance, rheumatoid arthritis when treated with antiinflammatory drugs. The selection optimally would require ICD-like criteria for Bryonia patients.

Although these types of studies are not of relevance for convincing representatives of conventional medicine, they are important for the complementary therapy under study as well as for the evolution of knowledge within this specific field of complementary medicine.

DISCUSSION

In this chapter, we focused on the selection of patients who are included in a clinical trial. Three categories were distinguished based on whether conventional and/or complementary criteria were used in the selection process. In summary:

Category	Selection criteria	
	Conventional	Alternative
1	Yes	No
2	Yes	Yes
3	No	Yes

With respect to the ongoing discussion between complementary medicine and conventional medicine on the efficacy of complementary therapeutic approaches, it is important to perform clinical trials of the second category. The proposed selection process is shown in Figure 9.2. Only after such a two-step selection procedure can a homogeneous group of patients be obtained on whom the effects of a standardized therapy can be evaluated. In such an evaluation maximum attention can be paid to the characteristic philosophy and the way of working, as well as to the diagnostic equipment used by the complementary practitioner.

One of the disadvantages is that a two-step selection of the research population results in small group sizes. In these circumstances one has to find alternatives for the traditional group design. One of the possibilities which remains to be explored is the single case design. Single case studies might be a useful research tool for investigating a very specific research question framed in relation to an individual patient (Aldridge 1988, Kazdin 1982). There is still little experience with these trials

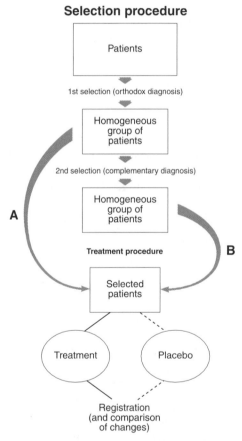

Figure 9.2 Procedure to select patients for inclusion in clinical trials. In the first selection step, a 'homogeneous' group of patients is formed using conventional diagnostic criteria. This group meets the criteria for a uniform conventional medical treatment to be studied in a clinical trial (arrow A). However, to participate in a trial in which the effect of a complementary therapy is studied, a second selection step should be performed. This twice-selected group now meets the criteria for a uniform complementary treatment (arrow B).

in the field of complementary medicine, although a number of examples have been published (e.g. Vincent 1990). Ernst (1998) recently suggested that single case studies should be used to decide whether a given treatment (which ideally has previously been tested for efficacy) is helpful for a given patient.

As a further important characteristic of the selection procedure, the degree of controllability was mentioned in the form of a black box (no control possible) and an open box (some form of control possible). In other words, are the readers able to assess whether or not the most optimal complementary treatment or remedy has been applied to the individual patient? In conventional medicine patients are usually selected according to well-defined criteria and protocols (such as the ICD-10 or DSM-IV criteria). Although a trial with rheumatoid arthritic patients can be conducted anywhere in the world, all rheumatologists will know which characteristic symptoms have been used to include patients in a clinical study. In general this consensus in the characterization of patients is absent in complementary medicine. For instance, in homeopathy many different schools exist, stressing the importance of different symptoms in the selection of remedies. In other words, not all homeopaths agree on the importance of symptoms that lead to the prescription of a certain remedy. Therefore, development of ICD-like criteria of the different patient typologies used in complementary medicine is of importance. Computer programs may help in the process of identification of a symptom pattern and remedy selection (Van Haselen & Fisher 1990). In addition, the patient–remedy score may be helpful in developing standardized selection criteria.

A number of examples were discussed and it was concluded that, in particular, the development of controllable selection criteria needs further research.

In line with the experience of Gibson et al (1980), Fisher (1986) and Jacobs et al (1997), it might be interesting to further develop the patient–remedy score (PRS), a special control instrument in homeopathic research that aims to quantify the confidence of the therapist in their prescription. Using this instrument, the validity of the principle of similars, the basis of homeopathy, could be verified. So in a clinical trial on homeopathy it might be useful to ask the prescriber for a kind of 'prescription confidence score' per patient. In principle, such a trial might even include patients across conventional diagnoses. The heterogeneous population of patients is treated individually and evaluated by correlating the PRS with the measure outcome variables. A positive correlation between a strong prescription confidence and positive outcome results (or the other way around: poor prescription confidence and negative outcome) would favor the principle of similars and hence the homeopathic treatment. It would be worthwhile to develop a generally accepted procedure for scoring the prescription confidence in homeopathy. In addition to the scales used by Gibson et al (1980) and Fisher (1986), Kramers (1998) introduced a four-point PRS with a quality/quantity balance:

1. similarity rather uncertain: quantity and quality of symptoms unsatisfactory
2. similarity debatable: quantity sufficient, quality limited; in this situation the homeopath generally identifies a number of possible remedies
3. similarity quite certain: quality sufficient, quantity limited ('a chair with three legs')
4. similarity certain: quality and quantity of symptoms satisfactory.

The need for the development of an alternative methodology for clinical trials in complementary medicine has been suggested several times. However, in our opinion the conventional methodological criteria are a useful starting point that can subsequently be adapted depending on the specific philosophy of the complementary therapy under study. Currently guidelines and recommendations on the conduct of clinical trials in the field of complementary medicine are available, including studies that incorporate the issue of, for instance, individualization in homeopathy (Kramers 1998, Kron et al 1998, Linde & Melchart 1998). In addition, guidelines for good-quality reporting of key methodological issues in scientific journals were published in a CONSORT statement (Begg et al 1996).

Based on the arguments proposed in this chapter we suggest that the issue of patient selection needs more attention and careful consideration.

REFERENCES

Aldridge D 1988 Single-case research designs. Complementary Medicine Research 3: 37–46
Aldridge D, Pietroni PC 1987 Clinical assessment of acupuncture in asthma therapy: discussion paper. Journal of the Royal Society of Medicine 80: 222–224
Begg C, Cho M, Eastwood S et al 1996 Improving the quality of reporting of randomized trials: the CONSORT statement. Journal of the American Medical Association 27: 637–639
Brigo B 1987 Le traitement homéopathique de la migraine: une etude de 60 cas, controlée en double aveugle (remède homéopathique vs. placebo) [Homeopathic treatment of migraine: a sixty case, double blind, controlled study (homeopathic remedy vs. placebo)]. Proceedings of the Congress of the Liga Medicorum Homoeopathica Internationalis 42: 318–329
Canter D 1987 A research agenda for holistic medicine. Complementary Medicine Research 2: 104–121
De Lange-de Klerk ESM, Blommers J, Kuik DJ, Bezemer PD, Feenstra L 1994 Effect of homoeopathic medicines on daily burden of symptoms in children with recurrent upper respiratory tract infections. British Medical Journal 309: 1329–1332
Ernst E 1998 Single-case studies in complementary/alternative medicine research. Complementary Therapies in Medicine 6: 75–78
Fisher P 1986 An experimental double-blind clinical trial method in homeopathy; use of a limited range of remedies to treat fibrositis. British Homoeopathic Journal 75: 142–147
Fisher P 1990 Research into homeopathic treatments of rheumatologic disease; why and how? Complementary Medicine Research 4(3): 34–40
Fisher P, Greenwood A, Huskisson EC, Turner P, Belon P 1989 Effect of homeopathic treatment on fibrositis (primary fibromyalgia). British Medical Journal 299: 365–366
Fung KP, Chow OKW, So SY 1986 Attenuation of exercise-induced asthma by acupuncture. Lancet 228: 1419–1421
Gibson RG, Gibson SLM, MacNeill AD, Buchanan WW 1980 Homeopathic therapy in rheumatoid arthritis; evaluation by double-blind clinical therapeutic trial. British Journal of Clinical Pharmacology 9: 453–459
Heron J 1986 Critique of conventional research methodology. Complementary Medicine Research 1: 12–22
Jacobs J, Jiménez LM, Gloyd SS, Gale JL, Crothers D 1994 Treatment of acute childhood diarrhea with homeopathic medicine: a randomized clinical trial in Nicaragua. Pediatrics 93: 719–725
Jacobs J, Malthouse S, Chapman E, Jiménez LM, Crothers D 1997 Childhood diarrhea; results from Nepal and combined analysis. Proceedings of the Congress of the Liga Medicorum Homoeopathica Internationalis 52: 81–83
Jingfeng C 1987 Toward a comprehensive evaluation of alternative medicine. Social Science and Medicine 25: 659–667
Jobst K, McPherson K, Brown V et al 1986 Controlled trial of acupuncture for disabling breathlessness. Lancet 228: 1416–1419

Kainz JT, Kozel G, Haidvogl M, Smolle J 1996 Homoeopathic versus placebo therapy of children with warts on the hands: a randomized, double-blind clinical trial. Dermatology 193: 318–320

Kazdin A 1982 Single case research designs: methods for clinical and applied settings. Oxford University Press, New York

Kleijnen J, Knipschild P, ter Riet G 1991 Clinical trials of homoeopathy. British Medicine Journal 302: 316–323

Kramers CW 1998 Klinische toetsing van de homeopathie; een leidraad voor onderzoekers [Clinical verification of homeopathy; a guideline for researchers]. Nearchus, Hemrik

Kron M, English JR, Gaus W 1998 Guidelines on methodology of clinical research in homeopathy. In: Ernst E, Hahn EG (eds) Homeopathy; a critical appraisal. Butterworth-Heinemann, Oxford, pp. 9–47

Kuzeff RM 1998 Homeopathy, sensation of well-being and CD4 levels: a placebo-controlled, randomized trial. Complementary Therapies in Medicine 6: 4–9

Leibrich J 1990 Measurement of efficacy: a case for holistic research. Complementary Medicine Research 4(1): 21–25

Levin JS, Glass TA, Kushi LH, Schuck JR, Steele L, Jonas WB 1997 Quantitative methods in research on complementary and alternative medicine; a methodological manifesto. Medical Care 35: 1079–1094

Linde K, Melchart D 1998 Randomized controlled trials of individualized homeopathy: a state-of-the-art review. Journal of Alternative and Complementary Medicine 4: 371–388

Lökken P, Straumsheim PA, Tveiten D, Skjelbred P, Borchgrevink CF 1995 Effect of homoeopathy on pain and other events after acute trauma: placebo controlled trial with bilateral oral surgery. British Medicine Journal 310: 1439–1442

Lynöe N 1989 Theoretical and empirical problems in the assessment of alternative medical technologies. Scandinavian Journal of Social Medicine 17: 257–263

Patel MS 1987 Problems in the evaluation of alternative medicine. Social Science and Medicine 25: 669–678

Pischinger A 1975 Das System der Grundregulation [The basic bioregulatory system]. Haug Verlag, Heidelberg

Reilly DT, McSharry C, Taylor MA, Aitchison T 1986 Is homeopathy a placebo response? Controlled trial of homeopathic potency, with pollen in hayfever as model. Lancet ii: 881–886

Straumsheim PA, Borchgrevink C, Mowinckel P, Kierulf H, Hafslund O 1997 Homeopatisk behandling av migrene [Homeopathic treatment of migraine]. Dynamis 2: 18–22

Van Haselen R, Fisher P 1990 Analysing homeopathic prescribing using the Read classification and information technology. British Homoeopathic Journal 79: 74–81

Vincent CA 1990 The treatment of tension headache by acupuncture: a controlled single case design with time series analysis. Journal of Psychosomatic Research 34: 553–561

Walach H 1998 Methodology beyond controlled clinical trials. In: Ernst E, Hahn EG (eds) Homoeopathy: a critical appraisal. Butterworth-Heinemann, Oxford, pp. 48–59

Walach H, Haeusler W, Lowes T et al 1997 Classical homeopathic treatment of chronic headaches. Cephalalgia 17: 119–126

Whitmarsh TE, Coleston-Shields DM, Steiner TJ 1997 Double-blind randomized placebo-controlled study of homeopathic prophylaxis of migraine. Cephalalgia 17: 600–604

10

Investigating the safety of complementary medicine

Edzard Ernst

INTRODUCTION

This chapter will challenge the widespread and much promoted belief that complementary medicine (CAM) is entirely free of risks. It will, moreover, stress that therapeutic risks must not be seen in isolation but in relation to demonstrable benefits. Finally, it will attempt to constructively show a way forward towards identifying existing risks, which is a necessary step towards maximizing CAM's safety.

RISKS OF COMPLEMENTARY THERAPIES

This is not the place to review all possible risks of CAM in full detail (readers interested in a more complete discussion of this topic are referred elsewhere (Ernst 2000f)). The area is too complex, the data are too numerous and the treatments too many to tackle this task within the constraints of this chapter. Instead, the following pages will provide pertinent and recent examples of direct and indirect risks related to CAM. The choice of these examples is based on neither the prevalence nor the severity of risks; rather, it is a random selection influenced by the author's previous work in this field.

Indirect risks

Even if a (mainstream or complementary) treatment existed that was completely free from risks, it would still be associated with indirect risks relating by and large to the (lack of) competence of (some) providers of that therapy (Ernst 1995). In CAM this is a particularly delicate issue because most CAM professions are not adequately regulated (e.g. some acupuncturists in the UK may have a very high standard of acupuncture training but, as this is not a necessary requirement for practice, there may be others who do not). In this situation it is inevitable that regulated health-care professions continue to voice concern and it is likely that lack of competence (rather than the intrinsic risk of an intervention) leads to harm. The medical literature holds many examples and variations of this basic theme. They include:

- hindering access to effective conventional treatments
- disregarding contraindications
- failing to diagnose treatable conditions
- (over)using potentially harmful or unreliable diagnostic techniques
- interfering with prescribed treatments.

Perhaps the most obvious indirect risk of CAM danger lies in the fact that some patients (or their parents) elect to abandon conventional therapies for serious diseases in favor of CAM. This can have fatal consequences (Coppes et al 1998, Oneschuk & Bruera 1999). Preliminary survey data suggest that a sizeable proportion of CAM providers advise their clients to reduce their prescribed medication (Moody et al 1998). In other instances clinicians may disregard contraindications or important precautions. An example is provided by US midwives advising their patients to use herbal remedies during pregnancy (Allaise et al 2000). For the vast majority of medicinal herbs, no adequate data exist for use in pregnancy. Thus any advice to use herbal treatment during pregnancy involves an incalculable risk.

Risks can also be brought about by CAM providers (over)using diagnostic techniques which, in turn, are burdened with serious risks; examples are the way some chiropractors employ X-ray diagnostics (Ernst 1998) or the use of unreliable 'alternative' diagnostic methods which carry a high risk of false-positive or false-negative results (Ernst 2000c).

Some CAM providers (e.g. chiropractors and non-medically qualified homeopaths) tend to advise their patients against any form of immunization, which can clearly constitute an indirect risk (Ernst 1997). If such advice is widely adopted, the population at large is at risk of losing its herd immunity. This, in turn, would constitute a significant danger to public health.

The attitude of the consumer towards complementary medicine may constitute a risk which is independent of CAM providers. When users of herbal remedies were interviewed about their behavior regarding an adverse effect of a herbal versus a synthetic 'over-the-counter' drug, the results suggested that about one quarter would consult their doctor for a serious adverse effect of a conventional medication while less than 1% would do the same in relation to a herbal remedy (Barnes et al 1998). A further indirect risk (largely unrelated to CAM providers but nevertheless associated with CAM) might lie in the plethora of lay books on CAM now available in every high street bookstore. Preliminary evidence suggests that this lay literature has the potential to put the health of the reader at risk if the advice from these books is being adhered to by seriously ill individuals (Ernst & Armstrong 1998).

Direct risks

Like all medicine, CAM is inevitably associated with various degrees of direct risk. Due to the wide range of interventions involved, the risks are extremely diverse so a few select examples will have to suffice.

Acupuncture

In most areas of CAM, no prospective studies of risks are available which are a precondition for defining incidence figures. Acupuncture is the laudable exception to

Table 10.1   The most frequently reported complications of acupuncture

Condition	Frequency
Bleeding (usually minor)	About 3%
Cardiac trauma	Low*
Contact dermatitis	Low*
Drowsiness	About 1%
Endocarditis	Low*
Erythema	Low*
Hepatitis	About 150 cases reported*
Local pain	About 1%
Perichondritis	Low*
Peripheral nerve injury	Low*
Pneumothorax	About 60 cases reported
Renal injury	Low*
Retained needle	Low* (except with Japanese acupuncture)
Septicemia	Low*
Spinal cord injury	Low*
Syncope	Considerable*

*Exact incidence figures are not known

this rule. Our current knowledge in this area is summarized in Table 10.1. When all adverse effects experienced by patients in a Japanese acupuncture clinic seen between November 1992 and October 1997 were recorded (Yamashita et al 1998), a total of 64 adverse events were noted. Thus incidence of risk was very low. Failure to remove the needles, dizziness, discomfort or perspiration (probably due to hypotension) were the most frequent hazards identified. No serious adverse events were noted.

A recent prospective investigation of ~25 000 acupuncture treatments carried out in the UK (White & Ernst 2000) shows that the most common minor adverse effects are bleeding (3%), aggravation of symptoms (1%) and pain during needling (1%). With the exception of one epileptic fit, no serious adverse effects were reported.

However, serious adverse events of acupuncture are on record (Ernst & White 1997) and continue to be reported (Ernst & White 1999, 2000). Perhaps the most worrying incidents relate to infection with hepatitis B due to the inadequate hygiene standards of acupuncturists (Walsh et al 1999).

Aromatherapy

Aromatherapists apply plant-based essential oils, usually by gentle massage techniques, to the body surface of their patients. A 39-year-old woman had a 10-week history of pruritic, erythematous lesions on her face and chest (James & Weiss 1997). She had been using aromatherapy for the past 2–3 years. Patch testing was positive for neomycin, fragrance mix and benzoylperoxide. Discontinuation of aromatherapy led to a rapid resolution of the allergic reaction. Similar cases of allergic contact dermatitis have been associated with tea tree oil (Kranke 1997) and black cumin oil (Agothos et al 1997) and many other topically applied HMPs (Ernst 2000d).

Herbal medicinal products (HMPs)

Toxicity St John's wort (SJW) has been repeatedly shown to be an effective herbal antidepressant (Williams et al 2000). It also has a most encouraging safety profile (Ernst et al 1998a). The adverse effects reported in clinical trials are invariably mild and transient: gastrointestinal symptoms (8.5%), dizziness/confusion (4.5%), tiredness/sedation (4.5%) and dry mouth (4.0%). Synthetic drugs used in comparative trials are burdened with significantly higher rates of adverse effects. Nevertheless, SJW is not totally free from potentially serious adverse effects.

A 35-year-old woman took ground whole SJW (500 mg/day) for her mild depression (Bove 1998). After 4 weeks she developed stinging pain on her face and the dorsum of both hands, symptoms which worsened with sun exposure. A diagnosis of subacute toxic neuropathy was made. After discontinuation of SJW, the symptoms gradually disappeared. Photoactive hypericins may have caused demyelination of cutaneous nerve axons which, in turn, was responsible for the symptoms.

A 47-year-old woman who suffered from nocturnal panic attacks and major depression was put on paroxetine and sertraline (Scheck 1998). After several months she complained of irritability, insomnia and anorgasmia; she discontinued this treatment and self-medicated a 0.1% tincture of SJW. Ten days later she noted racing and distorted thoughts, increased irritability, hostility, aggressive behavior and a decreased need for sleep. After discontinuing the SJW, her symptoms resolved within 2 days. Several further cases of mania associated with SJW have been reported recently (Nierenberg et al 1999).

Herb–drug interactions Compelling evidence from in vitro, preclinical and clinical investigations shows that SJW can lower the plasma levels of several conventional medications (Ernst 1999). The effect relates to interactions with theophylline, cyclosporine, oral anticoagulants, estrogens and probably many other drugs. It therefore has considerable clinical relevance. Its mechanism is as yet not fully understood and probably involves at least two pathways: hepatic enzyme induction via the cytochrome P450 system and induction of the transporter P-glycoprotein (Drewe 2000).

Ginkgo biloba has antiplatelet activity and could therefore interact with anticoagulants. A 78-year-old woman had been on warfarin since a coronary bypass 5 years previously (Matthews 1998). She started taking ginkgo biloba for 2 months and subsequently developed clinical signs consistent with a stroke. She was then diagnosed to have suffered an intracerebral hemorrhage. It is conceivable that the stroke was the result of over-anticoagulation induced by an interaction between ginkgo biloba and warfarin.

Herb–drug interactions are not confined to the above two HMPs but potentially relate to a very large range of medicinal herbs (Ernst 2000e). Table 10.2 gives examples of interactions associated with commonly used HMPs. So far only relatively few case reports have been documented (Ernst 2000b, Fugh-Berman 2000). It is likely that this situation will change dramatically as health-care professionals realise the possibility of herb–drug interactions.

Contamination and adulteration Contamination and adulteration are notorious and potentially very important problems with HMPs, particularly those from Third World countries (Table 10.3).

Table 10.2 Examples of (suspected) herb–drug interactions associated with commonly used HMPs

Name	Indication	May interact with	Nature of suspicion
Devil's claw	Rheumatic pain	Warfarin	Case report
Dong quai	Chinese herb used for a variety of indications	Warfarin	Case report
Evening primrose	Eczema, premenstrual syndrome, etc.	Phenytoin	Case report
Feverfew	Migraine prophylaxis	Aspirin	Theoretical consideration
Garlic	Hypercholesterolemia	Warfarin	Case report
Ginger	Nausea	Anticoagulants	Theoretical consideration
Ginkgo biloba	Dementia, intermittent claudication	Warfarin, aspirin, thiazide diuretics	Case report
Hawthorn	Congestive heart failure	Nitrates, cardiac glycosides	Theoretical consideration
Kava	Anxiety	Anxiolytics	Case report
Liquorice	Used in many Chinese herbal mixtures	Antihypertensives	Case report
Panax ginseng	Various	Phenelzine	Case report
Red clover	Menopause	Anticoagulants, digoxin, oral contraceptives	Theoretical consideration
St John's wort	Depression	Numerous drugs (see text)	Case reports
Valerian	Insomnia	CNS depressants	Theoretical consideration

Table 10.3 Contaminants that have been found in herbal medicines

Type of contaminant	Examples
Other pharmacologically active HMPs	Atropa belladonna, Digitalis, Colchicum, Rauwolfia serpentina, pyrrolizidine-containing plants
Microorganisms	Staphylococcus aureus, Escherichia coli (certain strains), Salmonella, Shigella, Pseudomonas aeruginosa
Microbial toxins	Bacterial endotoxins, aflatoxins
Pesticides, herbicides	Chlorinated pesticides (e.g. DDT, DDE, HCH-isomers, HCB, aldrin, dieldrin, heptachlor), organic phosphates, carbamate insecticides and herbicides, dithiocarbamate fungicides, triazin herbicides
Fumigation agents	Ethylene oxide, methyl bromide, phosphine
Radioactivity	Cs-134, Cs-137, Ru-103, I-131, Sr-90
Heavy metals	Lead, cadmium, mercury, arsenic

Some herbal remedies have been shown to contain undeclared amounts of *Digitalis lanata* (Slifman et al 1998). Patients taking such herbs have suffered from a serious overdose of cardiac glycosides with toxic serum digoxin levels as a result.

At least 100 cases of interstitial fibrosis of the kidneys were observed in Belgium in patients who had taken a Chinese HMP for weight loss. In this preparation *Stephania tetrandra* was inadvertently replaced by *Aristolochia fangchi* (Vanherweghem 1998, Van Ypersele de Strichou 1998). Several further such cases have been reported from other countries (Stengel & Jones 1998). Recently a histological investigation of the tissue samples from kidneys of these patients has shown an exorbitantly high rate of neoplasms (Nortier et al 2000). It is thus likely that Aristolochia species cause cancer.

A 49-year-old woman developed clinical signs of hepatitis and all usual causes of hepatitis were ruled out (Levi et al 1998). She had recently started to use a Chinese herbal tea to treat her eczema. Examination of the HMP showed that it contained *Aristolochia debilis* root and seven other medicinal plants. Like *Aristolochia fangchi*, *Aristolochia debilis* contains the highly toxic aristolochic acid and is therefore the likely cause of the toxic hepatitis.

When 73 samples of HMPs were examined in Croatia, fungal contamination was found to be abundant (Halt 1998). *Aspergillus flavus*, a known producer of aflatoxins, was present in 12 samples. Mycotoxins were found in seven of the samples analysed.

An outbreak of skin lesions affecting 20 patients from an Iranian village was reported (Sadjadi 1998). Then clinical signs led to the suspicion of anthrax infection. Patients had applied Kombucha mushroom topically and the skin lesions had developed 5–7 days later. Cultures from the skin lesions confirmed the presence of *Bacillus anthracis*.

In Taipei, 319 children aged 1–7 years were screened for increased blood lead concentrations (Cheng et al 1998). The consumption of Chinese HMPs was significantly correlated with blood lead levels ($P=0.038$). When 2803 subjects from Taipei were tested for blood lead levels, a history of using HMPs proved to be a major risk factor for increased concentrations of lead in the blood (Chu et al 1998).

When 260 Asian patent medicines on sale in California were analyzed, 7% contained undeclared pharmaceuticals. Of 251 samples, 24 products were demonstrated to contain at least 10 parts per million of lead, 36 contained arsenic and 35 contained mercury (Ko 1998).

Three cases of chronic arsenic poisoning with characteristic skin changes were reported from Singapore (Wong et al 1998). All patients had taken Chinese HMPs to treat their asthma. Two cases were diagnosed as suffering from cancers likely to be caused by this arsenic exposure.

Homeopathy

Homeopathic remedies are generally considered safe as their usually high dilution renders adverse effects unlikely. Yet low dilutions can cause allergic reactions. Several rare cases of adverse effects after homeopathy have been documented in the literature (Jonas & Ernst 1999). Moreover, homeopathic aggravations which are thought to occur in about 20% of patients could be viewed as a relevant safety issue from an orthodox point of view.

Hypnotherapy

An authoritative review of the potential risks of hypnosis reminds us that hypnotherapy is by no means free of adverse reactions (Baber 1998). Complications include amnesia, catharsis, paralysis, disorientation, literalness of response, accelerated transference and memory contamination. A further unwanted effect of hypnotherapy is the inability to dehypnotize the patient. A review of the literature lists several such cases and contributes two new incidents (Gravitz 1998).

Massage

A 51-year-old woman with a left ureteral stent to relieve the symptoms of a ureteral stricture consulted a therapist, who treated her with a deep body massage. The massage included the patient's abdomen, pelvis and lower back. Towards the end of the session she felt left flank pain and was incontinent. X-ray examination showed displacement of the stent. Surgical restoration of the stent quickly resolved her symptoms (Kerr 1997).

A 39-year-old woman with no relevant medical history underwent a deep body massage which included massage of the abdomen. Within 24 hours she experienced pain and nausea. She was admitted to hospital where anemia and a hematoma in the right hepatic lobe were diagnosed. A thorough investigation left the physical force of the massage as the most likely cause of the intrahepatic bleeding (Trotter 1999).

Qigong

The inappropriate application of qigong or the inability to terminate the exercise has been reported to cause minor, mostly short-lived symptoms (Lee 2000). In rare cases, this is associated with more severe abnormalities like violent behaviors. Qigong-induced mental disorder is a recognized complication of qigong in China where about 5% of the population practice this form of exercise.

Spinal manipulation

Several surveys have addressed the safety of spinal manipulation (SM). For instance, a questionnaire was sent to all 13 consultant neurologists in the Republic of Ireland (Lynch 1998). The 11 who responded reported a total of 16 patients with neurological complications after chiropractic SM within a period of 5 years. Cerebrovascular accidents were the most frequent problem. In 13 of the 16 cases, this had led to a persistent neurologic deficit. None of these cases would have emerged in the medical literature but for this survey. This exemplifies the suspicion of gross underreporting of adverse events after CAM.

In a survey of UK physiotherapists trained in SM, 19% reported that they had encountered complications of SM (Adams & Sim 1998). These related mostly to the upper spine and were mostly not serious. Our own survey of 686 general practitioners from the UK disclosed 28 serious adverse effects related to SM (Abbot et al 1998).

Case reports of serious adverse effects after SM continue to be published. Recent incidents are summarized in Table 10.4. In addition to these (probably rare) serious adverse effects (Di Fabio 1999), SM is associated with frequent (incidence ~50%) adverse effects of a more transient and mild nature (Senstad et al 1997).

THE RISK–BENEFIT CONCEPT

The above list of examples of direct and indirect risks is perhaps impressive (some CAM proponents would probably say alarmist) but also meaningless if not seen in the correct context. First, most of the above-quoted evidence is based on case reports. Such evidence is by definition limited due to the difficulties encountered in establishing a cause–effect relationship. Second, only very rarely (e.g. in the case of SJW or acupuncture) are we able to name sufficiently accurate incidence figures associated with direct risks (for indirect risks, such figures are anybody's guess). Clearly one complication after, for instance, massage therapy does not render massage a hazardous intervention (yet such a case indicates that there *may* be a problem and should compel us to investigate further, particularly when more such cases can be found in the literature). Third, and perhaps most importantly, the potential risks of a given therapy must not be seen in isolation but have to be viewed relative to its potential benefit. In other words, we should not look at risks alone but should attempt to carry out a risk–benefit assessment. Unfortunately, this is a difficult task at the best of times and in CAM it is impossible in the vast majority of cases. The reason is that for many complementary therapies, we know too little about either their risk or their benefit.

There are, of course, some exceptions. For instance, there is good evidence to demonstrate that acupuncture (White & Ernst 1999) and some herbal treatments

Table 10.4 Recent case reports of adverse events associated with spinal manipulation (SM)

First author	Indication for SM	Number of cases	Nature of adverse event	Location of SM	Therapist	Causality
Balblanc	Back pain	1	Cauda equina syndrome	Lumbar	Traditional healer	Likely
Lipper	Cervical pain	1	Brown Séquard syndrome due to contusion of the spinal cord	Cervical	Chiropractor	Fairly certain
Hillier	Neck pain	1	Vertigo, profuse vomiting	Cervical	Chiropractor	Certain
Ruelle	Low back pain	1	Thoracic epidural hematoma	Lumbar	Chiropractor	Certain
Hufnagel	Various	10	Stroke	Cervical	Physician	Certain
Leweke	Neck pain	1	Bilateral vertebral dissection	Cervical	Not known	Likely

(Ernst 2000a) are effective for a number of conditions. We can also now begin to estimate the risks of these treatments with an acceptable degree of certainty (see above). Thus we can be reasonably sure that these treatments are associated with a favorable risk–benefit profile when used for those conditions.

For other (important) situations this is sadly not the case. For instance, we know that SM is associated with a high frequency of minor and a lower but unknown frequency of serious risks (see above). There are authoritative, critical assessments of the benefit of SM for back pain (Assendelft et al 1996a). Thus one may have reasonable doubt that a risk–benefit analysis of SM would result in a convincingly positive verdict (Assendelft et al 1996b, Ernst & Assendelft 1998).

THE WAY FORWARD

The message that emerges from the above discussion is that the investigation of CAM's safety is as much a matter of urgency as is research into its effectiveness. Such research is not aimed at demonstrating how dangerous CAM can be (even though certain proponents of CAM insist on the perpetuation of this myth). On the contrary, such research could (and more often than not will) demonstrate how safe CAM really is (Ernst et al 1998a, White & Ernst 2000).

How should we research safety?

A central question therefore relates to which research methods are best suited for the investigation of CAM's safety (Ernst & Barnes 1998).

The 'test of time'

Long-standing traditional experience as it often exists in CAM can reveal much about short-term safety but it is not a reliable tool for detecting rare or delayed adverse effects. There are numerous reasons why the 'test of time' is notoriously unreliable (Ernst et al 1998b).

- A treatment might have changed over time (e.g. a change in the source of raw material or production process for an HMP can impact on its pharmacological properties).
- Traditional experience cannot be applied to all variations of a particular treatment category (e.g. some HMPs marketed today have no history of traditional use).
- New routes of administration are associated with risks (e.g. Hahnemann never advocated the administration of homeopathic remedies by injection).
- Interactions with treatments that did not exist until recently (e.g. the vast majority of today's drugs were not available during the time when traditional experience was generated).
- A given therapy may have been used safely for one indication but current use for other conditions may not necessarily be risk free.
- Today's users of CAM may have different characteristics from their traditional counterparts (e.g. different diets or concomitant diseases).

Thus the 'test of time' can represent useful supporting evidence but to mistake it for convincing proof is a naïve and potentially dangerous mistake which is worryingly prevalent in CAM.

Controlled clinical trials

Controlled clinical trials (CCTs) test the efficacy or effectiveness of therapeutic interventions and often generate useful data on frequent adverse effects. They are, however, of very limited value in identifying rare or delayed adverse effects. This is predominantly due to the normally small number of patients and the usually short duration of the treatment phases.

CCTs comparing a complementary with a conventional treatment (rather than placebo or no treatment) can generate useful, albeit preliminary data to demonstrate relative safety. This is particularly true if the two approaches are therapeutically equivalent. For example, SJW has been shown in such studies to be as effective as conventional antidepressant drugs for mild to moderate depression (Williams et al 2000). These CCTs have also demonstrated that SJW has a more favorable short-term adverse effect profile than conventional antidepressant drugs (Stevinson & Ernst 1999).

Spontaneous reporting schemes

Spontaneous reporting schemes are an essential element of postmarketing surveillance. They act as an early warning system for identifying adverse effects, allow comparisons of adverse effect profiles between similar therapies and ensure continual safety monitoring (De Smet 1997). However, underreporting renders such schemes notoriously unreliable. It has been suggested that less than 15% of all suspected adverse effects are being reported in the UK, for instance (Lumley et al 1986).

There are no reasons to assume that the problem of underreporting would be any less with regard to CAM and there is some indirect evidence suggesting that it might be more than in conventional medicine (Ernst & Barnes 1998). For the vast majority of complementary therapies, formalized spontaneous reporting schemes do not exist. Reporting of an adverse effect would require its detection by the consumer, reporting to a doctor or pharmacist, attribution of the event to CAM exposure and notification of this to the appropriate authorities. Deficiencies in any of these steps would inevitably lead to underreporting. It follows that spontaneous reporting schemes would be useful but not totally reliable in identifying safety problems in CAM.

Cohort studies

In cohort studies, groups of individuals are defined by the presence or absence of exposure to a suspected risk factor. Such investigations can be retrospective or prospective. In a retrospective cohort study, both exposure and outcome have already occurred when the study is initiated. The aim is to compare the frequency of the outcome (e.g. mortality) in exposed individuals with that in non-exposed individuals. In prospective cohort studies, exposed and non-exposed groups are identified at the start of the study. Follow-up over a sufficient length of time is essential. Cohort studies usually rely on easily measurable endpoints (e.g. mortality). Such outcome measures are likely to be too insensitive for CAM to yield relevant information. Thus their usefulness is limited.

Case-control studies

Case-control studies can be used to investigate whether a particular therapy is associated with a certain suspected adverse effect. For example, if acupuncture is suspected as the route of infection with hepatitis C virus (HCV), large numbers of HCV-infected individuals ('cases') would be compared with non-infected individuals ('controls') in terms of their use of acupuncture (Mitchitaka et al 1991). If HCV-infected individuals had used acupuncture to a significantly greater extent than had controls, a hypothesis of a causal link could be derived. Alternatively, one might compare all people using acupuncture within a given population (cases) with those who never had acupuncture (controls). If users of acupuncture had a higher prevalence of HCV-positive individuals than non-users, this would again generate a hypothesis of a cause–effect relationship.

Case-control studies can generate relevant findings, particularly if the association is made repeatedly in different samples and if it is biologically plausible. They cannot, however, prove causality. In the above example, the 'cases' might differ from the 'controls' in factors other than their use of acupuncture which could be of causal relevance. Nevertheless, the case-control method is a powerful (hypothesis-generating) tool for investigating safety.

Case registers

Two different types of case registers exist: either all individuals with a certain condition (e.g. HCV infection) are recorded or all individuals who receive a certain treatment (e.g. acupuncture) are registered. In the first instance, the prevalence of acupuncture use in HCV-infected individuals would be compared with that in a similar (but non-HCV infected) population. In the second instance, the prevalence of HCV infection in users of acupuncture would be compared with that in an otherwise similar sample of non-users.

Case registers are expensive and critically depend on registering all individuals. However, they are good methods for generating reliable incidence rates and should be considered for the investigation of risks of CAM.

Surveys

The use of a survey to investigate safety would typically involve sending a questionnaire to a (defined) sample of individuals in order to gather data on adverse effects. Surveys can generate useful data, although they must be interpreted with great caution. Survey data can only be related to *perceived* adverse effects, i.e. causality cannot be inferred; the population investigated is often ill defined (e.g. residents of a given area); many surveys yield low response rates which further limits their generalizability (responders usually differ systematically from non-responders);

and surveys usually collect data retrospectively which introduces recall bias. Thus, the accuracy and reliability of surveys are questionable. Unfortunately, much of what (we think) we know at present about the safety of CAM is based on surveys.

Outcome studies

Outcome studies (i.e. uncontrolled, prospective, observational studies) are popular in CAM as they are relatively easy to conduct and can be placed in a 'real-life' setting. Patients can be studied prospectively or retrospectively. The incidence of adverse effects can be ascertained either generally (e.g. by asking patients or therapists) or specifically (e.g. including specific diagnostic tests), and studies can have long or short follow-up periods.

Outcome studies must involve large samples of patients. Moreover, it is crucial that 100% of the incident adverse effects within the target sample are recorded. Whenever possible, a comparison should be made with a sample not exposed to the therapy under investigation (Waller et al 1992). If not, they are difficult to interpret. Outcome studies can provide useful information about the nature of adverse effects and their incidence. Furthermore, they may give indications as to predisposing (risk) factors and they are not prone to false-negative results. Thus, they are powerful tools for investigating the safety of CAM.

Systematic reviews

Systematic reviews include explicit statements of objectives and detailed descriptions of methods ensuring that all the evidence (according to predefined inclusion and exclusion criteria) is being reviewed. Depending on this methodology, they can be exclusive (e.g. CCTs only) or inclusive (e.g. including most or all of the type of investigation listed above).

Inclusive systematic reviews are the optimal methodology for summarizing and critically evaluating the safety profile of therapeutic interventions. Obviously, they are only possible if sufficient primary data are available in the first place. In CAM, few examples of systematic reviews of safety issues exist. Those that have been published (for example, Stevinson & Ernst 1999) have made important contributions to this area.

What can we do now?

Research along the lines suggested above is urgently required but such investigations are time and money consuming. In all likelihood, therefore, they will not be available in the foreseeable future. What can we do in the meantime? The answer to this obvious question is far from easy. Several suggestions do seem to be justified, nevertheless.

- Apply the highest standards to your own clinical practice.
- Ensure you are up to date with the most recent knowledge in your field.
- Be open to the possibility of adverse effects in your own clinical setting.
- Be meticulous in recording all details of suspected adverse effects.
- Report adverse effects to the appropriate authorities.

- Be cautious, particularly with highly vulnerable patients (e.g. young children, elderly individuals).
- Be aware of concomitant use of treatments.

Professional CAM bodies should begin to seriously consider monitoring adverse effects of their respective treatments. Amongst the various options for achieving this (see above), spontaneous reporting schemes similar to those used in mainstream medicine would be a valuable first step. The onus of demonstrating the safety of a given therapy unquestionably lies with those who employ and promote it.

CONCLUSION

Research into the safety of CAM is in its earliest infancy yet reliable information regarding the risks of CAM would be an essential precondition for the integration of CAM into conventional health care. The research methodologies for investigating safety issues of CAM are similar to those used in mainstream medicine. To rigorously apply these methods provides one of the biggest challenges that CAM faces today. Even though few CAM enthusiasts seem to agree, I continue to be convinced that researching the risks of CAM will not be to the detriment but ultimately to the credit of our field.

REFERENCES

Abbot NC, Hill M, Barnes J, Hourigan PG, Ernst E 1998 Uncovering suspected adverse effects of complementary and alternative medicine. International Journal of Risk and Safety in Medicine 11: 99–106

Adams G, Sim J 1998 A survey of UK manual therapists' practice of and attitudes towards manipulation and its complications. Physiotherapy Research International 3: 206–227

Agothos M, Breit R, Schatzle M, Steinmann A 1997 Allergic contact dermatitis from black cumin (*Nigella sativa*) oil after topical use. American Journal of Contact Dermatitis 36: 268–269

Allaire AD, Moos MK, Wells SR 2000 Complementary and alternative medicine in pregnancy: a survey of North Carolina certified nurse-midwives. Obstetrics and Gynecology 95: 19–23

Assendelft WJJ, Koes BW, Van Der Heijden GJMG, Bouter L 1996a The effectiveness of chiropractic for treatment of low back pain: an update and attempt at statistical pooling. Journal of Therapeutic and Physiological Therapeutics 19: 499–507

Assendelft WJJ, Bouter LM, Knipschild PG 1996b Complications of spinal manipulation: a comprehensive review of the literature. Journal of Family Practice 42: 475–480

Baber J 1998 When hypnosis causes trouble. International Journal of Experiment Hypnosis 44: 157–170

Balblanc J, Pretot C, Ziegler F 1998 Vascular complication involving the conus medullaris or cauda equina after vertebral manipulation for an L4–L5 disk herniation. Revue du Rhumatisme 65: 279–282

Barnes J, Mills SY, Abbot NC, Willoughby M, Ernst E 1998 Different standards for reporting ADRs to herbal remedies and conventional OTC medicines: face-to-face interviews with 515 users of herbal remedies. British Journal of Clinical Pharmacology 45: 496–500

Bove GM 1998 Acute neuropathy after exposure to sun in a patient treated with St. John's Wort. Lancet 352: 1121–1122

Cheng T, Wong R, Lin Y, Hwang Y, Hong J, Wang J 1998 Chinese herbal medicine, sibship, and blood lead in children. Occupational and Environmental Medicine 55: 573–576

Chu N, Liou S, Wu T, Ko K, Chang P 1998 Risk factors for high blood lead levels among the general population in Taiwan. European Journal of Epidemiology 14: 775–781

Coppes MJ, Anderson RA, Egeler RM, Wolff JEA 1998 Alternative therapies for the treatment of childhood cancer. New England Journal of Medicine 339: 846

De Smet PAGM 1997 An introduction to herbal pharmacovigilance. In: De Smet PAGM, Keller K, Hönsel R, Chandler RF (eds) Adverse effects of herbal drugs, vol 3, Springer-Verlag, Heidelberg

Di Fabio RP 1999 Manipulation of the cervical spine: risks and benefits. Physical Therapy 79: 50–65

Drewe J 2000 Mechanismen der Interaktionen mit Johanniskraut. Proceedings of the German Society of Clinical Pharmacology, Berlin, 16–17 June

Ernst E 1995 Competence in complementary medicine. Complementary Therapies in Medicine 3: 6–8

Ernst E 1997 Attitude against immunisation within some branches of complementary medicine. European Journal of Paediatrics 156: 513–515

Ernst E 1998 Chiropractors' use of X-rays. British Journal of Radiology 71: 249–251

Ernst E 1999 Second thoughts about safety of St. John's wort. Lancet 345: 2014–2016

Ernst E (ed) 2000a Herbal medicine. A concise overview for professionals. Butterworth Heinemann, Oxford

Ernst E 2000b Interactions between synthetic and herbal medicinal products. Part 2: a systematic review of the direct evidence. Perfusion 13: 60–70

Ernst E 2000c Iridology – not useful and potentially harmful. Archives of Ophthalmology 118: 120–121

Ernst E 2000d Adverse effects of herbal drugs in dermatology. British Journal of Dermatology 143: 923–929

Ernst E 2000e Possible interactions between synthetic and herbal medicinal products. Part 1: a systematic review of the indirect evidence. Perfusion 13: 4–6, 8–15

Ernst E 2000f Risks associated with complementary therapies. In: Dukes MNG, Aronson JK (eds) Meyler's side effects of drugs, 14th edn. Elsevier, Amsterdam

Ernst E, Armstrong NC 1998 Lay books on complementary/alternative medicine: a risk factor for good health? International Journal of Risk and Safety in Medicine 11: 209–215

Ernst E, Assendelft WJJ 1998 Chiropractic for low back pain. British Medical Journal 317: 160

Ernst E, Barnes J 1998 Methodological approaches to investigating the safety of complementary medicine. Complementary Therapies in Medicine 6: 115–121

Ernst E, White A 1997 Life-threatening adverse reactions after acupuncture? A systematic review. Pain 71: 123–126

Ernst E, White AR 1999 Indwelling needles carry greater risks than other acupuncture techniques. British Medical Journal 318: 536

Ernst E, White AR 2000 Acupuncture may be associated with serious adverse events. British Medical Journal 320: 513–514

Ernst E, Rand JI, Barnes J, Stevinson C 1998a Adverse effects profile of the herbal antidepressant St. John's Wort (Hypericum perforatum L.) European Journal of Clinical Pharmacology 54: 589–594

Ernst E, De Smet PAGM, Shaw D, Murray V 1998b Traditional remedies and the 'test of time'. European Journal of Clinical Pharmacology 54: 99–100

Fugh-Berman A 2000 Herb–drug interactions. Lancet 355: 134–138

Gravitz MA 1998 Inability to dehypnotize – implications for management. Hypnos 25: 93–97

Halt M 1998 Moulds and mycotoxins in herb tea and medicinal plants. European Journal of Epidemiology 14: 269–274

Hillier CEM, Gross MLP 1998 Sudden onset vomiting and vertigo following chiropractic neck manipulation. Journal of Postgraduate Medicine 48: 567–568

Hufnagel A, Hammers A, Schönle P-W, Böhm K-D, Leonhardt G 1999 Stroke following chiropractic manipulation of the cervical spine. Journal of Neurology 246: 683–688

James WD, Weiss RR 1997 Allergic contact dermatitis from aromatherapy. American Journal of Contact Dermatitis 8: 250–251

Jonas WB, Ernst E 1999 The safety of homeopathy. In: Jonas WB, Levin JS (eds) Essentials of complementary and alternative medicine. Lippincott Williams Wilkins, Philadelphia: 167–171

Kerr HD 1997 Ureteral stent displacement associated with deep massage. Wisconsin Medical Journal 12: 57–58

Ko RJ 1998 Adulterants in Asian patent medicines. New England Journal of Medicine 339: 847

Kranke B 1997 Allergy inducing potency of tea tree oil. Hautarzt 36: 268–269

Lee S 2000 Chinese hypnosis can cause qigong induced mental disorders. British Medical Journal 320: 803

Levi M, Guchelaar HJ, Woerdenbag HJ, Zhu YP 1998 Acute hepatitis in a patient using a Chinese herbal tea – a case report. Pharmacy World and Science 20: 43–44

Leweke F, Teschendorf U, Stolz E, Kern A, Hahn M, Dorndorf W 1999 Doppelseitige Dissektionen der Vertebralarterien nach chiropraktischer Behandllung der Halswirbelßule. Aktuelle Neurologie 26: 35–39

Lipper MH, Goldstein JH, Do HM 1998 Brown-Sèquard syndrome of the cervical spinal cord after chiropractic manipulation. American Journal of Neuroradiology 19: 1349–1352

Lumley CE, Walker SR, Hall GC, Staunton N, Grob PR 1986 The under-reporting of adverse reactions seen in general practice. Pharmaceutical Medicine 1: 205–212

Lynch P 1998 Incidence of neurological injury following neck manipulation. Irish Medical Journal 91: 130

Matthews MK 1998 Association of Ginkgo biloba with intracerebral haemorrhage. Neurology 5: 1933

Mitchitaka K, Horiike N, Ohta Y 1991 An epidemiological study of hepatitis C virus infection in a local district in Japan. Rinsho Bvori 39: 586–591

Moody GA, Eaden JA, Bhakta P, Sher K, Mayberry JF 1998 The role of complementary medicine in European and Asian patients with inflammatory bowel disease. Public Health 112: 269–271

Nierenberg AA, Burt T, Matthews J, Weiss AP 1999 Mania associated with St. John's wort. Biological Psychiatry 46: 1701–1708

Nortier JL, Muniz Martinez M-C, Schmeiser HH et al 2000 Urothelial carcinoma associated with the use of a Chinese herb (*Aristolochia fangchi*). New England Journal of Medicine 342: 1686–1692

Oneschuk D, Bruera E 1999 The potential dangers of complementary therapy use in a patient with cancer. Journal of Palliative Care 15: 49–52

Ruelle A, Datti R, Pisani R 1999 Thoracic epidural hematoma after spinal manipulation therapy. Journal of Spinal Disorders 12: 534–536

Sadjadi J 1998 Cutaneous anthrax associated with the Kombucha 'mushroom' in Iran. Journal of the American Medical Association 280: 1567–1568

Scheck C 1998 St. John's wort and hypomania. Journal of Clinical Psychiatry 59: 689

Senstad O, Leboeuf-Yde C, Borchgrevink C 1997 Frequency and characteristics of side effects of spinal manipulative therapy. Spine 22: 435–441

Slifman NR, Obermeyer WR, Aloi BK et al 1998 Contamination of botanical dietary supplements by *Digitalis lanata*. New England Journal of Medicine 339: 806–810

Stengel B, Jones E 1998 Insuffisance rénale treminale associée à la consommation d'herbes chinoises en France. Néphrologie 19: 15–20

Stevinson C, Ernst E 1999 Safety of Hypericum in patients with depression. CNS Drugs 11: 125–132

Trotter JF 1999 Hepatic hematoma after deep tissue massage. New England Journal of Medicine 341: 2019–2020

Vanherweghem JL 1998 Misuse of herbal remedies: the case of an outbreak of terminal renal failure in Belgium (Chinese herbs nephropathy). Journal of Alternative and Complementary Medicine 4: 9–13

Van Ypersele de Strihou C 1998 Chinese herb nephropathy or the evils of nature. American Journal of Kidney Disease 32: 2–3

Waller PC, Wood SM, Langman MJS et al 1992 Review of company post-marketing studies. British Medical Journal 304: 1470–1472

Walsh B, Maguire H, Carrington D 1999 Outbreak of hepatitis B in an acupuncture clinic. Communicable Disease and Health 2: 131–140

White A, Ernst E (eds) 1999 Acupuncture: a scientific appraisal. Butterworth-Heinemann, Oxford

White AR, Ernst E 2000 Survey of adverse events following acupuncture (SAFA). Forschende Komplementärmed 7: 56

Williams JW, Mulrow CD, Chiquette E et al 2000 A systematic review of newer pharmacotherapies for depression in adults: evidence report summary. Annals of Internal Medicine 132: 743–756

Wong ST, Chan HL, Teo SK 1998 The spectrum of cutaneous and internal malignancies in chronic arsenic toxicity. Singapore Medical Journal 39: 171–173

Yamashita H, Tsukayama H, Tanno Y, Nishijo K 1998 Adverse events related to acupuncture. Journal of the American Medical Association 280: 1563–1564

11

Systematic reviews and metaanalyses

Klaus Linde

INTRODUCTION

Every year more than two million articles are published in over 20 000 biomedical journals (Mulrow 1995). Even in speciality areas it is impossible to keep up to date with all relevant new information. In this situation systematic reviews hold a key position to summarize the state of actual knowledge. A review is called systematic if it uses predefined and explicit methods for identifying, selecting and assessing the information (typically research studies) deemed relevant to answer the particular question posed. A systematic review is called a metaanalysis if it includes an integrative statistical analysis (= pooling) of the included studies.

Within complementary medicine systematic reviews are of major relevance. This chapter gives an introduction on how to read and how to carry out a systematic review and discusses advances and limitations of this method.

THE PROTOCOL

A systematic review is, in principle, a retrospective study. Instead of a patient, the unit of investigation is the original research study (= primary study); for example, a randomized controlled trial. The retrospective nature limits the conclusiveness of systematic reviews. Nevertheless, the methods of retrospective studies should be defined as far as possible in advance.

The protocol of a systematic review should have subheadings similar to those in this chapter. To write a feasible and useful protocol it is necessary to have at least some basic ideas about what and how much primary research is available. Therefore, in practice the protocol of a systematic review often has to be developed in a stepwise approach where the methods are defined rather loosely in the early screening phase and then become more and more specific.

THE QUESTION

As in any research a clear and straightforward question is a precondition for a conclusive answer. A well-defined question for a systematic review on a treatment is, for example, whether garlic can lower cholesterol levels over placebo in patients with hypercholesterolemia. A question of this type already predefines the group of patients (those with hypercholesterolemia), the type of experimental (garlic) and control interventions (placebo) as well as the outcome of interest (serum cholesterol levels). Systematic reviews on such narrowly defined questions make sense particularly when a number of similar studies is available but their results are either not widely known or contradictory or if the number of patients in the primary studies is too small to detect relevant differences with sufficient likelihood.

In complementary medicine the number of studies on a particular topic is usually small. If the question is very narrow it might be that only a few or even no relevant trials can be identified. For example, a systematic review has been performed to assess whether there is evidence from randomized trials that cranberry juice is effective in the treatment of urinary tract infections (Jepson et al 1999). No trial met the inclusion criteria. While it can be easily concluded from such a review that there is no evidence, this is not very satisfying for reviewers or readers.

Sometimes it might be useful to ask broader questions; for example, 'is there evidence that cranberry juice can be beneficial in urinary tract infections?'. Such a review will give a more descriptive overview of probably rather inhomogeneous studies (regarding study design, outcomes, prevention or treatment, etc.). It will be more hypothesis generating than hypothesis testing.

Most available systematic reviews on complementary medicine have focused on treatment effects. But of course, it is possible to do systematic reviews on other topics; for example, the validity and reliability of diagnostic methods (Ernst 1999), side effects (Ernst et al 1998) or surveys regarding attitudes (Ernst et al 1995).

SEARCHING THE LITERATURE

An obvious precondition for a good systematic review is that the relevant literature is covered comprehensively. In conventional medicine the majority of research journals are listed in one or more of the electronic databases such as MEDLINE, EMBASE, Current Contents, etc. In complementary medicine the situation is much more difficult. The majority of journals in this area are not listed in these databases so a good literature search should use multiple sources (see Box 11.1). Although there are a number of complementary medicine databases, these are typically specialized on certain areas, difficult to access and to search.

A very effective and simple method is checking the references of identified studies and reviews relevant to the topic. This method often also identifies studies which are published only as abstracts, in conference proceedings or books. The problem of this method can be that studies with 'undesired' results are systematically undercited. Contacting persons, institutions or industry relevant to the field can help both in identifying new sources to search (for example, a specialized database which was unknown to you before) and obtaining articles directly. Finally, handsearching of journals, conference proceedings, etc. is a possibility although this often surpasses the time resources of reviewers.

Box 11.1 Sources for literature search in systematic reviews

- Searches in conventional databases (for example, MEDLINE, EMBASE, Current Contents, Cochrane Controlled Trials Register)
- Searches in specialized databases (for example, CISCOM = database of the Research Council of Complementary Medicine in London, HOMINFORM = database of the Glasgow Homeopathic Hospital, Phytodok = private database on herbal medicine in Germany)
- Screening of references of identified studies and review articles
- Contacting researchers, experts and institutions relevant to the field
- Contacting manufacturers/relevant industry
- Handsearching conference proceedings or relevant journals

A problem that has to be kept in mind is that specific complementary therapies and research activities might be concentrated in certain countries. A number of systematic reviews by native English-speaking researchers have been limited to studies published in English. Either they searched only sources which mainly identify English language literature or they explicitly excluded studies published in languages other than English. This may lead to misleading conclusions. For example, a large number of clinical trials on herbal extracts have been undertaken in Germany and have only been published in German. While the translation of articles of doubtful relevance is expensive, the obvious solution for such a problem is to try to include a person able to read the specific language in the research team.

In practice, the scrutiny of the literature search will depend strongly on the resources available. Reviews which are based on literature searches in only one or two of the mentioned sources should, however, be interpreted with great caution, keeping in mind that a number of relevant studies might have been missed.

Sometimes it can be difficult to obtain hard copies of potentially relevant studies, particularly if these have been published in small, foreign language journals or books not available in commonly accessible libraries. Personal contacts with researchers are often the only way to get hold of such studies.

A major problem pertinent to systematic reviews is publication bias (Dickersin et al 1987, Kleijnen & Knipschild 1992). Publication bias occurs when studies with undesired results (mostly negative) are less often published than those with desired results (mostly positive). Small negative or inconclusive studies are especially likely to be rejected. Publication bias typically leads to over-optimistic results and conclusions in systematic reviews. Very rarely, however, the opposite might occur. Some researchers in controversial areas of complementary medicine have had the experience that it was easier to get negative findings accepted by conventional medicine journals than positive findings.

Reviewers should try to find out whether unpublished studies exist. Informal contacts with researchers in the field is, in our experience, the most effective way to achieve this. However, it is often difficult to get written reports on these studies. Handsearching the abstract books and proceedings of research meetings is another potential way to identify otherwise unpublished studies.

There are no foolproof ways to detect and quantify publication bias (see Checking the Robustness of Results (below) for a method to estimate the influence). Every reviewer and all readers should always be aware of this risk.

SELECTING THE RELEVANT STUDIES

Selecting the studies for detailed review from the often large number of references identified from the search is the next crucial step in the review process. Readers should check carefully whether this process was transparent and unbiased.

A good systematic review of studies on diagnosis or therapy should explicitly define inclusion and exclusion criteria (Box 11.2). It has been outlined above that 'the question' of the review already crudely predefines these criteria. In the methods section of a systematic review they should be described in more detail. In the example of the review on garlic for cholesterol lowering, it should be stated above which cholesterol level patients were considered as hypercholesterolemic. Garlic can be applied in quite different ways (fresh, dried preparations, oil) and we have to know whether all of them were considered. Another selection criterion typically applies to the type of studies considered. For example, many reviews are limited to randomized trials. The measurement and reporting of predefined outcomes as inclusion criterion is of particular importance when a metaanalysis is planned. This often leads to the exclusion of a relevant proportion of otherwise relevant studies and the reader has to consider whether this might have influenced the findings of the review.

In practice, the selection process is mostly performed in two steps. In the first step all the obviously irrelevant material is discarded; for example, all articles on garlic which are clearly not clinical trials in patients with cardiovascular problems. To save time and money, this step is normally done by only one reviewer in a rather informal way. The remaining articles should then be checked carefully for eligibility by at least two independent (one does not know the decision of the other) reviewers. In the publication of a systematic review it is advisable to list the potentially relevant studies which were excluded and give the reasons for exclusion. A recent consensus paper on how metaanalyses should be reported recommended the use of flowcharts displaying the number of papers identified, excluded and selected at the different levels of the review and assessment process (Moher et al 1999). This makes the selection process transparent for the reader.

EXTRACTING INFORMATION

When a number of eligible studies have been identified, obtained and passed the selection process, relevant information has to be extracted. If possible, the extraction

---

Box 11.2 Inclusion and exclusion criteria for primary studies in systematic reviews

- Type of patients/participants (for example, patients with serum cholesterol <200 mg/dl)
- Type of studies (for example, trials with an explicit statement that allocation to groups was randomized)
- Type of intervention (for example, dried garlic monopreparations applied for at least 4 weeks in the experimental group and placebo in the control group)
- Type of outcomes (for example, trials had to present mean and standard deviations for serum cholesterol in experimental and control groups at baseline and at least another point in time 4 weeks or more after start of treatment)
- Other restrictions (for example, only trials published in English, published in a peer-reviewed journal, no abstracts, etc.)

should be standardized, for example by using a pretested form. The format should allow you to enter the data into a database and to perform basic statistical analyses. Another efficient method is to directly enter the data into a prestructured table. Regardless of what method is used, the reviewers must have a clear idea of what information they need for their analysis and what readers will need to get their own picture. Extraction and all assessments should be done by at least two independent reviewers. Coding errors are inevitable and personal biases can influence decisions in the extraction process. The coded information of the reviewers has to be compared and disagreements have to be discussed.

ASSESSING QUALITY

A major criticism of skeptics about metaanalysis (and to a lesser extent non-meta-analytic systematic reviews) is the garbage in, garbage out problem. The results of unreliable studies do not become more reliable by lumping them together. It has been shown in conventional and complementary medicine that less rigorous trials tend to yield more positive results (Lijner et al 1999, Linde et al, 1999, Schulz et al 1995). Sometimes it might be better to base the conclusions on a few, rigorous trials and discard the findings of the bulk of unreliable studies. This approach has been called 'best-evidence synthesis' (Slavin 1986). While it is sometimes considered as an alternative, it is in principle a subtype of systematic reviews in which defined quality aspects are used as additional inclusion criteria (see White et al 1997 as an example from complementary medicine).

However, the assessment of quality is difficult. The first problem is that quality is a complex concept. Methodologists tend to define quality as the likelihood that the results of a study are valid. This dimension of quality is sometimes referred to as internal validity or methodological quality. But a perfectly internally valid study might have fundamental flaws from a clinician's point of view if, for example, the outcomes measured are irrelevant for the patients, the patients are not representative of those commonly receiving the treatment, etc.

A second problem is that quality is difficult to operationalize in a valid manner. An experienced reviewer will gain a lot of subtle information on the quality of the study by reading 'between the lines', from omissions and small details. However, subjective, global ways to assess quality are not transparent and are prone to subjective biases.

Many systematic reviews on treatment interventions include some standardized assessments of internal validity. There is agreement that key criteria for the internal validity of treatment studies are random allocation, blinding and adequate handling of drop-outs and withdrawals. Often these and other criteria are combined in scores (see Moher et al 1995, 1996 for overviews) but the validity of such scores is doubtful (Jüni et al 1999). Whether the criteria are combined in scores or applied separately, the problems remain that the formalized assessment is often crude and that the reviewers have to rely on the information reported.

In conclusion, assessments of methodological quality are necessary but need to be interpreted with caution. The assessment of other dimensions of quality is desirable but the problems in the development of methods for this purpose (which have to take account of the specific characteristics of the interventions and conditions investigated) are even greater than for internal validity.

SUMMARIZING THE RESULTS

The clinical reader of a systematic review is mainly interested in its results. While the majority of readers will only look at the abstract and metaanalytic summary, the review also has to provide sufficient information for those who want to get their own idea of the available studies and their results. For example, in a review of acupuncture in headache, it will be relevant for specialists to know what type of headache was studied in each primary study, to have information on sex and age of the patients and where they have been recruited. Regarding the methods, they should know what the design was, whether there was some blinding, how long the patients were followed and whether follow-up was complete. They need details on the nature of the experimental (which acupuncture points, how many treatments, etc.) and the control interventions (type of sham acupuncture, etc.). And of course, they want to know which outcomes have been measured and what the results were. This detailed information is typically summarized in a table.

If the primary studies provide sufficient data the results are summarized in effect size estimates. Table 11.1 lists some of the most common measures.

Tables including a graphical display of the results are extremely helpful. Table 11.2 shows the standard display from a metaanalysis from the Cochrane Library, in this case on randomized trials of Hypericum extracts in patients with depressive disorders (Linde & Mulrow 1999). For each single study, the actual results in the groups

Table 11.1 Estimates commonly used to summarize the results of controlled trials

Estimate	Calculation	Advantages/Disadvantages
For dichotomous data (response, death, etc.)		
Odds ratio	$\dfrac{a \times d}{b \times c}$	Most widespread estimate in medicine/intuitively difficult to understand
Relative risk (rate ratio)	$\dfrac{a\,/\,(a + b)}{c\,/\,(c + d)}$	Easy to understand/problematic in case of very low or high control group event rates
For continuous data (blood pressure, enzyme activity, etc.)		
Weighted mean difference	$x_e - x_c$ weighted by $1\,/\,\text{variance}$	Easy to interpret/only applicable if all trials measure the outcomes with the same scale
Standardized mean difference	$\dfrac{x_e - x_c}{sd}$	Applicable over different scales/clinically difficult to interpret

a = number of patients with an event in the experimental group
b = number of patients without event in the experimental group
c = number of patients with an event in the control group
d = number of patients without event in the control group
x_e = mean experimental group
x_c = mean control group
sd = standard deviations (either of the control group or pooled for both groups)

Table 11.2 Example of the presentation of results in systematic reviews: treatment responders and rate ratios in randomized controlled trials of Hypericum extracts (modifed from Linde & Mulrow 1999)

Comparison: 01 Hypericum mono-preparations vs. placebo A. Dichotomous measures
Outcome: 01 Responder

Study	Hypericum n/N	Placebo n/N	RR (95% CI random)	Weight %	RR (95% CI random)
01 extract 1					
Halama 1991	10/25	0/25		1.1	21.00[1.30,340.03]
Hänsgen 1996	35/53	12/54		27.1	2.97[1.74,5.07]
Hübner 1993	14/20	9/20		24.8	1.56[0.89,2.73]
Lehrl 1993	4/25	2/25		3.4	2.00[0.40,9.95]
Schmidt 1993	20/32	6/33		13.9	3.44[1.59,7.44]
Sommer 1993	28/50	13/55		27.1	2.37[1.39,4.04]
Subtotal (95% CI)	111/205	42/212		97.4	2.44[1.80,3.30]
Chi-square 6.95 (df=5) P: 0.22 Z=5.80 P: <0.00001					
02 extract 2					
Osterheider 1992	0/23	0/24		0.6	1.04[0.02,50.43]
Quandt 1993	29/44	3/44		6.0	9.67[3.18,29.42]
Schlich 1987	15/25	3/24		6.0	4.80[1.59,14.50]
Schmidt 1989	10/20	4/20		7.3	2.50[0.94,6.66]
Witte 1995	34/48	25/49		24.9	1.39[1.00,1.93]
Subtotal (95% CI)	88/160	35/161		44.7	2.33[1.49,3.64]
Chi-square 15.86 (df=4) P: 0.00 Z=3.73 P: <0.00001					
03 other extracts					
Hoffmann 1979	19/30	3/30		4.7	6.33[2.09,19.17]
König 1993	29/55	31/57		11.6	0.97[0.69,1.37]
Laakmann 1998	24/49	16/49		10.0	1.50[0.92,2.46]
Philipp 1999	67/100	22/46		11.8	1.40[1.01,1.95]
Reh 1992	20/25	11/25		10.1	1.82[1.12,2.95]
Schrader 1998	45/80	12/79		9.3	3.70[2.12,6.46]
Subtotal (95% CI)	204/339	95/286		57.5	1.83[1.23,2.70]
Chi-square 35.76 (df=5) P: 0.00 Z = 3.01 P: < 0.00001					
Total (95% CI)	403/704	172/659		199.7	2.27[1.68,3.06]
Chi-square 58.57 (df= 16) P: 0.00 Z = 5.40 P: <0.00001					

```
          .1   .2        1      5   10
          favors placebo     favors hypericum
```

n = number of patients responding to treatment
N = number of patients

(here the number of patients responding/number of patients allocated to the group) compared are listed in columns two and three. In column four the effect estimate (in this case the ratio between the responder rates in treatment and control groups) and their respective confidence intervals for each study are presented graphically and in column six numerically. The boxes indicate the actual effect size estimates of the single trials while the horizontal lines represent the respective 95% confidence intervals (CI). The diamonds represent the pooled effect size estimates for the different extracts ('subtotal') and all extracts analyzed together ('total'). In the example, effects estimates right of the vertical line (which represents equal responder rates in treatment and control group) indicate superiority of Hypericum, those to the left superiority of the control treatment. However, the side representing superiority depends on the actual outcome measure. If the 95% CI does not include the vertical line the difference between treatment and control is statistically significant ($P < 0.05$). Column five gives the weight of each study in the pooled estimate which depends on sample sizes and variances. The chi-square, z- and P-values presented together with each pooled estimate are indicators of heterogeneity. A significant P-value here means that the results of the trials vary more than would be expected by chance alone. Possible reasons for heterogeneity are bias in some trials, varying patient characteristics in each trial, etc. Metaanalyses with indication of heterogeneity (as in the case of the Hypericum trials) have to be interpreted with special caution.

A number of computer programs for systematic reviews and metaanalysis are available (see Egger et al 1998 for review). Depending on the type of data and other characteristics of the data (for example, heterogeneity), different statistical techniques are adequate. Although the computer programs allow the novice to perform metaanalyses it is important to get guidance or advice from a statistician or an experienced reviewer if pooling of independent studies is an issue.

CHECKING THE ROBUSTNESS OF RESULTS

If possible, a systematic review should include sensitivity analyses to check the robustness of the results. For example, one can check whether the conclusions would be altered if only studies meeting defined quality criteria were included. Subgroup analyses (for example, on patients with major depression only) can also be of value but should be interpreted with caution, particularly if they were not predefined. Unfortunately, a considerable number of primary studies is needed to perform sensitivity and subgroup analyses in a meaningful manner.

Textbooks on systematic reviews recommend funnel plots as another means to investigate empirically for biases. A precondition for a funnel plot is a sufficiently large and clinically reasonably homogeneous group of studies (so that a single 'true' effect size is a plausible expectation). In funnel plots effect sizes of single studies are plotted against a measure of precision or sample size. The basic idea is that larger studies provide the more reliable estimates of treatment effects as they are less prone to random error (chance variation), within-study bias (larger studies tend to have better internal validity) and publication bias (larger studies are more expensive, known to more people and therefore more likely to be published regardless of the results). If the results of the small studies differ only due to chance variation, the resulting graph should resemble an inverted funnel. An asymmetric plot has long been interpreted as an indication of publication bias. However, the concept of 'small-study effects', including both elements of publication and within-study bias, is more accurate (Sterne et al 2000). Both the reviewer and the reader should consider an asymmetric funnel plot a red flag: the findings of the review might be biased!

WHO SHOULD DO SYSTEMATIC REVIEWS?

Many people grossly underestimate the amount of time needed to perform a rigorous systematic review. Protocol development, literature search, extraction, discussion of disagreements in coding and assessments, obtaining missing data from authors and analyzing are all time-consuming steps and a realistic timeline from start to completion of the final report is 12–24 months with repeated periods of intensive work. Of course, it is also possible to make systematic reviews faster but this will probably result in rather superficial work of doubtful utility.

Many systematic reviews on complementary medicine have been performed by research methodologists with limited experience on the interventions and conditions investigated. In my opinion, the research team for a systematic review should have competency in methodology, intervention and the condition under scrutiny to ensure that the results will be both methodologically sound and clinically relevant. As complementary therapies are often controversial and prejudices strong, it is desirable to include persons with different prejudices to make the review as balanced as possible. Many steps in retrospective studies such as systematic reviews include rather arbitrary decisions which leave space for personal bias to infect the results.

The Cochrane Collaboration is a worldwide network of researchers who perform, regularly update and disseminate systematic reviews of health-care interventions (Ezzo et al 1998). Within the collaboration there is also a group focusing on complementary medicine. Researchers who plan to do a systematic review should consider contacting the group (www.compmed.unmc.umaryland.edu/Compmed/Cochrane/Cochrane.htm).

HOW TO IDENTIFY EXISTING SYSTEMATIC REVIEWS

The most relevant sources for identifying existing systematic reviews are MEDLINE and the Cochrane Library. By using the term 'metaanalysis' as publication type and combining it with the clinical problem of interest, MEDLINE can be searched efficiently. Unfortunately, this database does not code 'systematic review' as a publication type. As a consequence, many systematic reviews which do not include a quantitative metaanalysis are misclassified while others are simply missed as they are not coded as 'metaanalysis'.

The Cochrane Library is a CD-ROM produced by the Cochrane Collaboration. It contains the full text of all reviews performed by the network as well as references and abstracts of a large number of other systematic reviews.

SHOULD WE BELIEVE THE RESULTS OF SYSTEMATIC REVIEWS?

This chapter should have made clear that while systematic reviews are of the utmost importance, they are prone to a number of biases. Even the best systematic review will be of limited value if the primary studies are flawed. It has been shown that the findings of very large clinical trials (which are considered as the ultimate gold standard to assess the merit of a treatment) differ in a considerable number of cases from those of metaanalyses on the same topic (LeLorier et al 1997). The large number of decisions in

---

Box 11.3 Questions to consider when reading a systematic review

- Was there a clearly defined question?
- Was the literature search comprehensive?
- Were inclusion and exclusion criteria defined and adequate?
- Was bias avoided in the process of selecting studies for inclusion in the review from the body of literature identified?
- Was the quality of the included studies assessed using relevant criteria?
- Have patients, methods, interventions and results of the included studies been described in sufficient detail?
- If the review included a metaanalysis, were the methods used adequate and the primary studies sufficiently comparable?
- Have the shortcomings of the review been discussed?
- Are the results relevant to clinical practice?

---

a systematic review can also have a relevant impact on the results. As a consequence, it should not be surprising that systematic reviews performed by different research groups sometimes come to conflicting conclusions (see, for example, Ernst & White 1998, Van Tulder & Irnich 1999, Van Tulder et al 1999 for commentaries).

Readers should check reviews carefully. Guidelines for critical appraisal are available (see Further Reading). Box 11.3 lists a number of questions to consider when reading systematic reviews.

Systematic reviews cannot replace original research. Particularly in complementary medicine, their conclusiveness will remain limited unless new, reliable primary studies become available.

REFERENCES

Dickersin K, Chan S, Chalmers TC, Sacks HS, Smith H 1987 Publication bias and clinical trials. Controlled Clinical Trials 8: 343–353

Egger M, Sterne JAC, Davey Smith G 1998 Meta-analaysis software. British Medical Journal 316 (available on the Internet http://www.bmj.com/archive/7126/7126ed9.htm)

Ernst E 1999 Iridology: a systematic review. Forschende Komplementärmed medizin 6: 7–9

Ernst E, White AR 1998 Acupuncture for low back pain: a meta-analysis of randomized controlled trials. Archives of Internal Medicine 158: 2235–2241

Ernst E, Resch KL, White AR 1995 Complementary medicine – what physicians think of it: a meta-analysis. Archives of Internal Medicine 155: 2405–2408

Ernst E, Rand JI, Barnes J, Stevinson C 1998 Adverse effects profile of the herbal antidepressant St. John's wort (*Hypericum perforatum* L.). European Journal of Clinical Pharmacology 54: 589–594

Ezzo J, Berman BM, Vickers AJ, Linde K 1998 Complementary medicine and the Cochrane Collaboration. Journal of the American Medical Association 280: 1628–1630

Jepson RG, Mihaljevic L, Craig J 1999 Cranberries for treating urinary tract infections (Cochrane Review). The Cochrane Library, Issue 1. Update Software, Oxford (CD-ROM)

Jüni P, Witschi A, Bloch R, Egger M 1999 The hazards of scoring the quality of clinical trials for meta-analysis. Journal of the American Medical Association 282: 1054–1060

Kleijnen J, Knipschild P 1992 Review articles and publication bias. Arzneimittel-forschung/Drug Research 42: 587–591

LeLorier J, Grégoire G, Benhaddad A, Lapierre J, Derderian F 1997 Discrepancies between meta-analysis and subsequent large randomized, controlled trials. New England Journal of Medicine 337: 536–542

Lijner JG, Mol BW, Heisterkamp S et al 1999 Empirical evidence of design-related bias in studies of diagnostic tests. Journal of the American Medical Association 282: 1061–1066

Linde K, Mulrow CD 1999 St John's wort for depression (Cochrane Review). The Cochrane Library, Issue 1. Update Software, Oxford (CD-ROM)

Linde K, Schulz M, Ramirez G, Clausius N, Melchart D, Jonas WB 1999 Impact of study quality on outcome in placebo-controlled trials of homeopathy. Journal of Clinical Epidemiology 52: 631–636

Moher D, Jadad AR, Nichol G, Penman M, Tugwell P, Walsh S 1995 Assessing the quality of randomized controlled trials: an annotated bibliography of scales and checklists. Controlled Clinical Trials 16: 62–73

Moher D, Jadad AR, Tugwell P 1996 Assessing the quality of randomized controlled trials – current issues and future directions. International Journal of Technology Assessment in Health Care 12: 196–208

Moher D, Cook DJ, Eastwood S, Olkin I, Rennie D, Stroup DF 1999 Improving the reporting of meta-analyses of randomised controlled trials: the QUORUM statement. Lancet 354: 1896–1900

Mulrow CD 1995 Rationale for systematic reviews. In: Chalmers I, Altman DG (eds) Systematic reviews. British Medical Journal Books, London, p. 1

Schulz FK, Chalmers I, Hayes RJ, Altman DG 1995 Empirical evidence of bias: dimensions of methodological quality associated with estimates of treatment effects in controlled trials. Journal of the American Medical Association 273: 408–412

Slavin RE 1986 Best-evidence synthesis: an alternative to meta-analysis and traditional reviews. Educational Research 15: 9–11

Sterne JAC, Egger M, Davey Smith G 2001 Investigating and dealing with publication and other bias. In: Egger M, Davey Smith G, Altman DG (eds) Systematic reviews in healthcare: meta-analysis in context. British Medical Journal Books, London

Van Tulder MW, Irnich D 1999 Journal Club commentaries on Ernst E, White AR: Acupuncture for low back pain. Fordizinsch Komplementärmed 6: 155–157

Van Tulder MW, Cherkin DC, Berman B, Lao L, Koes BW 1999 Acupuncture for low back pain. The Cochrane Library, Issue 1. Update Software, Oxford (CD-ROM)

White AR, Resch KL, Ernst E 1997 Smoking cessation with acupuncture? A 'best evidence synthesis'. Forsch Komplementärmedizin 4: 102–105

FURTHER READING

Introductions to systematic reviews

Chalmers I, Altman DG (eds) 1995 Systematic reviews. British Medical Journal, London

Cooper H, Hegdes LV (eds) 1994 The handbook of research synthesis. Russel Sage Foundation, New York

Egger M, Davey Smith G, Altman DG (eds) 2001 Systematic reviews in healthcare: meta-analysis in context. British Medical Journal Books, London

Light RJ, Pillemer DB 1984 Summing up – the science of reviewing research. Harvard University Press, Cambridge, MA

Mulrow C, Cook D (eds) 1998 Systematic reviews – synthesis of best evidence for health care decisions. American College of Physicians, Philadelphia

Mulrow C, Oxman A (eds) 1997 The Cochrane Collaboration handbook. The Cochrane Library. Update Software, Oxford (CD-ROM)

Pettiti DB 1994 Meta-analysis, decision analysis and cost-effectiveness analysis. Oxford University Press, Oxford

Guidelines for critical appraisal of review articles

Greenhalgh T 1998 How to read a paper. British Medical Journal Books, London

Oxman AD, Cook DJ, Guyatt GH 1994 User's guides to the medical literature. VI. How to use an overview. Journal of American Medical Association 272: 1367–1371

12

Economic evaluation of complementary therapies

John Brazier   Anne Morgan

INTRODUCTION

Complementary therapies are increasingly available on the NHS (Zollman & Vickers 1999) and are beginning to compete with conventional medicine for scarce NHS resources. It has been suggested that complementary therapies may be cheaper than conventional treatments in many situations or where there is an extra cost, it offers good value for money. These claims need to be supported by evidence if they are to be accepted by health-care providers. Australia and Canada, for example, have produced guidelines on conducting economic evaluations of new technologies. In the UK, the National Institute for Clinical Excellence (NICE) makes recommendations on the use of new and established technologies and prepares guidance for the NHS. Its recommendations are based on a full appraisal of the clinical effectiveness *and* the cost effectiveness of interventions. The NHS is expected to use NICE guidelines to ensure that decisions to adopt one therapy rather than another will promote an efficient and equitable use of NHS resources (Box 12.1). Health economics plays an important role in this process because it is concerned with efficiency and equity and has a set of techniques for assessing relative efficiency by comparing the costs *and* benefits of competing alternatives, known as economic evaluation.

There are a variety of techniques available for conducting economic evaluations in complementary therapy studies. Despite the methodological problems in this area the goal of performing a full economic evaluation is within the reach of most health service researchers. This chapter describes the basic principles of economic evaluation, the different types of evaluation and the circumstances under which the various analytical tools are appropriate. In addition, consideration is given to some of the practical issues in undertaking an economic evaluation.

Box 12.1 Some key terms

Economic efficiency is achieved when the maximum benefit is obtained from given NHS resources

Equity is concerned with how fairly health-care costs and benefits are distributed

---

WHAT IS AN ECONOMIC EVALUATION?

An economic evaluation compares both costs and outcomes of two or more alternative therapies (Drummond et al 1997). To report costs alone is not an economic evaluation. At the same time, most forms of economic evaluation only make sense where one intervention is compared with the next best alternative. The purpose is to provide information to aid decision making about which therapies to adopt within a fixed health-care budget.

THE PRINCIPLES OF ECONOMIC EVALUATION

To perform an economic evaluation the following steps are recommended by Drummond et al (1996). The **study question** needs to be important in terms of resource implications, it should consider both costs and outcomes of the competing alternatives, and the perspective of the study should be clearly stated: that is, the viewpoint (NHS, patients or society) from which the evaluation is undertaken. The **alternative interventions** to be included for comparison in the study need to be fully described and the choices justified (e.g. is it really the next best alternative?).

The type or types of **economic evaluation** (see Box 12.2) to be undertaken must be stated and justified. There are at least four to choose from though in practice it may be necessary to plan for more than one (see below). The techniques of economic evaluation mainly differ in the way in which health benefits are measured and hence the policy questions they are designed to answer. Cost-minimization analysis (CMA) and cost-effectiveness analysis (CEA) implicitly assume that a particular health-care objective is worthwhile and attempt to answer the question

---

Box 12.2 Economic evaluation techniques

Cost-minimization analysis seeks to establish which is the least cost alternative, but is only a technique of economic evaluation if it can be shown that the alternatives achieve identical outcomes.

Cost-effectiveness analysis considers what is the best method of achieving a given objective usually measured in 'natural' units and presents results in terms of cost per unit of effect (e.g. cost per positive cancer detected or cost per symptom-free day).

Cost-utility analysis compares the costs of alternative health-care programs with their utility, usually measured in terms of quality-adjusted life-years.

Cost-benefit analysis compares the benefits with costs of a health-care program, where all the benefits are valued in money terms, including health improvement.

'What is the most efficient way of achieving this goal?'. Cost-utility analysis (CUA), on the other hand, can be used to inform the question 'What is the most efficient way of spending a given health-care budget?'. And hence whether or not NHS resources should be diverted towards one intervention and if so, how much. Finally, there is cost-benefit analysis (CBA), which in principle can answer the big question 'Is this program worthwhile for society as a whole?'.

Although not recognized as a technique of economic evaluation, there is a more pragmatic approach known as cost-consequences analysis (CCA) which simply presents the costs and benefits of competing alternatives without attempting a formal analysis as described in Box 12.2. This is often the case where health outcomes, although clinically important, are not suited to a formal economic analysis.

Costs need to be described in terms of the resources consumed by each intervention, such as the number of therapy sessions, and the value of those resources such as therapist fees, rental of premises and the price of any prescribed treatment. Quantities of resources used and their unit costs should be reported separately and the methods for estimating each need to be stated clearly. Costing will be discussed in more detail under Practical Issues.

For many reasons individuals prefer receiving benefits earlier rather than later and delaying costs for as long as possible. It is important, therefore, that the **time period** over which costs and benefits are measured is clearly stated and justified. Costs and benefits often need to be adjusted by a procedure known as **discounting** when they are spread over a period of years. To illustrate how discounting works, Drummond et al (1997) use as an example the case where two programs require different outlays over 3 years, as shown below.

Year	Cost of program A (£000s)	Cost of program B (£000s)
1	5	15
2	10	10
3	15	4

Simply adding the two cost streams shows program B to have a lower cost than A. However, by adjusting for the differential timing of costs by discounting future costs to present values, program B is shown to be more costly than A. If P = present value, F_n = future cost at year n and r = the discount rate, then

$$P = \frac{F_1}{(1+r)} + \frac{F_2}{(1+r)^2} + \frac{F_3}{(1+r)^3}$$

If the discount rate is 5% the present value of A = £26.79 and the present value of B = £26.81. For a discussion of choice of discount rate for use in adjusting costs and benefits, see Drummond et al (1997).

Consideration needs to be given to any **uncertainty** surrounding data estimates of costs and benefits. For example, if estimates are taken from a sample of the population, standard statistical methods can be used. If on the other hand cost data have been extrapolated, sensitivity analysis is more appropriate. This approach examines the impact on the evaluation results of using a range of estimates.

Although a randomized controlled trial is often regarded as the gold standard for producing results on clinical efficacy, it is not always the most appropriate vehicle for conducting economic evaluation. A trial may not collect results for long enough to assess the full costs or benefits of an intervention or the artificial context of a trial may be unrealistic. In these circumstances, **modeling** can be used to fill in the gaps and to handle the inevitable uncertainties which exist for many of the key parameters.

The **evaluation results** should be presented in a clear and generalizable way. A decision maker is not usually concerned with all or nothing but options for incremental expansion or contraction of program. In other words, the question is likely to be 'What would be the costs (and benefits) of having a little more or a little less of a service in this area?'. A primary care group, for example, might be considering adding chiropractic, acupuncture or physiotherapy sessions to existing services for patients presenting with low back pain. The additional costs of introducing these sessions will vary with location depending on local factors such as the supply of relevant practitioners and existing demand for their services. Consequently, the results of an economic evaluation undertaken in one location cannot be universally applied to all settings. It is important therefore that disaggregated data should be presented along with summary measures such as cost-effectiveness ratios.

PRACTICAL ISSUES IN AN ECONOMIC EVALUATION

Study question

Care needs to be given to formulating the study question. Once it is established that the resource implications of the new intervention are such that a full economic evaluation is warranted, the alternative therapies for comparison must be selected. A new treatment, for example, is often compared with the most widely used alternative, although the most cost-effective alternative available is the preferred comparator. Complementary therapies are often added onto conventional therapies so it may be appropriate to compare a standard therapy, for back pain for example, with and without additional therapy, such as acupuncture. If in practice there is currently no service provided for the condition in question then the comparator should be a 'do nothing' option. This may well be the case for certain conditions in many developing countries. Economists recommend that a societal perspective be adopted when considering costs and benefits so that the values of all are used, even though ethical arguments can be put forward for using the values of patients or taxpayers only. This makes the perspective of the study explicit and also allows separate analyses to be performed by societal subgroups such as the NHS, patients or social services.

Choosing the economic evaluation technique

Although it is recommended that the type of economic evaluation be chosen at the outset, it is often difficult to decide on the appropriate technique until the results are known. For example, a cost-effectiveness analysis may change to a cost-

---

Box 12.3 Cost definitions

Opportunity cost is the value of that which must be given up to acquire or achieve something.
Marginal cost (or benefit) is the cost (or benefit) of the next unit of service provided.

---

minimization analysis if the health outcomes are found to be the same for both interventions. Similarly, if two interventions are found to have similar costs and intervention A is more effective than intervention B then intervention A is obviously dominant and should be chosen. It is more often the case, however, that the new intervention will be found to be both more effective and more costly and in such situations a CUA or CBA is required, though a less formal way of dealing with the trade-offs would be a cost-consequences approach.

Costing

Any decision to use resources to satisfy a particular health-care demand, such as acupuncture for low back pain, involves sacrificing the opportunity of using the same resources to satisfy other health-care demands, such as primary care counseling services for depression. It is this sacrifice or 'opportunity cost' that economic evaluation aims to estimate and compare with treatment benefits.

For all economic evaluations, costs must be identified, measured and valued for each alternative therapy. The identification of costs will be determined by the perspective of the study: that is, the point of view from which the study is undertaken. It is usually recommended to take a societal view but a more limited viewpoint is easier for costing purposes and legitimate provided it is made explicit. All identified resources need to be measured in natural units such as number and length of acupuncture sessions, number of general practitioner surgery visits or number of days taken off work with back pain. Ideally these resources would then be valued using their opportunity cost. This requires, among other things, the marginal cost of the resources to be used rather than the average cost. The marginal cost, or cost of the next unit of service provided, may be quite different from the average which is simply total cost divided by quantity. The average cost of a day in hospital, for example, may give a very misleading impression of the consequences of reducing length of stay for a particular group of patients. Market prices are often poorly related to actual cost. However, average values, including market values (such as therapists' fees), are often used instead for practical reasons and can only be approximations. Table 12.1 shows how Thomas et al (1999) plan to measure and value resources in their study into acupuncture for low back pain.

The first column identifies the resources to be measured. Since this study is taking a societal perspective the relevant costs are thought to be those borne by the NHS and patients. In the second and third columns the measurement of resources is described. For example, the number and length of acupuncture sessions provide will be quantified using records kept by acupuncturists. Columns four and five describe the valuation method, which in the case of acupuncture sessions will be standard charges, and the data source for these charges will be the practitioners themselves.

Table 12.1 Measurement and valuation of resources used by patients in the trial (from Thomas et al 1999)

Resource	Measurement	Data source	Valuation method	Data source
Acupuncture	No. and length of sessions	Records kept by acupuncturists	Standard charges	Practitioners in study, supplemented by data from elsewhere
Primary care				
GP consultation	No. of visits to and by GPs	GP notes	Cost per contact	Netten & Dennett 1996
Drugs	Drugs prescribed	"	Cost of drugs to NHS	British National Formulary
Hospital				
Outpatient clinic attendances	No. of attendances	Patient questionnaire schedule and hospital records	Cost per attendance	Local hospital finance departments
Physiotherapy	No. of sessions	"	Cost per session	"
A & E attendances	No. of attendances	"	Cost per attendance	"
Admissions	Length of stay	"	Cost per diem by speciality	"
Other NHS services				
Physiotherapy	No. of sessions	Patient questionnaire	Cost per session	Netten & Dennett 1996
Non-NHS services				
Chiropractic	"	"	"	Data from national survey estimates (publication in preparation)
Osteopathy	"	"	"	"
Acupuncture	"	"	"	"
Patient time				
Treatment time	Time spent using services	Patient questionnaire	Cost per minute	Dept of Transport
Work time	Time off work	"	Gross earnings plus employment costs	National average earnings

Measures of benefit

The economic techniques described earlier differ mainly in terms of the way in which benefits are measured. A simple cost-minimization analysis is required when health outcomes are the same. A North American study, for example, compared outcomes and costs of care for acute low back pain among patients of primary care practitioners, chiropractors and orthopedic surgeons (Carey et al 1995). The authors found that while clinical outcomes (time to functional recovery, return to work and complete recovery) were similar among the various practitioners, health service costs were lowest for patients seen by primary care practitioners. Unfortunately, only health service costs were considered. Furthermore, patients were not randomly assigned to practitioners and consequently the validity of the clinical results is questionable. Cost-minimization analysis can only confidently be performed when good evidence of equal effectiveness exists.

A cost-effectiveness analysis requires one unambiguous objective of treatment alternatives such as years of life gained. In studies of complementary therapies problems arise in finding a clear objective measure of outcome since many of the conditions for which complementary therapies are sought are often chronic rather than life threatening. Health-related quality of life measures are more relevant to such patient groups than biomedical measures. However, many measures of health-related quality of life are not suitable for use in formal economic evaluations (Brazier & Dixon 1995).

Economists have attempted to solve this problem by combining quality and quantity of life in a single index of health benefit, such as the quality-adjusted life-year (QALY) to allow cost-utility analysis to be performed. In theory this is an extremely useful technique for investigating complementary therapies: that is, where health-related quality of life, rather than mortality, is the most important outcome (Drummond et al 1997). In addition, one of the reasons CUA was developed was to address the problem of having more than one outcome of interest. To produce QALYs, individuals' preferences or values are used to score health states. Health state values can be elicited directly from patients but this requires substantial time and cognitive effort and many clinicians believe it creates an unnecessary burden on patients. Another alternative, and one which requires little effort, is a preference-based measure, which is a standardized health state classification with a preexisting set of valuations.

These instruments are not without their critics but methodological research in this field is continuing and is aimed at improving the practicality, validity and reliability of instruments available to researchers (Brazier & Deverill 1999). Thomas et al (1999) are using the Bodily Pain dimension of the General Health Static Profile (SF-36) as the primary outcome measure, in their study of acupuncture for low back pain. In addition, there will also be an opportunity to estimate QALYs from the larger SF-36. Alternatively, researchers can develop their own descriptions of health states or health experience following an intervention through qualitative patient interviews if questionnaires do not include aspects of the illness or treatment which are thought to be important to patients. This may be useful in investigating complementary therapies where, for example, processes of care may have a considerable influence on patient preferences (Brown & Sculpher 1999).

Table 12.2   Measures of benefit

Technique	Benefits
Cost-minimization analysis	Requires outcomes to be shown to be the same
Cost-effectiveness analysis	Requires one unambiguous health outcome
Cost-utility analysis	Requires a single index of health benefit, e.g. QALY
Cost-benefit analysis	Requires all benefits to be valued in monetary terms

By using the same unit of account, such as money, to value both benefits and costs CBA is conceptually the most powerful technique in economic evaluation. In practice, however, the problem is how to value length and quality of life in money terms. The values individuals place on goods and services are normally indicated by their maximum willingness to pay for them. In health care, however, market values are regarded as inadequate measures of society's values. Economists have therefore either attempted to adjust market values for these imperfections or conducted 'willingness to pay' experiments where individuals are asked what they would be willing to pay for a specified improvement (Drummond et al 1997). The main criticisms of this approach are the hypothetical nature of the question and that responses will depend in part on existing income distributions, which the NHS may wish to ignore. It could, for example, lead to the 'diseases of affluence' receiving a higher weighting because of the higher incomes of sufferers.

EXISTING ECONOMIC EVALUATIONS OF COMPLEMENTARY THERAPY

A literature search of EMBASE, CAM Citation Index and NHS Centre for Reviews and Dissemination found very few economic evaluations of complementary therapies. Most studies estimated the use (and sometimes the cost) of complementary therapies in general or for specific conditions. The reader should be aware that often the terms cost-effectiveness and cost-benefit analysis appear in the title of journal articles to describe studies which are limited to costings which is not the way they are used in health economics (see definitions in Box 12.2).

Despite methodological shortcomings Carey et al (1995) have described the costs and consequences of different interventions for back pain. Because outcomes were similar for all interventions it was, in effect, a cost-minimization analysis. Meade et al (1995) found that patients of chiropractors showed a 29% improvement in the total score of the Oswestry Low Back Pain Questionnaire compared to those receiving outpatient management but that higher proportions of chiropractic patients sought further treatment for their back pain. Unfortunately, no attempt was made to attach costs to the additional treatment and hence no economic evaluation performed.

CONCLUSION

The recent reforms in the NHS have meant that health economics has played and will continue to play an important part in evaluating new and existing technologies. Given that many complementary therapies are now being provided by the NHS, these alternative treatments must compete with conventional therapies for scarce resources. Economic evaluation in health care is a way of comparing costs and benefits of treatments. The chosen technique will depend on the question posed and the study results. Cost-benefit analysis measures benefits in monetary units and can be used to compare programs within the NHS and beyond. Given the difficulty in valuing benefits in such a way, health economists have mostly settled for addressing what are regarded as lower level efficiency questions. They make an initial assumption that the program is worthwhile and go on to consider the best means of achieving a given objective. Cost-effectiveness and cost-minimization analyses quantify health outcomes in natural units, which are, for the most part, objective biomedical measures. The limitation of these types of study is that they can only compare interventions with the same clinical outcomes. Cost-utility studies, on the other hand, use a single index measure of health outcome that combines quality and length of life. These allow programs to be assessed and, in theory, ranked according to their cost per marginal QALY gained. There are practical and methodological difficulties involved in measuring benefits for economic evaluations. However, these difficulties are not insurmountable and should not preclude the researcher from designing and carrying out full economic evaluations of complementary therapies.

Economic evaluation is a framework for systematically examining the costs and benefits of options and explicitly taking account of the necessary value judgments, as well as technical judgments, in choosing between them. This approach would seem particularly relevant to the expanding area of the technology of complementary medicine, with the large array of alternative means to help people achieve a better life.

Learning points

- **Economics** is concerned with making the most of society's resources.
- The **opportunity cost** of an activity is the sacrifice in terms of the benefits foregone from not allocating resources to the next best activity.
- **Complementary therapies** must compete with conventional therapies for scarce NHS resources.
- **Economic evaluation** is a comparative study of the costs and benefits of health-care interventions.
- The main difference between **economic evaluation techniques** is in the measure of benefit.

REFERENCES

Brazier J, Deverill M 1999 Obtaining the 'Q' in QALYs: a comparison of five multi-attribute utility scales. ScHARR discussion paper 99/1. University of Sheffield
Brazier J, Dixon S 1995 The use of condition specific outcome measures in economic appraisal. Health Economics 4: 255–264
Brown J, Sculpher M 1999 Benefit valuation in economic evaluation of cancer therapies: a systematic review of the published literature. Pharmacoeconomics 16(1): 17–31
Carey TS, Garrett J, Jackman A et al 1995 The outcomes and costs of care for acute low back pain among patients seen by primary care practitioners, chiropractors and orthopaedic surgeons. New England Journal of Medicine 333(14): 913–917

Drummond M, Jefferson T, on behalf of the BMJ Economic Evaluation Working Party 1996 Guidelines for authors and peer reviewers of economic submissions to the BMJ. British Medical Journal 313: 275–283

Drummond M, O'Brien B, Stoddart GL, Torrance GW 1997 Methods for the economic evaluation of health care programmes, 2nd edn. Oxford University Press, Oxford

Meade TW, Dyer S, Brawne W, Frank AO 1995 Randomised comparison of chiropractic and hospital outpatient management for low back pain: results from extended follow up. British Medical Journal 311: 349–351

Thomas K, Fitter M, Brazier J et al 1999 Longer term clinical and economic benefits of offering acupuncture to patients with chronic low back pain assessed as suitable for primary care management. Complementary Therapies in Medicine 7: 91–100

Zollman C, Vickers A 1999 ABC of complementary medicine. What is complementary medicine? British Medical Journal 319: 693–696

FURTHER READING

Drummond M, O'Brien B, Stoddart GL, Torrance GW 1997 Methods for the economic evaluation of health care programmes. Oxford University Press, Oxford.

Mooney G 1991 Economics, medicine and health care, 2nd edn. Harvester/Wheatsheaf, Brighton

Thomas KJ, Fitter M, Brazier J et al 1999 Longer term clinical and economic benefits of offering acupuncture to patients with chronic low back pain assessed as suitable for primary care management. Complementary Therapies in Medicine 7: 91–100

The therapies

This section deals with a broad range of very specific therapies. The aim of each chapter is to review the research literature within a specific therapeutic area and then to draw from that information inferences and suggestions as to how research in areas such as herbal medicine or homeopathy can and should be developed. The second section draws on the principles outlined in the first but allows the authors to develop much more specific strategies about future research within each specific therapy.

Herbal medicine

Simon Mills

INTRODUCTION

Herbal medicines, or phytomedicines (to give them their modern European name), are closer to conventional drugs than other complementary medical approaches. Herbs are traditional pharmaceuticals: the very word 'drug' derives from old German and Dutch words for 'dried herb'. In many countries phytomedicines are even orthodox pharmaceuticals, prescribed alongside modern drugs by doctors and dispensed or supplied primarily by pharmacists. It is only in the USA among developed countries that legislation has established herbs as 'dietary supplements' and thus removed them formally from the medical scene.

All this means that of complementary treatments, herbal medicines are perhaps the most obvious to regulating authorities and in Europe especially (but not in the USA) are subject to the same legislative controls and standards of quality, safety and efficacy as other medicines. Manufacturers of herbal medicinal products in Europe therefore have long been used to negotiating their research agenda in the orthodox forum.

Long experience of herbal medicine in a modern pharmaceutical culture, however, confirms that they have particular distinguishing features. They do not fit exactly into the modern framework. Herbal medicines consist of many chemical constituents with complex pharmacological effects on the body. They have been used continuously for many decades or centuries, often in ways much different from those of modern medical prescribing.

There is often serious discomfort in meeting the research requirements of legislators. While new clinical trials are being published at an increasing rate and there has long been a surprising quantity of studies in German and other European scientific literature not easily accessed in American or English databases, there are still huge gaps in the evidence base and most clinical studies are judged as not ideally rigorous. For proprietary herbal products, the efficacy requirement is substantial.

THE FORMAL REQUIREMENTS OF EFFICACY

Although preliminary assessments of efficacy can be obtained through the results of in vitro testing and experiments on animals, authorities licencing new medicines for public use require evidence of their effect on human beings. Only carefully planned clinical trials that clearly minimize experimental bias are able to satisfy these requirements.

Most herbal remedies can call on a tradition of popular use which has in practice allowed licence holders to submit relevant bibliographic evidence in reviewing their earlier historical 'licences of right'. Nevertheless, this has been a reluctant concession by licencing authorities and in reviews of licences there is the prospect that additional evidence will be required. This would be at the less demanding Phase IV or post-marketing level of scrutiny (EC 1989a) but still involves conventional clinical trials.

The requirements for the conduct of any clinical trials have been clearly defined by European regulators.

A clinical trial is any systematic study of medicinal products in human subjects whether in patients or non-patient volunteers in order to discover or verify the effects of and/or identify any adverse reaction to investigational products, and/or study their absorption, distribution, metabolism and excretion in order to ascertain the efficacy and safety of the products . . . Evaluation of the application for marketing authorization shall be based on clinical trials . . . designed to determine the efficacy and safety of the product under normal conditions of use . . . Therapeutic advantages must outweigh potential risks. (EC 1989a)

All test procedures shall correspond to the state of scientific progress at the time and shall be validated procedures; results of the validation studies shall be provided. (EC 1989b)

The clinical particulars to be provided pursuant to point 8 of Article 4 (2) of Directive 65/65/EEC must enable a sufficiently well-founded and scientifically valid opinion to be formed as to whether the medicinal product satisfies the criteria governing the granting of marketing authorization. Consequently, an essential requirement is that the results of all clinical trials should be communicated, both favourable and unfavourable. (EC 1989c)

Clinical statements concerning the efficacy or safety of a medicinal product under normal conditions of use which are not scientifically substantiated cannot be accepted as valid evidence. (EC 1991)

METHODOLOGICAL DISCRETION IN ESTABLISHING EFFICACY FOR HERBS

It is not the researchers or the suppliers of herbal medicinal products who can determine how they establish their case. Discretion as to the validity or credibility of any research method rests with three main bodies: the licencing authority, the ethics committee and the independent author of the expert report.

The licencing authority has had its position set out above and reiterated in the establishment of the European Agency for the Evaluation of Medicinal Products (EMEA) (EC 1993): the EMEA is to adopt 'transparent' procedures in licencing medicines, to give detailed reasons for all negative decisions, to grant appeal rights and to publish decisions. (EC 1990a) It will interpret the regulations, in conjunction with medical and scientific advice, so as to establish 'a standard by which clinical trials are designed, implemented and reported so that there is a public assurance that the data are credible, and that the rights, integrity and confidentiality of subjects are protected'. (EC 1990b) The establishment of a Working Group on Herbal Medicinal Products within the EMEA has refocused the conventional procedures on herbs rather than amended them.

The ethics committee is an essential referee in all research involving human subjects. It has a mandatory role in protecting the interests of subjects and other study participants. The role of the ethics committee is also firmly entrenched in the appropriate legislation as 'an independent body, constituted by medical professionals and non-medical members, whose responsibility is to verify that the safety, integrity and human rights of the subjects participating in a particular trial are protected, thereby providing public reassurance . . .' (EC 1990b). Subjects must not be entered into the trial until the relevant ethics committee(s) has issued its favorable opinion on the procedures and documentation (EC 1990b); it is unethical to enlist the cooperation of human subjects in trials which are not adequately designed.

The expert report has an important role before the licencing authority, determined by Article 2 of European Directive 75/319/EEC. There are several required for each medicine licence application, including for clinical documentation. This latter 'shall consist of a critical evaluation of the investigations carried out on animals and human beings and bring out all the data relevant for evaluation . . .'. It is produced by a suitably qualified and experienced (and formally independent) person and 'the pertinence of the different trials to the assessment of safety and the validity of methods of evaluation shall be discussed in the expert report' (EC 1991).

CONTROLLED CLINICAL TRIALS FOR HERBAL MEDICINES

There is little doubt that orthodox evidence requirements are appropriate for most herbal medicines consumed by the public. Over-the-counter (OTC) herbal use in Europe far outstrips practitioner prescription, probably by a factor of more than 20:1 (IMS/Phytogold 1998). For researching OTC label indications for discrete medicinal products, in which individual responses to remedies are not the critical issue, the double-blind controlled clinical trial is clearly the most applicable method. In addition, as the 'patient' is in many cases not being diagnosed professionally and is determining his or her own treatment and prognosis, self-assessment questionnaires are often an appropriate measure of progress. These are not expensive to administer. Also, as this is often 'outpatient' medicine research costs can be saved as close clinical supervision may not always be necessary thoughout the trial.

There are, however, practical problems in pursuing good clinical research in herbal medicine.

• Herbal medicine in the West can boast few teaching hospitals or research institutes, nor support from public resources. Industrial investment has been limited to a few larger manufacturers used to working in a pharmaceutical culture. In most parts of the sector the necessary infrastructure is lacking. Neither can the costs of undertaking research studies easily be justified commercially: it is difficult to patent herbs and the size of the market for any individual product is only occasionally comparable to that for any patentable conventional drug.

• The indications often claimed for herbal medicines include many without robust outcome measures. As many are destined for the self-medication OTC market, they are by definition directed at lesser degrees of morbidity where hard measures are elusive. By contrast, most synthetic OTC medicines on the market have 'switched' from prescription status and have acquired their efficacy evidence on harder clinical indications and in hospital or similar settings. Without hard or acceptably validated outcome measures, with more variable and lower grade symptoms among the patient population, with a greater likelihood of self-limiting or other spontaneously changing conditions, clear treatment effects are thereby harder to establish. The result is often the need to recruit large patient samples and to devise particularly artificial exclusion criteria to constrain sample variability. All this places extra logistic demands on those wishing to set up effective clinical trials for these products.

• Herbs are complex medicines, occupying an unusual position as being medicines with many of the characteristics of vegetables. Being a complex of pharmacologically active chemicals, the whole package will have different properties from that of any single constituent acting alone. Knowing the action of the latter will not itself be predictive of the effect of the former, particularly if the experimental evidence is based on work done on laboratory animals (see below). It is therefore rare to find the satisfactory preclinical evidence often required by ethics committees for approval of major clinical studies.

Although contributing only a small part to the public's use of herbal medicines, the herbal practitioner, or phytotherapist, notes further limitations of the controlled clinical study. Such practitioners may emphasize more strongly than in conventional medicine the individuality of their treatments and often mix a number of individual herbs in a prescription. They might point out that conventional clinical trials involve the homogenization of the patient population so that only an average effect is confirmed. Clinical trial data will help with, but still not answer, the basic question 'Is this drug going to be good for this patient?'. It is also likely that genuinely important benefits for a minority of the population will be overlooked.

There are also certain cases where satisfactory blinding will always be difficult. In particular, it will always be impossible to blind for the effects of bitters or other prominent-tasting agents on oral consumption; these have played important parts in the claims of traditional herbal medicine. There will as always be a role for the good single-blind study, especially if other elements are rigorously controlled.

Nevertheless, the controlled clinical trial is a notably flexible instrument. With an adequate investment structure a significant section of the herbal medicinal market could be clearly evaluated in the public interest. The increasing rate of publication of rigorous clinical trials on herbal products in the scientific literature highlights the potential for a stronger evidence base in conventional terms.

THE MEASUREMENT OF TRANSIENT CLINICAL EFFECTS

There is one application of the controlled clinical trial that could be particularly appropriate for assessing the impact of traditional herbal treatments: observing physiological responses to treatments in human subjects rather than direct effects on morbidity.

Traditional views of herbal remedies emphasize their primary influence on transient body functions, e.g. they are classed as diaphoretics, expectorants, circulatory stimulants, diuretics, digestive stimulants, laxatives and so on. In other words, contrary to common belief, many herbs may have almost immediate results on the body. It is possible to devise methods by which such effects can be detected. Activity on biological markers, physiological functions and tissue or fluid constitution can be monitored directly in healthy or morbid populations and could provide much useful information on the effects on the body of herbal products. With advances in non-invasive monitoring technologies it is possible to conceive of important trials in human subjects, in both observational and controlled studies.

Against such ideas, it has been pointed out that measures of efficacy tend to be based on a medicine's effects on morbidity or mortality. 'Surrogate parameters' may be acceptable but would restrict possible indications as labeled claims. It would need to be argued in each individual case, with the support of other medical evidence, that a verified effect in changing some physiological parameter would be likely to have an effect on morbidity or mortality.

METHODOLOGICAL ALTERNATIVES FOR CLINICAL TRIALS IN HERBAL MEDICINE: THE ESCOP DEBATE

Although the above section focuses on conventional research methodologies, the actual submissions for herbal medicines will inevitably include a broad range of other evidence. As well as 'pivotal' randomized controlled clinical trials there is potential scope seen for accumulating other studies as supporting evidence, perhaps enabling the number of different pivotal trials to be reduced in any licence application, especially given that these are for well-established traditional remedies.

As part of a wide-ranging research program funded by the European Commission between 1992 and 1996 and conducted by ESCOP (the European Scientific Cooperative on Phytotherapy), a review of efficacy requirements was conducted. Participants in the review represent accomplished authors of published research literature on phytomedicines, in toxicology, pharmacognosy and phytochemistry as well as in clinical efficacy studies. In a wide-ranging brief, these discussions also included consideration of alternatives to the conventional randomized control trial. The following section on three alternative clinical trial options summarizes responses to a proforma survey, as well as a series of wide-ranging discussions about research trial methodologies (Mills 1998).

Historical controlled trials

The fact that phytomedicines often derive from a long tradition of use has led many to consider ways to apply historical use to modern research (this topic is referred to later in this chapter).

Historical controls are harder to establish as reliable.

- Baseline and clearly defined outcome data to establish treatment effect are usually absent.
- There are seldom concurrent comparisons recorded between treatments.
- Analyses of historical control studies have shown that the placebo effect is consistently underestimated.
- By definition it is hard to correct the deficiencies in historical data. Much more promising is to start again with such observations, to generate 'new' historical data by rigorously designing prospective observational studies.

Observational studies

In some cases, attempting controlled clinical studies may prove fruitless. Such cases include, for example:

- rare diseases
- where there are many clinical complexities
- for cases where blinding is impossible
- rigorous scrutiny of possible adverse effects.

In these circumstances careful observations of non-controlled clinical events may be the best or even only feasible source of evidence.

There is another way in which observational studies are an appropriate method for the study of herbal medicines. A persistent tradition is that these medicines may support self-corrective functions in the body, perhaps more readily than synthetic pharmaceuticals. This claim cannot be validated but modern insights into the behavior of complex dynamic systems suggest that new perspectives on the behavior of the human being as an ecosystem may be productive. It is apparent in this case that different research methodologies are required. These should:

- have regard to global behavior of the system rather than particular variables in isolation
- aim to measure quantifiable components of health, rather than of morbidity, mortality or other indicators of disease
- involve minimal intervention.

Again observational rather than controlled studies are appropriate. Non-invasive monitoring of physiological functions may be applied (as above), perhaps coupled with patient self-rated questionnaires, clinical observations of overall behavior and epidemiologic methods, to establish as far as possible what actually happens to living patients when they seek treatments.

Routine collection of patient and clinical data at a teaching clinic is feasible, for example, including self-rating questionnaires for general health and target conditions, perhaps combined with a number of other non-invasive observations, compared with general remission rates. With computer technology there are precedents to show that it is possible to accrue considerable quantities of useful observational data by involving patients and practitioners in simultaneous recording of treatments and questionnaire-derived outcomes (using simple touch-screen check-box entry forms, for example).

To satisfy basic standards of research rigor for observational studies, however, it is important formally to set up clear experimental criteria prospectively, as follows.

- A protocol with full prospective description of the study is required before studies are commenced.
- There should be no bias in subject selection; during a given period of time all the subjects meeting the conditions should be admitted to the project.
- Clear description of the condition is mandatory (using quantitative and semi-quantitative parameters).
- Only one treatment may be provided for each diagnosis at a time or only one treatment may be used per indication.
- The description of the herb must be precise; the same applies to the duration of therapy and dosage. All drugs and treatments administered to the subject concomitantly (including treatments of other diseases) must be recorded.
- In addition to efficacy, compliance and adverse events must be documented.
- The observations are to be made by the same person prior to and after treatment.
- Incomplete records should be discarded.
- It should be possible to compare empirical reports to other reports on the same subject.
- Therefore all terms should be carefully defined and reproducible and validated standard computer or other forms should be used.

Although it is difficult to establish cause and effect in observational or field studies, or specifically to separate specific from non-specific treatment effects, there are a number of ways in which observational studies could productively be used in herbal research. For example:

- to set up controlled studies by monitoring matched groups where blinding or other ideals are impracticable
- to have individual practitioners generating longitudinal case studies, with standardized report forms, to address the question usually ignored in controlled clinical studies – the effect of long-term treatments
- to audit clinical practice and generate new hypotheses; with computerized data input (as above) and sufficient quantities of data, even complex and multiple prescription patterns can be evaluated
- to generate safety data.

Such information, however, suffers from one clear problem: it is rarely subject to independent validation or review, so includes partisan judgments. Its use without supporting controlled data in determining efficacy of treatment is therefore limited. Nevertheless, in combination with other trials, such studies could provide very useful information.

Single case studies

The main charge against single case studies is that they cannot credibly select out real effects from confusing variables, specific from non-specific treatment effects and so on. Further investigation of such research, however, shows both that it can have more credibility than might be supposed and that it is not a soft option.

A good single case study design can be very rigorous. It includes providing as many points of view on the event as possible, clarifying operational definitions and recycling observed data around the researchers (including the patient as co-researcher) for checking and possible refutation. It is possible to conduct double-blind, placebo-controlled studies in a series of such individual case studies with each patient being his or her control. These could allow a useful database of reliable case histories to be assembled over the years, as both an educational and a research exercise.

Perhaps most importantly, the single case study is the raw caseload of each practitioner. A routine of rigorously collating studies is a commendable continuing education exercise that may encourage practitioners to become more active in the generation of efficacy data.

USING TRADITIONAL EVIDENCE

The persistent theme running through any discussion on the efficacy of herbal medicine is that it has been used consistently over centuries and millennia. It is claimed with some justification that at least some value will have been distilled out by this vast store of human bioassay data, especially as there would have been little room for sentiment and idealism in the life-and-death situations that prevailed through most of herbal use.

However, without a rigorous screening the record of traditional use can appear as little more than a motley primitive hotchpotch of folk fancies. The review of historical methodologies highlights some limitations but the power of cultural placebo alone renders any individual observation almost worthless. What is needed is the identification of themes, a structure for assessing traditional claims. Fortunately this is now possible.

The pharmaceutical pillars of traditional herbal medicine

Clinical insight into the traditional record leads to the realization that from the very earliest and most primitive accounts of herb use, humans classified the plant material into relatively consistent pharmaceutical categories. The classification was based on subjective properties of taste or appearance and the immediate impact they made on consumption. These categories, encountered repeatedly in the ethnobotanical records, became the basis of core therapeutic principles in the classic texts of China, India, Graeco-Roman Europe, Islam and almost all other written traditions. Many of these categories survive today as recognizable phytochemical groups. Below they are referred to as 'archetypal' plant constituents. They constitute a primal pharmaceutics of surprising potency. It had to be: there was usually no other choice. Going to a traditional herbal practitioner was often a most robust experience!

The pharmaceutical principles of traditional medicine provide a potentially robust correlation with modern phytomedical research, provided the latter can be linked to these phytochemical subgroups; in other words, provided both the scientific and the traditional data relate to the same common elements in

Table 13.1 Pharmaceutical categories

Archetypal phytochemical subgroup and common sources	Subjective impact and application in traditional medicine of plants rich in this subgroup	Confirmed pharmacological activity
Acrid, 'pungent' principles (hot spices), e.g. in cayenne, ginger, peppers	Hot, heating, increasing warmth to diseased tissues, preventing food poisoning in hot climates, sustaining febrile response in fever management, topical to arthritis and other subdermal inflammations	Thermogenic (Kawada et al 1988) and metabolic stimulant (Doucet & Tremblay 1997) (involving catecholamine release and possibly reflex irritation, e.g. from vanilloid receptors on C-fibres (Biro et al 1997)), increased gastric secretions (Desai et al 1977), prophylactic against some food poisoning, pain relief (Rains & Bryson 1995), increase in absorption of other nutrients and agents (Bano et al 1991)
Alkaloids, e.g. in opium, henbane, belladonna, datura, hemlock, psylocibin, tobacco	Poisonous, neuroactive, analgesic, sedative, psychoactive	Neuroactivity prominent among disparate group, a major pharmaceutical dispensary of its own
Anthraquinone and other laxatives, e.g. in senna, cascara, aloes	Laxative, topically anti-inflammatory	Laxative (Mascolo et al 1998), anti-inflammatory (Anton & Haag-Berrurier 1980)
Aromatic (essential) oils, e.g. in cinnamon, cardamon, fennel, rosemary and other kitchen spices	Aromatic and warming, settling digestion, stimulating digestion in debilitated states, warming treatment for bronchial congestions	Carminative (Giachetti et al 1988), spasmolytic (Reiter & Brandt 1985), antiinflammatory (Albring et al 1983), antiseptic (Pattnaik et al 1997), expectorant (Dorow et al 1987), diuretic (Stanic et al 1998)

Table 13.1 (continued)

Archetypal phytochemical subgroup and common sources	Subjective impact and application in traditional medicine of plants rich in this subgroup	Confirmed pharmacological activity
Bitters, e.g. in wormwood, chicory, hops, coffee, angostura, quinine bark, condurango	Bitter, stimulant to appetite and digestion, cholagogue, cooling effect in fever management, prevention and treatment of enteric infections, tonic	Systemic or local gastric responses shown (Wolf & Mack 1956), digestive stimulant (Wegener 1998)
Cardioactive glycosides, e.g. in foxglove, lily-of-the-valley, ouabain	Arrow poisons, in small doses for the treatment of dropsy	Toxic, positive inotropic and negative chronotropic myocardial stimulant
Cyanogenic glycosides, e.g. in wild cherry bark, bitter almonds, apricot kernels	Bitter, aroma of almonds, toxic, antitussive, sedative	Sedative, antitussive effects likely
Emetics, e.g. in ipecacuanha, squills	Emetic, expectorant in subemetic doses	Emetic, reflex expectorant in subemetic doses
Fibre, e.g. in flaxseed, psyllium	Bulking, bowel regulator, demulcent (like mucilages)	Bulking laxative (Stevens et al 1987), hypocholesterolemic (Roberts et al 1994), improving glucose tolerance (Frati-Munari et al 1989)
Flavonoids and anthocyanidins, e.g. in hawthorn, citrus peel, grapes, elderflower	Color, fever management, digestive modulator, wound remedies, cough/cold	Antioxidant (Tournaise et al 1993), vasculoprotective (Keli et al 1996, Knekt et al 1996), antiinflammatory (Pelzer et al 1998), vasculoactive (Le Devenat et al 1997), antitumor, estrogenic activity

Mucilages, e.g. in slippery elm, marshmallow, plantains	Slimy, emollient, demulcent, soothing to wounds and abrasions, reducing coughing due to dry irritability, soothing upper digestive inflammations	Physical basis for soothing properties demonstrated (Rafatullah et al 1994), antitussive (Nosalova et al 1992)
Resins, e.g. in myrrh, Tolu balsam, balm of Gilead, mastic, propolis	Sticky, antiseptic, stimulating defensive activity on exposed mucosa	Antiinflammatory (Al-Said et al 1986)
Saponins, e.g. in ginseng, licorice, astragulus, helonias root, wild yam	Lather in water, sweet taste, emetic-expectorant, tonics and gynecological remedies	Steroidal molecules with various competitive, modulating effects on steroidal receptors and functions postulated (Baker 1995), expectorant (Boyd & Palmer 1946), hypocholesterolemic (Oakerfull & Sidhu 1990), aid digestion of nutrients (Gee & Johnson 1988)
Sulphur-containing volatiles, e.g. in garlic, horseradish, mustards	Hot, odiferous, heating, warming and clearing bronchial congestion, antipathogenic, topically counterirritant	Antimicrobial (Pulverer 1968), antitumor (Verhoeven et al 1997), hypocholesterolemic, antiatherogenic (Reuter 1995), rubefacient and vesicant
Tannins, e.g. in oak, witchhazel	Astringent, making leather, wound cautery, antiinflammatory in upper digestive tract, reducing reflex diarrhea in gastroenteritis	Astringent (crosslinks exposed protein molecules) (Lamaison et al 1990), styptic (Akah 1988, Root-Bernstein 1982) and protective (Maity et al 1995), antioxidant (Haslam 1996)

comparable contexts (it is important, for example, that dosage and pharmacokinetic criteria in the scientific studies are consistent with traditional application).

The most consistently encountered pharmaceutical categories are listed below, with the traditional experience of the category as a whole followed by the established modern pharmacological assessment. There are obviously as many variations on these themes as there are plants included within them but the properties listed predominate across each category.

Modern endorsement of traditional use

There are many other cases where otherwise fragmentary scientific insights can illuminate and validate traditional practices and vice versa. The unusual traditional practices in the growth and preparation of kava, the early use of salicylate-rich willow bark as antipyretic and antiinflammatory, the widespread use of licorice sticks as dentifrices, the 3000-year-old use of psoralen-rich plants in the treatment of vitiligo in India, the use in ancient Egypt of a treatment for angina pectoris based on visnagin and khellin have all been validated by modern research and modern lessons learnt. Modern ethnopharmacological studies show countless examples where pharmacological activity can be demonstrated in traditional remedies and practices. Such correlations are clearly interesting; in effect, the early reputation provides the 'human bioassay data', the clinical evidence before the preclinical studies, rather than the other way around as is usual in modern pharmaceutical research.

Combining traditional and modern research?

As with the case for the pharmaceutical archetypes, it means that combining two or more otherwise incomplete data sources can provide much more evidence for efficacy than either used alone. The evidence will remain circumstantial until subjected to rigorous controlled studies but applying the law-court principle 'on the balance of probabilities', compared to the level of intelligence considered necessary to inform the world of corporate decision making and particularly in the case of the health-care practitioner struggling to find a way through the vicissitudes of everyday clinical practice, looking for potential answers to intractable difficulties, then this sort of evidence may be considered very good indeed.

Reliable sources of traditional use

There are a few key documents that could be treated as resources for those seeking a coherent view of traditional practices. These are recommended as being anthropological accounts of traditional use rather than interpretations of these.

British Herbal Medicine Association 1983 The British Herbal Pharmacopoeia 1983. BHMA, Bournemouth

Perry LR 1980 Medicinal plants of East and Southeast Asia. Massachusetts Institute of Technology Press, Cambridge, MA

Vogel VJ 1970 American Indian Medicine. University of Oklahoma Press

Lassak EV, McCarthy T 1983 Australian medicinal plants. Methuen Australia

PRECLINICAL STUDIES FOR HERBAL MEDICINE

In addition to providing a second guess on the veracity of traditional reputations, laboratory studies can cast light on some of the persistent puzzles in herb use. Some of the more relevant questions follow.

Pharmacokinetic issues

Any rationale for herbal medicine is likely to be based on the activity of many plant chemical constituents. There are fundamental technical questions raised in building a rational case for herbal therapeutics. The following might usefully form the basis of pharmacokinetic research questions which in turn could provide important information for quantifying efficacy and underpinning clinical research proposals.

- In what ways are plant constituents likely to interact in the gut and body tissues to affect bioavailability and activity? (Obvious interactions are between essential oils, mucilages, tannins, resins, alkaloids, saponins, minerals and complex carbohydrates.)
- What is known of hepatic action on plant constituents, both in terms of the results of the 'first-pass effect', as plant constituents move into the tissues from the digestive tract, and the impact of enterohepatic recycling?
- Following from both the above, what plant-derived constituents are likely to reach the systemic circulation (an answer to this question is an essential requisite for meaningful tissue culture experiments – see below)?
- How do changes in pharmaceutical preparation affect the bioavailability and activity of plant constituents? For example, do alcoholic extracts have significantly different actions from the aqueous extracts generally dominant in traditional practice?

With new biochemical monitoring technology it is feasible that some of these answers could be obtained non-invasively in healthy human subjects. This would provide more useful answers than the traditional reliance on animal experiments.

Cell and tissue cultures

As part of the modern move to find alternatives to animal experimentation, increasing attention is being paid to techniques for assessing the effects of drugs on cultures of cells, tissues and organs in vitro. Conventional drug research is switching in this direction for preliminary screening in drug discovery programs and there is also a move for at least initial toxicological testing.

The advantages are in the opportunity for the direct observation of the action of an agent on target cells with some reduced ethical difficulties (although the sacrifice of animals is often necessary to supply short-lived organ and tissue samples).

The problems are the limited application of such observations to the in vivo situation and the need to confirm any in vitro findings anyway; from the point of view of herbal research, there is the additional problem that it is impossible at this stage to reproduce that balance of plant constituents that will actually reach internal tissues (after digestion, absorption and the 'first-pass' hepatic effect). Difficulties are increased by the desirability of using tissues most closely mimicking the real situation, i.e. mammalian organ cultures (rather than the easier to culture amphibian tissues or the less sophisticated cell lines).

Table 13.2 Levels of evidence

Level	Type of evidence
Ia	Meta-analysis of randomized controlled trials
Ib	At least one randomized controlled trial
IIa	At least one well-designed controlled study without randomization
IIb	At least one other type of well-designed quasi-experimental study
III	Well-designed non-experimental descriptive studies, such as comparative studies
IV	Expert committee reports or opinions and/or clinical experiences of respected authorities

Table 13.3 Types of herbal evidence

	Types of evidence	Comments
	● Popular claims and reputations; non-systematized ethnobotanical records	Impossible to rule out possibility that non-specific effects including placebo account for all claimed effect
	● In vitro studies of plant constituents in isolation	Almost no bearing on effect of plant in clinical context
	● In vivo studies of plant constituents in isolation	Very little bearing on effect of plant in clinical context, especially if based on injections
III	● Systematized observations of traditional use; systematized practitioner accounts; case research studies	Valuable resource for further studies and can validate other conclusions; however, insufficient basis for rigorous single efficacy alone
IIb	● In vitro studies of archetypal phytochemical subgroups recognized in traditional medicine or whole plant extracts	Potentially supportive and illuminative for propositions based on established pharmaceutical practices; however, correspondences limited to topical activity as oral consumption will largely change plant properties and bioavailabilities; dosage also usually a significant issue; however, as routine assays of activity, a helpful tool in preliminary screening
IIb	● In vivo studies of archetypal phytochemical subgroups recognized in traditional medicine or whole plant extracts	Potentially more value than in vitro studies but studies on intravenous or intraperitoneal injections rarely applicable to human oral consumption; mg/kg dose rates also often too high for therapeutic inferences; interspecies differences always a confounding factor
IIb	● Open clinical trials with human subjects	Variable value depending on rigor of study; confounded by relatively strong non-specific effects in most cases
III	● Records of traditional and practitioner use of remedies rich in archetypal phytochemical subgroups recognized in traditional medicine	Useful ethnobotanical records providing a direct link between traditional pharmaceutical insights and modern research

III	● Records of consistent patterns of traditional use at distant locations and cultures around the world	The most conclusive information from traditional use, although transmission of information is possible in some cases
IIa	● Controlled clinical trials	Any attempt to reduce confounding variables in clinical observations will reduce the impact of non-specific treatment factors in the recorded outcome; value obviously depends on methodological rigor; many of the early studies on herbal remedies were relatively weak
Ib	● Double-blind randomized placebo- or other controlled clinical trials	Still the gold standard and often well suited to studying herbal remedies; apart from problems of logistics and lack of patent protection, the main difficulties are with establishing reliable outcome measures for many of the low-morbidity indications for these treatments and the usual high recruitment therefore necessary
Ia	● Rigorous meta-analysis of controlled clinical trials	These are being published for an increasing number of herbal medicines marketed in Europe; they vary in rigor; the mean balance of conclusion is modestly positive

Nevertheless, in vitro techniques could provide valuable supplementary information to other research, as in the following suggested projects.

● The influence of herbal extracts on epithelial tissue cultures (e.g. gastric, enteric and tracheal tissues); such findings could inform pharmacokinetic calculations for herbal dosage.
● Observations on the biotransformation of plant constituents using liver cultures.
● Alteration in the migratory behavior and internal metabolism of macrophages as a result of exposure to herbal extracts.
● Non-specific observations (as in gerontological research) on cell migrations, length of interphase, longevity and other pointers to in vitro cell health.

AN EVIDENCE BASE FOR HERBAL MEDICINE

In summary of this chapter, a hierarchy of the evidence often presented for the efficacy of herbs can be set out. This may be correlated in part with the levels of evidence proposed in 1992 by the US Agency for Health Care Policy and Research as shown in Table 13.2.

These levels can be appended to the hierarchy of types of herbal evidence in Table 13.3 (and are entered in the left hand column).

REFERENCES

Akah PA 1988 Haemostatic activity of aqueous leaf extract of *Ageratum conyzoides* L. International Journal of Crude Drug Research 26(2): 97–101

Albring M, Albrecht H, Alcorn G, Lücker PW 1983 The measuring of the antiinflammatory effect of a compound on the skin of volunteers. Methods and Findings in Experimental and Clinical Pharmacology 5: 575–577

Al-Said MA, Ageel AM, Parmar NS et al 1986 Evaluation of mastic, a crude drug obtained from *Pistacia lentiscus*, for gastric and duodenal anti-ulcer activity. Journal of Ethnopharmacology 15: 271–278

Anton R, Haag-Berrurier M 1980 Therapeutic use of natural anthraquinone for other than laxative actions. Pharmacology 20 (suppl 1): 104–112

Baker ME 1995 Endocrine activity of plant-derived compounds: an evolutionary perspective. Proceedings of the Society for Experimental Biology and Medicine 208: 131–138

Bano G, Raina RK, Zutshi U et al 1991 Effect of piperine on bioavailability and pharmacokinetics of propranolol and theophylline in healthy volunteers. European Journal of Clinical Pharmacology 41(6): 615–617

Biro T, Acs G, Acs P et al 1997 Recent advances in understanding of vanilloid receptors: a therapeutic target for treatment of pain and inflammation in skin. Journal of Investigative Dermatology Symposium Proceedings 2(1): 56–60

Boyd EM, Palmer ME 1946 The effect of quillaia, senega, squill, grindelia, sanguinaria, chionanthus and dioscorea upon the output of respiratory tract fluid. Acta Pharmacologica 2: 235–246

Desai HG, Venugopalan K, Philipose M et al 1977 Effect of red chilli powder on gastric mucosal barrier and acid secretion. Indian Journal of Medical Research 66(3): 440–448

Dorow P, Weiss Th, Felix R et al 1987 Effect of a secretolytic and a combination of pinene, limonene and cineole on mucociliary clearance in patients with chronic pulmonary obstruction. Arzneimittel-Forschung 37(12): 1378–1381

Doucet E, Tremblay A 1997 Food intake, energy balance and body weight control. European Journal of Clinical Nutrition 51(12): 846–855

EC 1989a Rules governing medicinal products in the European Community Volume III: guidelines on the quality, safety and efficacy of medicinal products for human use. Part 4 Clinical documentation. EC, Brussels

EC 1989b Rules – Part 2 Chemical, pharmaceutical and biological testing of medicinal products. EC, Brussels

EC 1989c Rules – Part 4A General requirements. EC, Brussels

EC 1990a Future system for the free movement of medicinal products in the European Community. COM(90) 283 final. EC, Brussels, p 23

EC 1990b CPMP Working Party on Efficacy of Medicinal Products: good clinical practice for trials on medicinal products in the European Community. III/3876/88-EN. EC, Brussels

EC 1991 Commission Directive 91/507/EEC:4F: Clinical efficacy and safety. EC, Brussels

EC 1993 Council Regulation (EEC) No. 2309/93 of 22nd July 1993: Community procedures for the authorisation and supervision of medicinal products for human and veterinary medicinal products. EC, Brussels

Frati-Munari AC, Flores-Garduno MA, Ariza-Andraca R et al 1989 Effect of different doses of *Plantago psyllium* mucilage on the glucose tolerance test. Archives of Investigative Medicine (Mexico) 20(2): 147–152

Gee JM, Johnson IT 1988 Interactions between hemolytic saponins, bile salts and small intestinal mucosa in the rat. Journal of Nutrition 118: 1391–1397

Giachetti D, Taddei E, Taddei I 1988 Pharmacological activity of essential oils on Oddi's sphincter. Planta Medica 63: 389–392

Haslam E 1996 Natural polyphenols (vegetable tannins) as drugs: possible modes of action. Journal of Natural Products 59: 205–215

IMS/PhytoGold 1998 Herbals in Europe. IMS SelfMedication International, London

Kawada T, Sakabe S, Watanabe T et al 1988 Some pungent principles of spices cause the adrenal medulla to secrete catecholamine in anesthetized rats. Proceedings of the Society for Experimental Biology and Medicine 188(2): 229–233

Keli SO, Hertog MG, Feskens EJ 1996 Dietary flavonoids, antioxidant vitamins, and incidence of stroke: the Zutphen study. Archives of Internal Medicine 156(6): 637–642

Knekt P, Jarvinen R, Reunanen A et al 1996 Flavonoid intake and coronary mortality in Finland: a cohort study. British Medical Journal 312(7029): 478–481

Lamaison JL, Carnat A, Petitjean-Freytet C 1990 Teneur en tanins et activité inhibitrice de l'élastase chez les Rosacae. Annales de Pharmaceutiques Françaises 48(6): 335–340

Le Devehat C, Khodabandehlou T, Vimeux M et al 1997 Evaluation of haemorheological and microcirculatory disturbances in chronic venous insufficiency: activity of Daflon 500 mg. International Journal of Microcirculation 17 (suppl 1): 27–33

Maity S, Vedasiromoni JR, Ganguly DK 1995 Anti-ulcer effect of the hot water extract of black tea (*Camellia sinensis*). Journal of Ethnopharmacology 46: 167–174

Mascolo N, Capasso R, Capasso F 1998 Senna. A safe and effective drug. Phytotherapy Research 12: S143–S145

Mills SY 1998 The efficacy of herbal medicinal products. 2) Research questions and methods. Discussion paper with the ESCOP Research Committee and European Phytotherapy Research Group. European Journal of Phytotherapy. Issue 2. http://www.ex.ac.uk/phytonet/phytojournal/

Nosalova G, Strapkova A, Kardosova A et al 1992 Antitussive wirkung des extraktes und der polysaccharide aus eibisch (*Althaea officinalis* L., var. *robusta*). Pharmazie 47: 224–226

Oakenfull D, Sidhu GS 1990 Could saponins be a useful treatment for hypercholesterolaemia? European Journal of Clinical Nutrition 44: 79–88

Pattnaik S, Subramanyam VR, Bapaji M et al 1997 Antibacterial and antifungal activity of aromatic constituents of essential oils. Microbios 89(358): 39–46

Pelzer LE, Guardia T, Osvaldo JA et al 1998 Acute and chronic antiinflammatory effects of plant flavonoids. Farmaco 53(6): 421–424

Pulverer G 1968 Benzylsenföl: ein breitbandantibiotikum aus der kapuzinerkresse. Deutsche Medizinische Wochenschrift 93: 1642–1649

Rafatullah S, Al-Yahya MA, Al-Said MS et al 1994 Gastric anti-ulcer and cytoprotective effects of *Cyamopsis tetragonolaba* ('Guar') in rats. International Journal of Pharmacognosy 32(2): 163–170

Rains C, Bryson HM 1995 Topical capsaicin. A review of its pharmacological properties and therapeutic potential in post-herpetic neuralgia, diabetic neuropathy and osteoarthritis. Drugs and Aging 7(4): 317–328

Reiter M, Brandt W 1985 Relaxant effects on tracheal and ileal smooth muscles of the guinea pig. Arzneimittel-Forschung 35(1A): 408–414

Reuter HD 1995 *Allium sativum* and *Allium ursinum*: Part 2 Pharmacology and medicinal application. Phytomedicine 2(1): 73–91

Roberts DCK, Truswell AS, Bencke A et al 1994 The cholesterol-lowering effect of a breakfast cereal containing psyllium fibre. Medical Journal of Australia 161: 660–664

Root-Bernstein RS 1982 Tannic acid, semipermeable membranes and burn treatment. Lancet 2: 1168

Stanic G, Samarzija I, Blazevic N 1998 Time-dependent diuretic response in rats treated with juniper berry preparations. Phytotherapy Research 12: 494–497

Stevens J, Levitsky DA, Van Soest PJ et al 1987 Effect of psyllium gum and wheat bran on spontaneous energy intake. American Journal of Clinical Nutrition 46: 812–817

Tournaire C, Croux S, Maurette MT et al 1993 Antioxidant activity of flavonoids: efficiency of singlet oxygen (1 delta g) quenching. Journal of Photochemistry and Photobiology B – Biology 19(3): 205–215

Verhoeven DTH, Verhoeven H, Goldbohm RA et al 1997 A review of mechanisms underlying anticarcinogenicity by brassica vegetables. Chemico-Biological Interactions 103: 79–129

Wegener T 1998 Anwendung eines trockenextraktes augentianae luteae radix bei dyspeptischem symptomkomplex. Zeitschrift für Phytotherapie 19: 163–164

Wolf S, Mack M 1956 Experimental study of the action of bitters on the stomach of a fistulous human subject. Drug Standards 24(3): 98–101

14

Homeopathy

Harald Walach   Wayne B Jonas

INTRODUCTION

Research into homeopathy has boomed in recent years. When our interest in homeopathy began 20 years ago, hardly anybody worked in that field. There were very few academic institutions showing interest and research into homeopathy was a backyard sector of research, carried out by a few at the fringe, viewed with suspicion by those in the centre. This has changed somewhat. There is at least some public money available for research now, a couple of academic institutions have started to show more interest and even respectable journals have started publishing high-quality research. Forging ahead brings the danger of forgetting about history and repeating mistakes, especially because the history of recent homeopathic research is as yet mostly unwritten and the original sources often hidden in specialized journals. The great danger here is reinventing the wheel.

This chapter is therefore written from the perspective of those who have tried to understand homeopathy and to do research in several areas of homeopathy for nearly 20 years now. Its aim is to point out some paths which have already been trodden and abandoned as blind alleys and others which seem to be more promising. In this paper we will sketch out the central issues, isolate promising avenues for future research and warn about traps. We will not cover all - primary studies in depth and secondary reviews and metaanalyses will be the main emphasis, as well as some landmark studies which can teach lessons. Our perspective is that of researchers and scientists, committed to the values of the scientific inquiry, with a warm interest in homeopathy. We would love to see homeopathy scientifically accepted or at least respected. But we can live in a world without it, should it be found not to contribute to health and the treatment of disease.

After a short introduction to homeopathy and its history we will cover the major aspects of mostly clinical research. Basic research into fundamental principles of homeopathy, both physicochemical and biological, together with some major hypotheses we will only touch upon briefly, together with a word about homeopathic remedy provings. We will close with what we believe to be the agenda for the next decade, if homeopathy wants to become part of the public sector of health care or even be taken seriously by the scientific establishment.

HISTORY

Homeopathy was formulated by the German pharmacist and doctor Samuel Hahnemann (1755–1843) when in 1796 he published his ideas in a paper called 'New principle of how to find the remedial powers of remedies' (Hahnemann 1811). The true medicine, he claimed, should follow what he called the 'law of similars': like should be cured by likes (similia similibus curentur). This principle is in fact quite old and can be found in the *Corpus Hippocraticum*, a collection of Greek texts. It was known by the great Roman physician Galen and extensively used by Paracelsus, the German physician and natural philosopher of the Renaissance (Walach 1986).

Thus, the law of similars was well known in the history of medicine before Hahnemann; Hahnemann's discovery was how to use it. He gave medicinal substances of his day – often poisonous plants or toxic substances like belladonna or quicksilver – to volunteers (in the beginning his family and students, so they probably were reluctant volunteers) and studied the symptoms which those subjects suffered. This he called *Arzneimittelprüfung*, which has been somewhat clumsily translated into English as 'remedy proving'; a better proposal is homeopathic pathogenetic trial (HPT) (Dantas 1996), since in such a trial the pathogenesis (and especially symptoms) of a substance in the human organism is studied. Hahnemann then applied the substances in cases of illness which had a similar appearance. Thus the law of similars and its operationalization in HPTs is the first pillar of homeopathy (Jonas & Jacobs 1996, Walach 1994, 1997).

The method of proving remedies in healthy subjects was not Hahnemann's invention. The same suggestion had been made by others, like the well-known Swiss physician and scholar Albrecht von Haller (Walach 1992). But Hahnemann's genuine discovery was the second pillar of homeopathy, the principle of potentization. Hahnemann was a keen observer and a very good pharmacologist. He knew about the toxicity of the substances which were used in his day and with which he started his HPTs. Therefore he sought to diminish their potentially dangerous effects while at the same time retaining their power to affect the human organism. Hence he diluted them successively and shook them vigorously in between the steps of dilution. It is unclear why Hahnemann shook the remedies. Although he was not an alchemist, the early chemistry of his time still held mixtures of materialism and magical thinking. This procedure he called 'potentization' or 'dynamization' because he observed that the substances which had been prepared this way were even more effective, both in HPTs by bringing out symptoms and in clinical use.

While at first Hahnemann mainly used 'low' potencies, i.e. dilutions up to the 6th or 8th centesimal dilution (C6 – a preparation made by diluting the stock substance six times), he later experimented with so-called 'high' potencies up to C30 (dilution of the stock solution 30 times) and more. This corresponds to a dilution of 10^{-60}, which obviously is far beyond Avogadro's number (the amount of molecules in one mole of solution, roughly 6×10^{23}). Although this was not known to Hahnemann, he suspected as much, saying that these high potencies have an effect due to their 'spirit-like' nature, not because of the substance administered.

While in principle, homeopathy could be practised entirely without the much-debated high potencies by solely relying on the similia rule (Jütte 1997, Van Wijk & Wiegant 1994, 1997), and in effect has been practised this way in Germany since the turn of the last century (Donner 1935) when high potencies fell into disrepute, in practice homeopathy has become tied to the usage of high potencies. Many famous and efficient homeopaths claimed and keep claiming that high potencies are effective.

Theoretically, the similars rule could easily be incorporated into the canon of modern medicine and in fact it is being used in allergy medicine. Also, it is known that modern drugs often produce paradoxical effects, just as Hahnemann had observed (Coulter 1980, Eskinazi 1999, Schüppel 1990, Teixeira 1999). It is notoriously difficult, however, to integrate the potentization principle into modern scientific views (Morgan 1992) and indeed, it is the potentization principle which has engendered fierce opposition to homeopathy through the ages. It is a major challenge to come up with an explanation for the possible effects of ultramolecular potencies beyond Avogadro's number, if homeopathy ever wants to be taken seriously (Morgan 1992).

During his long career Hahnemann discovered that, although his remedies were quite effective, the cures were not always stable and long-lasting. He found that some patients required new prescriptions again and again, which made them somewhat better but did not cure them. But definite cure was Hahnemann's declared aim (Hahnemann 1979). He thus developed his theory of chronic diseases, stating that in some cases diseases had been so entrenched in the organism that they lay mostly dormant and in cases of strain or stress would awake to an acute stage (Hahnemann 1983). This in fact was an early type of the modern concept of a diathesis-stress model of disease, where an underlying disposition combined with some triggering factors are seen to give rise to actual symptoms. It is this theory that the so-called constitutional prescribing is derived from which interprets a disease as part of an underlying chronic condition, if it is recurring.

Hahnemann never succeeded in convincing the medical establishment of his system. Although he had some followers and some important persons supported him, by and large the establishment was hostile, partly because he was a choleric character who had difficulty living in peace with others and respecting others' opinions in the same way as he expected them to respect his. There were also economic reasons for the resistance to homeopathy. Hahnemann urged every physician to make his own remedies, a practice that would threaten the livelihood of the pharmacies. In addition, a full homeopathic history took a long time, cutting into the number of patients that could be seen by a physician.

Very soon camps of friends and foes were established. Some extraordinary success of homeopaths brought publicity to the therapy and the support of the public, which in the end was decisive (Jütte 1998). Radetzky, the marshal general of the Austrian army, was cured by homeopathy as was the famous violinist Paganini. During the epidemics of cholera which swept Europe during the middle of the 19th century homeopaths were much more successful in saving lives. While in some conventional hospitals up to 74% of the patients died, in homeopathic clinics the figure was 4–11% (Glaz 1991, Leary 1994, Scheible 1994).

Homeopaths and the public usually attributed these successes to the use of homeopathic remedies but historical analyses and modern data (Gaucher et al 1993, 1994) show that what was decisive was the fact that homeopaths did not apply dehydration and bloodletting, which were the main interventions of conventional medicine in those days and were usually fatal.

Thus, the historical rise of homeopathy in Europe was due more to avoiding harmful measures than introducing radical cures. That is not to say that homeopathy was ineffective but that part of the historical victory of homeopathy is due to the inappropriateness of the conventional approach rather than to homeopathy's specific superiority. Homeopaths nowadays often claim that they are effective in cases of chronic diseases where conventional treatment is useless. While it might be true that there could be some specific or non-specific therapeutic efficacy in homeopathy, refraining from invasive intervention, which is a vital part of homeopathic theory, could also be an important factor.

Be that as it may, historically homeopathy has outlived many rival approaches which had been more powerful and were more favored by the medical establishment (Schwanitz 1983). This in itself poses a historical question to be resolved. An argument has been advanced that many medical interventions survived for centuries which were unproven and even harmful, like bloodletting (Ernst et al 1998). But this argument lacks a genuine historical understanding. While bloodletting and comparable measures were theoretically derived from the then accepted medical mainstream theory and thus had broad support, homeopathy was always on the defensive and had to fight its way against a powerful medical orthodoxy. History in the end is unrelenting against ideas and movements which do not contain some aspect of truth and reality. This is the hermeneutic principle of *Wirkungsgeschichte*, which can be rendered as 'history of effective ideas' (Gadamer 1975). Whatever is effective has something to it which refuses to be swept away by the passage of time. Whatever has outlived its usefulness is carried away. We have witnessed the decline of Marxist theory and practice. Medicine has witnessed the decline of many harmful or ill-founded interventions and theories. Homeopathy may be wrong in its theory but it certainly seems to offer some practical usefulness. And this in itself is a challenge to understand. If there were no usefulness and practical effectiveness, homeopathy would have died out long ago. The Northern American and Canadian renaissance of homeopathy, when it was as good as dead in those countries in the middle of the 20th century, is an especially fascinating phenomenon (Connor 1998, Schmidt 1994). This fact, among others, seems to indicate what is at the core of homeopathy's appeal: the often-reported therapeutic successes which impress the consumers and the public.

What is it that makes homeopathy so attractive that it managed to survive major medical conceptual revolutions fairly unscathed? What is it about this strange method, which is practised basically the same way as Hahnemann conceived it nearly 200 years ago, that it can afford to ignore most of what is considered essential today (Hess 1993) and yet attracts people and obviously satisfies them to some degree? Why do well-educated doctors, who, after all, have gone through orthodox training, decide to invest a lot of money, effort and time in studying such an outlandish theory and practice? Why does homeopathy arouse such passions when it is discussed? Homeopathy is a challenge and the major part of this chapter deals with how this challenge has or has not been met as yet.

BASIC RESEARCH
Biological

Basic research should provide us with a stable, replicable model – biological, in vitro or otherwise – which could be used to demonstrate the biological effects and investigate mechanisms of serially agitated high dilutions (SAHD). This area has a long history of research, ever since the work of Lilli Kolisko with wheat seedlings, which had been grown in different potencies of silver nitrate (Kolisko 1923). It is also the area with the longest history of failures. It is not the purpose of this chapter to critically review all of this research; there are several competent reviews available (Kollerstrom 1982, Linde et al 1994, Scofield 1984, Vallance 1998, Vickers 1999). However, a number of important observations relevant to developing a research strategy arise from this area. The most frequent observation is that there are often interesting initial results, highly significant, seemingly clearcut, with often rather simple experimental paradigms. But when probed for stable, independent replicability, not one has so far been proved so robust that the effects would be reproducible even by a believer, let alone a skeptic (Vickers 1999).

There has been a series of well-conducted research studies mainly in the field of hormesis (using low but not ultra-low doses). These are summarized in Van Wijk & Wiegant (1994, 1997). Hormesis refers to the fact that very low but still material doses of a toxic substance can induce repair mechanisms in the cell, which protects the cell from damage from such substances applied in higher dose. This research shows that there might be a possible biological basis to the similia rule. It remains to be seen whether such effects would also occur with SAHD beyond Avogadro's number.

Probably the only experimental model of SAHDs today which seems promising, because it has been replicated by a number of independent labs and even skeptical ones, is an immunological model (Belon et al 1999, Cherruault et al 1989, Hadjaj et al 1993, Sainte-Laudy & Belon 1993, 1996, 1997, Sainte-Laudy et al 1986). In that model basophil granulocytes are studied. Massive doses of IgE are used to trigger degranulation and histamine is used to produce an inhibitory effect in serial dilutions up to C19 (a dilution beyond Avogadro's number). In its most recent report (Belon et al 1999), this research was conducted by four independent labs. Mean degranulation was 48.8% with SADH of potentized histamine and 41.8% with control. This is a result which is significant if the results are pooled ($P < 0.0001$) and three out of the four experiments were independently significant. Work is still ongoing. Should this model prove replicable in the hands of independent researchers, this would be a milestone for homeopathy.

Meanwhile we can repeat the conclusion of Vickers' review (Vickers 1999): it is time for basic research to stop wasting energy in new paradigms. It is necessary to follow up the promising ones and see whether they can be made independently reproducible. As long as this has not been the case a conservative and critical observer must conclude that the effects reported so far are not stable enough to validate such an exotic idea as the biological activity of substances diluted beyond the realm where molecules can be expected to be present and active. The challenge still stands: what is the difference between homeopathic substances and controls?

What is needed in future research is not the 201st extravagant and creative model which shows impressive biological effects and could be potentially telling about homeopathic clinical effects but is either so difficult and expensive that it is unlikely to be repeated by anyone or so unbelievable that no widely read mainstream journal would publish it. What is needed is a very simple biological model, which can show robust, reproducible effects of such highly diluted SAHDs. In addition, we should ask why it is that so often impressive results are obtained on initial investigation, even in properly controlled trials, only to fade on repeated attempts. Usually this means that there are important variables influencing the results that are not being addressed. These variables may be quirky 'artefacts' of the experimental method or due to other influences that must be accounted for in a model of homeopathic action (Jonas 2000). In either case, such variables may need to be considered before any replicable model of homeopathy can be developed.

Physical

A thorough review of research on physical aspects of SAHDs up to 1992 was conducted by Weingärtner (1992). None of the claims reported in the literature, including NMR results, proved replicable and robust, although the author found some stunning anomalies. A rigorously conducted study with promising results has not been followed up or repeated independently (Demangeat et al 1992) and where other reports have been submitted to independent tests, they have failed so far (Walach et al 1998b). In reality, the amount of expertise devoted to this area is striking and has produced some unusual findings (even in well-conducted studies) but no area has been tested sufficiently to be able to make clear decisions clearly as negative or positive. Various theories and experimental approaches have been summarized (Endler & Schulte 1994, Schulte 1999, Schulte & Endler 1998) but none so far can cover all phenomena or is empirically tested well enough to support any of the bold claims put forward by homeopathic enthusiasts (Vithoulkas 1980).

CLINICAL RESEARCH

When in 1997 Linde and colleagues published their metaanalysis of clinical trials studying homeopathic interventions and found an odds ratio of 2.45 (with a confidence interval (CI) from 2.05 to 2.93) for all studies and 1.66 (CI 1.33–2.08) for the studies with a sufficiently good methodology, homeopaths beamed and critics scolded (Vandenbroucke 1997). It seemed clear that homeopathy is not only placebo. What has been overlooked by homeopaths and underlined by critics is the fact that the review did not find enough evidence for supporting homeopathic practice in a specific disease, since not enough replications existed.

Since then more studies have been published which have been summed up in a second metaanalysis by the same group (Linde & Melchart 1998) which, however, has escaped the attention of most authors, it seems. In this analysis only trials of individualized homeopathy were included, which theoretically should be the ones with the stronger effects. This analysis also showed a significant, albeit smaller effect of RR = 1.62 (CI 1.17–2.23). This significant effect vanished if only the methodologically sound trials were taken into account. Thus, the evidence seems to mount against homeopathy as results from methodologically sound trials keep accumulating (Linde et al 1999).

There are complications when conducting reviews that look for disease replications with classical homeopathy, however, in that selection of the 'correct' homeopathic remedy is not the same as finding the right allopathic diagnosis used for repeated comparisons. The practice of individual practitioners is heterogeneous which increases the variability across trials. If such heterogeneity could be reduced by non-classical (standardized clinical) approaches to homeopathy, these might be the best models to study homeopathy's effects on specific diseases.

The evidence from metaanalyses is only one leg on which an evidence base rests. The other is multiple replications. There have been some research paradigms in clinical research which have been replicated. One series of positive replications were the trials of David Reilly from Glasgow (Reilly & Taylor 1985, Reilly et al 1986, Taylor et al 2000). He used a simple model: patients suffering from allergic rhinitis because of grass pollen allergy were provided with ahomeopathic preparation of mixed grass pollen C30. It could be shown that they had significantly fewer symptoms than the controls in a pilot and in the main study. In a follow-up study which used a slightly different regimen, patients suffering from allergic asthma were provided with high dilutions of the allergogenic substance in C30 (Reilly et al 1994). They suffered significantly fewer symptoms than the controls. The pooled results of these three studies overwhelmingly rule out the thesis that the homeopathic interventions could have been identical with placebo. The challenge is to reproduce these results in a large and simple trial, independent of the original researcher. Two such trials have been conducted. The first one (Taylor et al 2000) was an independent replication by Morag Ann Taylor, a co-worker of David Reilly, in 51 allergic rhinitis patients. She found a significant effect in the objective parameter (nasal peak flow), but not in the subjective one (visual analog score of symptom severity) which was the significant parameter in all other studies. The second one was conducted by a consortium coordinated by George Lewith, which is only published as an abstract as yet (Lewith 2000). In this study 242 patients with asthma sensitive to house dust mite received a single split dose of the allergen in a C30 potency and then were monitored over the course of 16 weeks. The most important result of this study seems to be that, although the time courses of the two experimental groups were statistically different, there was no improvement in the treated group. Thus, although there was a clear difference between the groups, it is not a replication of the former results in the strict sense. Comparable studies in Norway with potentized birch pollen in subjects allergic to birch pollen were unable to demonstrate clear-cut effects (Aabel 2000, Aabel et al 2000).

More promising results arose from a series of trials of individualized homeopathy in childhood diarrhea (Jacobs et al 1993, 1994, 2000). A pilot study demonstrated promising if not significant results while a main study in children in Nicaragua yielded a significant effect. The study has subsequently been repeated by different doctors, although directed by the same team of researchers, in Nepal. The effects are again significant and of the same magnitude (Jacobs 2000). However, the significant effect was seen at a different time compared to the other trials. The effect size of all three trials was remarkably similar, showing a reduction in diarrhea days between 0.66 and 0.76 days over placebo. From this it was possible to more accurately calculate power requirements to adequately test this therapy and condition. As it turns out an adequate trial needs over 200 subjects, something rarely found in homeopathic trials. Again, an independent replication and sufficient funding for a larger sample size might clarify the picture.

Probably the most extensively replicated model is the application of Galphimia glauca 6 × in allergic rhinitis. There have been 11 trials altogether which have been summed up in a metaanalysis (Wiesenauer & Lüdtke 1996). They were all conducted by the same primary researcher but used different groups of physicians to deliver the therapy. While placebo rates were very high and ranged between 52% and 79%, the pooled effect of the homeopathic treatment had a rate ratio of 1.25 and thus was significantly different from placebo. This clinical model is typical of homeopathy at a comparatively low level of similarity (Van Wijk & Wiegant 1994) and seems to be quite robust. Again, an independent replication (by a different principal investigator) would be helpful here.

One of the flagship studies in classical individualized homeopathy was the migraine study by Brigo & Serpelloni (1987, 1991). In that study, which has been termed 'the best result in the migraine literature' with the implication that this itself would make it unbelievable (Diener 1994), 60 patients with migraine whose symptoms matched one of a set of chosen remedies received either homeopathy or placebo. Number of attacks and pain ratings were drastically reduced after 3 months of treatment, yielding a highly significant result. This result was so promising that it inspired three direct or indirect replications which have been conducted independently of each other. The first one, which was a close replication, could show only weak effects just approaching significance (Whitmarsh et al 1997). Our own study tried to broaden the outlook by taking in 98 patients not only with migraine but also with other types of chronic headaches and applied classical, individualized homeopathy unrestrictedly (Walach et al 1997a). Final evaluation was conducted after 3 months of treatment and open treatment and close observation were carried on for another year in 19 patients. There was no difference between homeopathic treatment and placebo, placebo being even slightly better than homeopathy, and there were no hints in the data that a larger group of patients or a longer observation period would have yielded a different result. Interestingly, this is one of the methodologically tight studies, which at the same time yielded the worst result for homeopathy in the literature. Another study was conducted in Norway in 68 migraine patients, using individualized homeopathy (Straumsheim et al 1997). Pain diaries showed no difference, but the neurologist rating, which normally would be considered an insensitive parameter, was significantly in favor of homeopathy. This leaves the study with an inconsistent result. Thus, the history of research in migraine and headache with the largest number of independent studies gives the impression that the strong initial result is not reproducible, interestingly similar to the pattern in basic research.

Another model with independent replication was the application of Arnica 30 × to prevent delayed-onset muscle soreness in runners and in experimental models. Two studies in runners of the Oslo marathon were promising, if not conclusive (Tveiten et al 1991, 1998). A replication in the London marathon failed (Vickers et al 1998). Two reviews of other Arnica studies had a negative result (Ernst & Barnes 1998, Ernst & Pittler 1998) and were criticized (Dean 1998). Another review, which is much more comprehensive and identified 40 studies, found that 13 studies (i.e. 35%) reported a significant result while 10 more show a significant tendency (Lüdtke & Wilkens 1999). Thus the majority of the studies support a possible effect of Arnica. The models are so divergent, however, that no common quantitative measure can be derived. The effects of Arnica in an experimental model of muscle soreness have been very weak and an estimated 300 subjects would have to be studied to detect such effects, (Vickers et al 1997).

Ileus was another target of repeated studies of homeopathy. In that model subjects after abdominal surgery received homeopathic Opium and Raphanus C6 and the time to transit was measured. Initial pilot studies were promising. A large-scale national study in France was not able to reproduce the initial results (Groupe de Recherche 1989, Mayaux et al 1988). The initial results were so strong, however, that a pooled analysis still yields significant results (Barnes et al 1997).

Another area with mixed replications is rheumatology. While two initial studies of homeopathy in rheumatoid arthritis were positive (Gibson et al 1978, 1980), an independent study failed to confirm these results (Andrade et al 1991). In fibromyalgia there has been a positive trial of the homeopathic remedy Rhus tox (Fisher et al 1989), following a negative one in osteoarthritis (Shipley et al 1983). But so far nobody seems to have taken up this lead.

The evidence from clinical studies, then, is still inconclusive, depending on one's outlook. If one takes a critical stance and wants to see multiple, independent replications the evidence for homeopathy shrinks to a few well-researched syndromes like Galphimia in pollinosis, Opium in ileus and possibly potentized allergogenic substances in atopic allergies. If one is optimistic and looks to the overall evidence from metaanalyses, the picture is brighter and homeopathy appears to be different from placebo. However, it should be borne in mind that sensitivity analyses show that the methodologically sound studies of classical individualized homeopathy yield, unexpectedly, the worst results.

The suspicion has been voiced that the lack of effect in those modern trials is due to confounding effects – toothpaste, coffee, diet and other factors antidoting homeopathy – or due to patients being unresponsive because of conventional drugs. The consequence would be to conduct a study which includes all these elements as exclusion criteria. Such a study, unknown to most, has been conducted (Remy et al 1995, Siebenwirth 1995, Siebenwirth & Rakoski 1997). A heroic homeopath tried to conduct a study of classical homeopathy in atopic dermatitis with a long list of criteria geared to exclude whatever could be hindering homeopathic effects, in patients who were willing to abstain from cortisone. Despite a lot of local media coverage and a huge area of possible respondents and screening of many hundreds of patients, only some 30 patients could be included and the study was stopped after 3 years, because there was no chance of finishing it according to protocol. The evaluation yielded not even a trend in favor of homeopathy but showed impressive remissions with placebo. Anyone thinking of doing the definitive trial of homeopathy should make contact with the author of that study first.

Clinical trials so far have tried to answer one single question: Is homeopathy different from placebo? This is the question of absolute efficacy. The effort of some 100 trials has not really succeeded in answering this question. The answer rather seems to converge to the point that it is more difficult to show a difference between homeopathy and placebo, the tighter controlled the study is and the closer it tries to come to homeopathy as it is practiced. In many ways the absolute question of whether all homeopathy is placebo or not is not one that can be answered by clinical trials, especially if one includes complex and chronic diseases in that mix.

Asking such a question is in principle like asking if surgery is better than placebo which, of course, can only be answered in the particular, not the general. Unless homeopathy is tested with simple, repeatable models, clinical trials are probably not sensitive enough to answer the general question of placebo. Even with proven drugs, such as H2-blockers in the treatment of gastric and duodenal ulcers, the variability of placebo healing rates is from 0% to 100% (Moerman 2000). If one adds a mix of heterogeneous conditions into a pool of studies the variability is so great as to make power calculations meaningless (Egger et al 2000).

A better approach may be the use of simple and short-term clinical conditions. The most investigated clinical study models in homeopathy are of Galphimia glauca for hayfever (Wiesenauer & Lüdtke 1996), Opium, Raphanus, Arnica or China for postoperative ileus (see Linde et al 1997 for review) and homeopathic immunotherapy (HIT) for allergic rhinitis (Taylor et al 2000). These trials have their own problems, however, for they do not address the system of homeopathy as it is practiced. For example, the remedy Galphimia and the HIT approach are rarely used by homeopaths and postoperative ileus is hardly ever addressed with homeopathy in daily practice.

It may well be the case that a blinded trial of individual homeopathy is internally invalid (Walach 1996). The blinding of doctors is usually employed in simple therapeutic strategies: giving a drug or not giving it; giving it in one dose or in another. But in homeopathy doctors have to make complex decisions, based on the presentation of the patient. In blinded trials they have the extra insecurity that the patient may be on placebo. They may start making inferences from the symptom picture the patient presents with. And consequently the attributions of the doctors may direct their conduct and therapeutic decisions. Patients, on the other hand, may withhold important information knowing they might be given placebo. As a consequence, blinding may be an inappropriate strategy for studying classical homeopathy but only applicable in research models which are simple and do not call for complex decisions on the part of the doctor. Hardly anybody has asked the question of effectiveness: Is homeopathy as effective as standard treatment? And we do not even know what improvement average patients can expect when they walk into the clinic of a homeopathic doctor, since no thorough prospective cohort studies or documentations exist, apart from currently ongoing studies (Güthlin et al 1998, Walach et al 1996, 1997b,c, 1998a, Witt et al 1998).

HOMEOPATHIC REMEDY PROVINGS

Remedy provings or homeopathic pathogenetic trials (HPT) are the basis of homeopathy, since it is in those trials that the symptoms are elicited which are then used therapeutically. Homeopaths are quite sure that the symptoms which were observed by Hahnemann and his followers can only be due to the powers of the medicinal substance, as Hahnemann stipulated this in his *Organon*. Hardly anybody has studied this. In the area of HPTs, which really are experimental studies, there are two general thrusts. The first line of research is meant to bring out a rich symptom picture which is useful for therapy (Riley 1994, 1995, Sherr 1994, Wehmeyer et al 1996). It aims at maximizing variability and does not distinguish whether the symptoms observed are due to placebo or not. If the symptoms are useful for choosing a remedy in an ill patient who is then cured, this is taken as an indirect validation of the symptom as a true remedy symptom in the first place. The other line of research asks whether the symptoms observed in a HPT are due to placebo or not (Walach 1992, 1993).

A review of HPTs shows a lack of awareness in homeopathic researchers about methodological issues like blinding or good reporting standards of HPTs (Dantas 1996, Dantas & Fisher 1998, Dantas et al 2001). The few HPTs which explicitly addressed the question of whether symptoms observed with a homeopathic remedy are different from placebo were not successful in demonstrating a difference (Clover et al 1980). This is no surprise, since it is a common experience of proving directors old or new that the best and most useful symptoms are also experienced by placebo provers or even by persons who are not taking a remedy at all, like family members or friends.

Modern provings inappropriately mix two types of research approaches, each with different goals: qualitative research and attributional clinical research. In qualitative research the goal is to bring out the rich subtleties of the remedy administration and its experience, looking for dramatic, repeated (in single individuals) and occasionally similar symptoms across patients. The validity of the symptom picture is later determined in clinical practice, not necessarily in other provers. In attributional research the goal is to determine statistically if there are quantitatively different symptom counts between groups on the remedy and controls. These are fundamentally different (and both worthy) goals that need to be examined in separate studies, not mixed into single studies which then do not address either goal adequately (Jonas 1996a).

OPEN QUESTIONS AND PRIORITIES FOR FUTURE RESEARCH

If one accepts that homeopathy is a type of placebo then this seems to end the debate: why bother to study it at all? But then, what does 'placebo' mean here? If we look at HPTs, for instance, and see how subjects experience very strange, hitherto unknown symptoms which belong to the remedy picture, although they are ingesting placebo, this should set us thinking.

Our suggestion would be that we should be asking different questions than whether homeopathy is different from placebo. These questions include: How effective is homeopathy compared with other treatments? What is the baseline chance of patients improving or being healed under homeopathic treatment? What are good prognostic indicators for success in homeopathic treatment? How stable are treatment effects? How much does success with homeopathy cost compared to conventional treatment? What are the risks of side effects in homeopathy weighed against the odds of improvement? None of these questions has been asked until now, let alone answered, but they are worth pursuing. The fixation of homeopaths and researchers on the placebo question has kept them from looking at more interesting areas (Jonas 1996b, Walach 1998). Certainly, the placebo question is interesting in itself but imagine the following scenario. Suppose we find out that homeopathy is not different from placebo – a subtle kind of placebo, so to speak – but that, in comparison with standard treatment, it is at least as effective or in places even more effective. (In fact, a recent systematic review indicates this may be so (Jonas 1998).) Suppose the placebo effect is not a fixed entity but variable. And suppose that self-healing, which allegedly is triggered by homeopathy, is just a nicer word for placebo (Reilly 1998, 2000a,b). So the bottom line would be that homeopathy is a clever way of triggering self-healing, certainly a cheaper and less dangerous one than other approaches, maybe even a more effective one or one that is at least as effective as other approaches. But the rate of self-healing brought about by homeopathic remedies is just about the same as that using placebos, as long as the whole homeopathic procedure is employed. Suppose this were the end of the story. Would it matter to patients? Would it matter to doctors? Would it matter to the public? Would it matter to purchasers? Would it matter to scientists and researchers? Would it matter to the manufacturers of homeopathic remedies? It is probable that patients would be rather indifferent towards the mechanisms which trigger self-healing.

So our main suggestion is to stop treating the placebo question as the only important and relevant factor. We should rather look at whether therapeutic effects of homeopathy as it is practiced are sizeable enough to worry about, whether they are worth our efforts and public money. We need comparison standards for answering these questions. Comparison with placebo in all circumstances, we contend, is not useful. We should aim at comparisons with previous disease history in well-documented cohort studies and randomized waiting-list controlled studies. We should aim at comparisons with standard treatments. We should look at cost, outcomes and side effects. And we should argue for a program of research on placebo effects in general. For it is the prejudice of the pharmacological era which implants the idea that only pharmacologically specific effects may be called efficacy. It would be our bet that homeopathy will lose the battle for specific effects, if it does not very soon change gear. This is not to give up all scientific standards. Indeed, very rigorous research methods are essential for answering the questions just suggested. It does, however, mean shifting emphasis and asking different questions. After all, scientific methods are ways of answering questions. Asking the wrong question will not provide us with right answers. Asking different questions, in practical terms, would mean starting different types of studies. We suggest that some of the following studies could be a main focus of any research agenda in homeopathy.

- Observational and cohort studies to determine the general effects of homeopathy.
- Combined with an analysis of large sets of prognostic factors on doctors and patients, among them personality traits, measures of expectancy, hope, self-involvement, sympathy.
- Randomized comparison studies to determine effectiveness compared with alternative treatments.
- Quasi-experimental comparison studies in natural, self-selected groups to find out about the importance of self-selection.
- Combined with measures of cost and safety.
- Studies of biological activity of SAHDs or the question of whether homeopathic dilutions are placebos should be delegated to stable, basic research models.
- Those who still believe in the superiority of homeopathy over placebo in clinical trials should try to replicate one of the promising positive results reported above and book a good therapist for the time after the trial.

Awareness that the triggering of self-healing responses is an important therapeutic intervention in itself could bring the breakthrough for homeopathy, not the demonstration of hitherto elusive specific effects of SAHDs. This at least would be something which homeopathy has in common with other branches of medicine. It would seem wise to take up the commonalities with conventional medicine and not focus on the gulf between the two approaches.

Several studies have now shown that across studies there is a high correlation ranging from $r = 0.6$ to $r = 0.8$ between placebo and pharmacological interventions in conventional treatment (Kirsch & Sapirstein 1998, Walach & Maidhof 1999). That means that in clinical conventional trials the effect which is due to the specific pharmacological effects is rather weak if seen against the commonalities of natural history, expectation and the self-healing response, which is always present. This shows that so-called 'non-specific' effects and self-healing are important in the therapeutic contribution even of conventional approaches.

This could be used as a bridge of understanding and common interest, which could make homeopathy an interesting partner to learn from for conventional therapists, rather than the outlandish, silly and ill-founded quackery that it has been perceived as by the majority of medical specialists ever since Hahnemann. If that could be achieved then the spectre of Hahnemann which has brought only discord would be laid to rest and a new cooperative era of investigation using research that matters to patients could be advanced.

REFERENCES

Aabel S 2000 No beneficial effect of isopathic prophylactic treatment for birch pollen allergy during a low-pollen season: a double-blind, placebo-controlled clinical trial of homeopathic Betula 30c. British Homeopathic Journal 89: 169–173

Aabel S, Laerum E, Dølvik S, Djupesland P 2000 Is homeopathic immunotherapy effective? A double-blind, placebo-controlled trial with the isopathic remedy Betula 30c for patients with birch pollen allergy. British Homeopathic Journal 89:161–168

Andrade LEC, Ferraz MB, Atra E, Castro A, Silva MSM 1991 A randomized controlled trial to evaluate the effectiveness of homoeopathy in rheumatoid arthritis. Scandinavian Journal of Rheumatology 20: 204–208

Barnes J, Resch KL, Ernst E 1997 Homeopathy for postoperative ileus? A meta-analysis. Journal of Clinical Gastroenterology 25: 628–633

Belon P, Cumps J, Ennis M et al 1999 Inhibition of human basophil degranulation by successive histamine dilutions: results of a European multi-centre trial. Inflammation Research 48 (Suppl 1): S17–S18

Brigo B, Serpelloni G 1987 Le traitement homéopathique de la migraine: une étude de 60 cas, controlée en double aveugle (remède homopathique vs. placebo). Journal of the Liga Medicorum Homoeopatica Internationalis 1: 18–25

Brigo B, Serpelloni G 1991 Homoeopathic treatment of migraines: a randomized double-blind controlled study of sixty cases (homoeopathic remedy versus placebo). Berlin Journal on Research in Homoeopathy 1: 98–106

Cherruault Y, Guillez A, Sainte-Laudy J, Belon P 1989 Etude mathémathique et statistique des effets de dilutions successives de chlorhydrate d'histamine sur la réactivité des basophiles humains. Bio-Sciences 7: 63–72

Clover A, Jenkins S, Campbell AC, Jenkins MD 1980 Report on a proving of Pulsatilla 3x. British Homoeopathic Journal 69: 134–149

Connor JTH 1998 Homoeopathy in Victorian Canada and its twentieth-century resurgence: professional, cultural and therapeutic perspectives. In: Jütte R, Risse GB, Woodward J (eds) Culture, knowledge, and healing. European Association for the History of Medicine and Health Publications, Sheffield, pp 111–138

Coulter HL 1980 Homeopathic science and modern medicine. North Atlantic Books, Richmand, VA

Dantas F 1996 How can we get more reliable information from homoeopathic pathogenetic trials? A critique of provings. British Homoeopathic Journal 85: 230–236

Dantas F, Fisher P 1998 A systematic review of homoeopathic pathogenetic trials ('provings') published in the United Kingdom from 1945 to 1995. In: Ernst E, Hahn EG (eds) Homoeopathy: a critical appraisal. Butterworth Heinemann, London, pp 69–97

Dantas F, Fisher P, Walach H, Wieland F, Poitevin B 2000 Homoeopathic remedy provings. An international review. British Homoeopathic Journal (in preparation)

Dean M 1998 Out of step with the Lancet homeopathy meta-analysis: more objections than objectivity? Journal of Alternative and Complementary Medicine 4: 389–398

Demangeat JL, Demangeat D, Gries P, Poitevin B, Constantinesco A 1992 Modification des temps de relaxation RMN à 4 MHz des protons du solvant dans les très hautes dilutions salines de silice/lactose. Journal de Medecine Nucleaire et Biophysique 16: 135–145

Diener HC 1994 Demands and reality of the homeopathic migraine therapy [German]. Medizinische Klinik 89 (suppl 1): 79

Donner F 1935 Answering the question of high potencies [German]. Allgemeine Homöopathische Zeitung 183: 81–105

Egger M, Davey SG, Altman DG 2000 Systematic Reviews in Health Care: Meta-analysis in Context. BMJ Books, London

Endler PC, Schulte J (eds) 1994 Ultra high dilution. Physiology and physics. Kluwer Academic Publishers, Dordrecht

Ernst E, Barnes J 1998 Are homoeopathic remedies effective for delayed-onset muscle soreness? A systematic review of placebo-controlled trials. Perfusion 11: 4–8

Ernst E, Pittler MH 1998 Efficacy of homeopathic arnica. A systematic review of placebo-controlled clinical trials. Archives of Surgery 133: 1187–1190

Ernst E, De Smet PAGM, Shaw D, Murray V 1998 Traditional remedies and the 'test of time'. European Journal of Clinical Pharmacology 54: 99–100

Eskinazi D 1999 Homeopathy re-revisited. Is homeopathy compatible with biomedical observations? Archives of Internal Medicine 159: 1981–1987

Fisher P, Greenwood A, Huskisson EC, Turner P, Belon P 1989 Effect of homoeopathic treatment on fibrositis (primary fibromyalgia). British Medical Journal 299: 365–366

Gadamer HG 1975 Truth and method. Fundamentals of philosophical hermeneutics [German]. Mohr, Tübingen

Gaucher C, Jeulin D, Peycru P, Pla A, Amengual C 1993 Cholera and homoeopathic medicine. The Peruvian experience. British Homoeopathic Journal 82: 155–163

Gaucher C, Jeulin D, Peycru P, Amengual C 1994 A double blind randomized placebo controlled study of cholera treatment with highly diluted and succussed solutions. British Homoeopathic Journal 83: 132–134

Gibson RG, Gibson SLM, MacNeill AD, Buchanan WW 1978 Salicylates and homoeopathy in rheumatoid arthritis: preliminary observations. British Journal of Clinical Pharmacology 6: 391–395

Gibson RG, Gibson SLM, MacNeill AD, Buchanan WW 1980 Homoeopathic therapy in rheumatoid arthritis: evaluation by double-blind clinical therapeutic trial. British Journal of Clinical Pharmacology 9: 453–459

Glaz VG 1991 Hahnemann's theory in Russia. British Homoeopathic Journal 80:231–233

Groupe de Recherche et d' Essais Cliniques en Homéopathie 1989 Evaluation de deux produits homéopathiques sur la reprise du transit après chirurgie digestive. Un essai controlé multicentrique. Presse Médicale 18: 59–62

Güthlin C, Walach H, Heinrich S, Esser P 1998 Outcome research in complementary medicine: an evaluation concept and first results (abstract) [German]. In: Bullinger M, Morfeld M, Ravens-Sieberer U, Koch U (eds) Medical psychology in a changing health system: identity, integration and interdisciplinarity. Congress of the German Society for Medical Psychology. Pabst Science Publishers, Lengerich, p 74

Hadjaj B, Cherruault Y, Sainte-Laudy J 1993 Control of basophil degranulation. International Journal of Biomedical Computing 32: 151–159

Hahnemann S 1811 Pure pharmaceutical science: first part [German]. Arnold, Dresden

Hahnemann S 1979 Organon of healing art, 6th edn [German]. Hippokrates, Stuttgart

Hahnemann S 1983 Chronical diseases: their characteristic nature and homeopathic healing. Arnold, Dresden

Hess V 1993 Samuel Hahnemann and semiotics [German]. In: Jütte R (ed) Jahrbuch des Instituts für Geschichte der Medizin der Robert Bosch Stiftung. Steiner, Stuttgart, pp 177–204

Jacobs J, Jiminez LM, Gloyd S, Carares FE, Gaitan MP, Crothers D 1993 Homoeopathic treatment of acute childhood diarrhoea. British Homoeopathic Journal 82: 83–86

Jacobs J, Jimenez LM, Gloyd SS, Gale JL, Crothers D 1994 Treatment of acute childhood diarrhea with homeopathic medicine: a randomized clinical trial in Nicaragua. Pediatrics 93: 719–725

Jacobs J, Jimenez LM, Malthouse S, Chapman E, Crothers D, Masuk M, Jonas WB 2000 Homeopathic treatment of acute childhood diarrhea: results from a clinical trial in Nepal. Journal of Alternative and Complementary Medicine (in press)

Jonas WB 1996a Homeopathic provings: reproduction of the subjective? Journal of the American Institute of Homeopathy 8(4): 178–181

Jonas WB 1996b Homeopathy: cause or consequence? In: Chasworth J (ed) The ecology of health: identifying issues and alternatives. Sage, Thousand Oaks: pp. 285–296

Jonas WB 1998 A systematic review of the quality of controlled clinical trials in homeopathy. Abstracts of the 8th International Cochrane Colloquium, Baltimore, MD. October 25, p. 221

Jonas WB 2000 Anomalies in the anomalous: last gasp or light at last? [guest editorial.] British Homoeopathic Journal 89: 103–104

Jonas WB, Jacobs J 1996 Healing with homeopathy: the complete guide. Warner Books, New York

Jütte R 1997 200 years of the simile-principle: magic, medicine, metaphor [German]. Allgemeine Homöopathische Zeitung 242: 3–16

Jütte R 1998 The paradox of professionalisation: homeopathy and hydrotherapy as unorthodoxy in Germany in the 19th and 20th century. In: Jütte R, Risse GB, Woodward J (eds) Culture, knowledge, and healing. European Association for the History of Medicine and Health Publications, Sheffield, pp 65–88

Kirsch I, Sapirstein G 1998 Listening to prozac but hearing placebo: a meta-analysis of antidepressant medication. Prevention and Treatment: http://journals.apa.org/prevention 1: 2a

Kolisko L 1923 Physiological and physical proof of the effectiveness of smallest entities [German]. Verlag 'Der kommende Tag', Stuttgart

Kollerstrom J 1982 Basic scientific research into the 'low-dose effect'. British Homoeopathic Journal 71: 414–447

Leary B 1994 Cholera 1854: update. British Homoeopathic Journal 83: 117–121

Lewith G 2000 A double-blind, randomised, controlled clinical trial of ultramolecular potencies of house dust mite in asthmatic patients (abstract). Forschende Komplementärmedizin 7: 46

Linde K, Melchart D 1998 Randomized controlled trials of individualized homeopathy: a state-of-the-art review. Journal of Alternative and Complementary Medicine 4: 371–388

Linde K, Jonas WB, Melchart D, Worku F, Wagner H, Eitel F 1994 Critical review and meta-analysis of serial agitated dilutions in experimental toxicology. Human and Experimental Toxicology 13: 481–492

Linde K, Clausius N, Ramirez G, Melchart D, Eitel F, Hedges LV, Jonas WB 1997 Are the clinical effects of homoeopathy placebo effects? A meta-analysis of placebo controlled trials. Lancet 350: 834–843

Linde K, Scholz M, Ramirez G, Clausius N, Melchart D, Jonas WB 1999 Impact of study quality on outcome in placebo-controlled trials of homeopathy. Journal of Clinical Epidemiology 52: 631–636

Lüdtke R, Wilkens J 1999 Clinical trials of Arnica in homeopathic preparations [German]. In: Albrecht H, Frühwald M (eds) Jahrbuch. Carl und Veronica Carstens-Stiftung. KVC Verlag, Essen, pp. 97–112

Mayaux MJ, Guihard-Moscato ML, Schwartz D, Benveniste J 1988 Controlled clinical trial of homoeopathy in postoperative ileus (letter). Lancet 5: 528–529

Moerman DE 2000 Cultural variations in the placebo effect: ulcers, anxiety, and blood pressure. Medical Anthropology Quarterly 14: 51–72

Morgan PP 1992 Homeopathy – will its theory ever hold water? Canadian Medical Association Journal 146: 1719–1720

Reilly D 1998 Is homoeopathy a placebo response? What if it is? What if it is not? In: Ernst E, Hahn EG (eds) Homoeopathy: a critical appraisal. Butterworth Heinemann, London, pp 118–129

Reilly D 2000a Creating therapeutic consultations. In: The placebo response: biology and belief in clinical practice. Churchill Livingstone, London

Reilly D 2000b Can a placebo make you blush? Advances in Mind-Body Medicine (in press)

Reilly D, Taylor MA 1985 Potent placebo or potency? A proposed study model with initial findings using homeopathically prepared pollens in hayfever. British Homoeopathic Journal 74: 65–75

Reilly D, Taylor MA, McSharry C, Aitchinson T 1986 Is homoeopathy a placebo response? Controlled trial of homoeopathic potency with pollen in hayfever as a model. Lancet 18: 881–886

Reilly D, Taylor MA, Beattie NGM, Campbell JH, McSharry C 1994 Is evidence for homoeopathy reproducible? Lancet 344: 1601–1606

Remy W, Rakoski J, Siebenwirth J, Ulm K, Wiesenauer M 1995 Classical homeopathic therapy of eczema constitutionalis atopica. Plan of a prospective randomized, placebo controlled double blind study at the Dermatological Clinic and Outpatients' Clinic of the TU Munich [German]. Allergologie 18: 246–252

Riley DS 1994 Contemporary drug provings. Journal of the American Institute of Homeopathy 87(3): 161–165

Riley DS 1995 History of homoeopathic drug provings. Paper presented at the Homoeopathic Pharmacopea Convention of the United States, Philadelphia

Sainte-Laudy J, Belon P 1993 Inhibition of human basophil activation by high dilutions of histamine. Agents Actions (Special Conference Issue) 38C: 245–247

Sainte-Laudy J, Belon P 1996 Analysis of immunosuppressive activity of serial dilutions of histamine on human basophil activation by flow cytometry. Inflammation Research 45 (suppl 1): S33–S34

Sainte-Laudy J, Belon P 1997 Application of flow cytometry to the analysis of the immunosuppressive effect of histamine dilutions on human basophil activation: effect of cimetidine. Inflammation Research 46 (suppl 1): S27–S28

Sainte-Laudy J, Haynes D, Gershwin G 1986 Inhibition effects of whole blood dilutions on basophil degranulation. International Journal of Immunotherapy 2: 247–250

Scheible KF 1994 Hahnemann and the cholera. Historical viewing and critical evaluation of homeopathic therapy compared to conventional treatment [German]. Hang, Heidelberg

Schmidt JM 1994 Development of homeopathy in the United States [German]. Swiss Journal of the History of Medicine and Sciences 51: 84–100

Schulte J 1999 Effects of potentization in aqueous solutions. British Homoeopathic Journal 88: 155–160

Schulte J, Endler PC (eds) 1998 Fundamental research in ultra high dilution and homoeopathy. Kluwer, Dordrecht

Schüppel R 1990 Principles of homeopathy in conventional medicine [German]. Deutsches Journal für Homöopathie 9: 3–7

Schwanitz HJ 1983 Homoeopathic and Brownianism [German]. Gustav-Fischer-Verlag, Stuttgart

Scofield AM 1984 Homoeopathy and its potential role in agriculture. A critical review. Biological Agriculture and Horticulture 2: 1–50

Sherr J 1994 The dynamics and methodology of homoeopathic provings. Dynamis Books, West Malvern

Shipley M, Berry H, Broster G 1983 Controlled trial of homoeopathic treatment of osteoarthritis. Lancet 8316: 97–98

Siebenwirth J 1995 Effectiveness of classical homeopathic therapy of eczema constitutionalis atopica [German]. Jahrbuch Karl und Veronica Carstens-Stiftung 1: 94–103

Siebenwirth J, Rakoski J 1997 Classical homeopathic therapy of eczema [German]. Der Hautarzt 48(suppl 1): S22

Straumsheim PA, Borchgrevink CF, Mowinkel P, Kierulf H, Hafslund O 1997 Homeopatisk behandling av migrene. En dobbelt-blind, placebonkontrollert studie av 68 pasienter. Dynamis 2: 18–22

Taylor MA, Reilly D, Llewellyn-Jones RH, McSharry C, Aitchison TC 2000 Randomized controlled trial of homeopathic versus placebo in perennial allergic rhinitis with overview of four trial series. British Medical Journal 321: 471–476

Teixeira MZ 1999 Similitude in modern pharmacology. British Homoeopathic Journal 88: 112–120

Tveiten D, Bruseth S, Borchgrevink CF, Lohne K 1991 Effekt av Arnica D30 ved hard fysisk anstrengelse. Tidsskrift for Den Norske Laegeforening 111: 3630–3631

Tveiten D, Bruset S, Borchgrevink CF, Norseth J 1998 Effects of the homeopathic remedy Arnica D30 on marathon runners: a randomized, double-blind study during the 1995 Oslo marathon. Complementary Therapies in Medicine 6: 71–74

Vallance AK 1998 Can biological activity be maintained at ultra-high dilution? An overview of homeopathy, evidence, and Bayesian philosophy. Journal of Alternative and Complementary Medicine 4: 49–76

Van Wijk R, Wiegant FAC 1994 Cultured mammalian cells in homoeopathy research. The similia principle in self-recovery. Universiteit Utrecht, Faculteit Biologie, Utrecht

Van Wijk R, Wiegant FAC 1997 The similia principle in surviving stress: mammalian cells in homeopathy research. Universiteit Utrecht, Faculteit Biologie, Utrecht

Vandenbroucke JP 1997 Commentary: homoeopathy trials: going nowhere. Lancet 350: 824

Vickers A 1999 Independent replication of pre-clinical research in homoeopathy: a systematic review. Forschende Komplementärmedizin 6: 311–320

Vickers A, Fisher P, Smith C, Wyllie SE, Lewith GT 1997 Homoeopathy for delayed onset muscle soreness: a randomised double blind placebo controlled trial. British Journal of Sports Medicine 31: 304–307

Vickers A, Fisher P, Smith C, Wyllie SE, Rees R 1998 Homoeopathic Arnica 30X is ineffective for muscle soreness after long distance running: a randomized, double-blind, placebo-controlled trial. Clinical Journal of Pain 14: 227–231

Vithoulkas G 1980 The science of homoeopathy. Grove Press, New York

Walach H 1986 Homoeopathy as basic therapy. Plea for the scientific respectability of homeopathy [German]. Haug, Heidelberg

Walach H 1992 Scientific homeopathic remedy proving. Double-blind crossover study of a homeopathic high potency compared to placebo [German]. Haug, Heidelberg

Walach H 1993 Does a highly diluted homoeopathic drug act as a placebo in healthy volunteers? Experimental study of Belladonna C30. Journal of Psychosomatic Research 37: 851–860

Walach H 1994 Provings: the method and its future. British Homoeopathic Journal 83: 129–131

Walach H 1996 Blinding in clinical trials of homeopathy? [German] In: Hornung J (ed) Research methods in complementary medicine. About the necessity of methodological renewal. Schattauer, Stuttgart, pp 1–16

Walach H 1997 The pillar of homoeopathy: remedy provings in a scientific framework. British Homoeopathic Journal 86: 219–224

Walach H 1998 Methodology beyond controlled clinical trials. In: Ernst E, Hahn EG (eds) Homoeopathy: a critical appraisal. Butterworth Heinemann, London, pp 48–59

Walach H, Maidhof C 1999 Is the placebo effect dependent on time? In: Kirsch I (ed) Expectancy, experience, and behavior. American Psychological Association, Washington DC, pp 321–332

Walach H, Brednich A, Heinrich S, Esser P 1996 The test procedure of the Innungskrankenkasse on acupuncture and homeopathy. Evaluation concept and first experiences [German]. Forschende Komplementärmedizin 3: 12–20

Walach H, Gaus W, Haeusler W et al 1997a Classical homoeopathic treatment of chronic headaches. A double-blind, randomized, placebo-controlled study. Cephalalgia 17: 119–126

Walach H, Güthlin C, Heinrich S, Esser P 1997b Effects of homoeopathy and acupuncture – a longitudinal documentation study. International Society for Technology Assessment in Health Care, Barcelona, p 124

Walach H, Schüller S, Heinrich S, Esser P 1997c The test phase of the Innungskrankenkassen on acupuncture and homoeopathy (abstract). Forschende Komplementärmedizin 4: 121

Walach H, Güthlin C, Heinrich S, Esser P 1998a Effects of acupuncture and homeopathy: a prospective documentation. Intermediate results. Alternative Therapies in Health and Medicine 4: 105

Walach H, Van Asseldonk T, Bourkas P et al 1998b Electric measurement of ultra-high dilutions – a blinded controlled experiment. British Homoeopathic Journal 87: 3–12

Wehmeyer A, Heger M, Riley DS 1996 Homeopathic remedy provings – basics and reality [German]. In: Hornung J (ed) Research methods in complementary medicine. The necessity of methodological renewal. Schattauer, Stuttgart, pp 32–43

Weingärtner O 1992 Homeopathic potencies. Dream and reality in the search for a therapeutically effective component [German]. Springer, Berlin

Whitmarsh TE, Coleston-Shields DM, Steiner TJ 1997 Double-blind randomized placebo-controlled study of homoeopathic prophylaxis of migraine. Cephalalgia 17: 600–604

Wiesenauer M, Lüdtke R 1996 A meta-analysis of the homeopathic treatment of pollinosis with Galphimia glauca. Forschende Komplementärmedizin 3: 230–234

Witt C, Lüdtke R, Baur R, Willich SN 1998 Observational study of patients in homeopathic general practice [German]. In: Albrecht H, Frühwald M (eds) Jahrbuch der Carl und Veronica Carstens-Stiftung. KVC Verlag, Essen, pp 144–150

Witt C, Lüdtke R, Weber K, Chigne M, Baur R, Willich SN 1999 Observational study of patients in homeopathic general practice: interim report [German]. In: Albrecht H, Frühwald M (eds) Jahrbuch Carl and Veronica Carstens-Stiftung. KVC Verlag, Essen, pp 187–193

15

Manual therapies

Alan C Breen

INTRODUCTION

Manual therapies are as old as civilization. So fundamental is physical contact between human beings that it is not surprising that its reduction to the level of scientific enquiry is something of a task. Variations in treatments, patients and circumstances are endless and the problem is augmented by the fact that manual interventions are seldom applied in isolation from other social issues.

Research into treatments can be broadly grouped into those which investigate outcomes and those which investigate natural history or underpin diagnostic assessments. Both are essential to clinical evaluation. This chapter will review current methods of evaluating manual treatments with emphasis on research which is intended to be generalizable. This is not, however, to deny the importance of qualitative research and its value in providing direction and relevance.

After a brief acknowledgment of historical context, we will explore the research designs currently advocated for studying natural history of conditions and the potential benefits and harms of manual therapy. We will then consider the design of studies which set out to appraise such work, with an exercise in systematic review for the interested reader. The chapter ends with a look at how the issues raised have been dealt with in the production of one national clinical practice guideline for the management of acute back pain, for the precedent it sets for the future of research in this field.

HISTORICAL OVERVIEW

Until recently, its apparent 'defiance of science' has denied manual therapy a place in conventional health care. This, however, is changing. Research methodologies are emerging to cope with much of the heterogeneity surrounding physical treatments. Outcome measures which address quality of life have come forward

(Staquet et al 1998) and the main conditions for which such treatment is sought have been identified (Burton 1981, Foster et al 1999, Pedersen 1994). All of this helps to define the questions which scientific enquiry might usefully apply to the field of manual medicine. It is, however, a radical departure from the very recent status quo.

In ancient times the provision of a bonesetter in a Roman army camp would, in all probability, have been uncontested whereas today a variety of professions compete for recognition in the provision of manual therapies for patients with skeletal disabilities. This is perhaps a consequence of the growing professionalization of medicine. In the case of manual medicine, this arose mainly through the rapid emergence of chiropractic, osteopathy and the musculoskeletal arm of physiotherapy into a health-care field already dominated by orthopedic surgeons and other physical medicine specialists. The ensuing market rivalries have had harmful as well as beneficial effects for patients. While there has been a considerable development of treatment techniques and their applications, important research questions have often been obfuscated by competing interpretations of the issues.

RESEARCH DESIGNS

Studies of natural history

By the latter half of the 20th century, public resources had begun to be applied to investigate the socioeconomic impact of musculoskeletal problems. Health and social security statistics revealed the rising costs in lost working days, lost production and health care related to back pain.

Government groups initially made attempts to gather evidence about treatments for these problems (Cochrane 1979, NINCDS 1976) before realizing the importance of natural history as a prerequisite (AHCPR 1994, CSAG 1994, Spitzer 1995). Such studies revealed, for example, that patients who are allowed to become chronic have a diminishing likelihood of ever returning to productive employment and that depression and behavioral change are just as likely to be consequences as causes of chronic disability. In addition, much of the health impact is hidden in recurrent attacks, which are either not reported or spread across different carers (Thomas et al 1999).

These issues tend to call for cohort studies (as opposed to single case or case series studies), which investigate prospectively and with the necessary follow-up. Larger numbers of patients are needed for these studies than may be necessary for a clinical trial. Indeed, there is no advantage in using a randomized trial for addressing such questions.

Box 15.1   Attributes of studies of assessment and natural history

- Prospective cohort study
- Sample relevant to research question
- At least 100 cases
- At least 1 year follow-up

Clinical trials

If, on the other hand, the need is to determine the effectiveness of a therapy, there is no substitute for trying it out. The problems lie in making such trials fair. With this in mind, researchers came to appreciate the importance of randomization and control groups. Without the first, competing treatment arms lack equality of the chance to prevail. Without the second, there is no benchmark from which to measure effectiveness. Despite early recognition of these prerequisites, many of the early clinical trials of physical treatments for musculoskeletal problems had neither adequate numbers of subjects to detect differences nor outcome measures which were sufficiently reliable and responsive.

The solutions to these problems were relatively late in coming. Advances in statistical methods enabled the calculation of sample sizes and made the issue of the number of subjects needed to detect clinically important differences a crucial one (Jaeschke et al 1989). Equally important was the ability of the measures of treatment outcome to detect differences. Until the rigor and responsiveness of the available outcome measures improved, scientists wanting to conduct clinical trials of manual treatments were either handicapped by less than ideal tools (and at greater expense) or compelled to conduct limited trials. The more successful researchers were often those who chose the latter. Most of those who launched clinical trials sacrificed follow-up. Others kept the number of treatment arms to a minimum and instinctively tried to recruit respectable numbers.

Lack of knowledge about the natural history of complaints initially made trial design difficult. For example, one back pain trial (Coxhead et al 1981) used a crossover design in which treatment groups were exchanged after a short period (as often happens in drug trials). Unfortunately, and as we now know, most acute episodes resolve within a few weeks but recur, making long-term effects of treatment extremely important and crossover designs problematical (Thomas et al 1999). However, it was the issue of long-term chronicity which made follow-up of at least 1 year an important quality criterion for trials.

Choices and limitations in trial design

Some practitioners of manual therapy have tended to reject conventional trial methodologies on the basis that they do not adequately allow for the number of important variations, either in treatments or in patients. It was (and still is) held that often the very presence of a trial environment can itself influence results unacceptably – either by affecting response to treatment or by limiting its relevance because of the number of patients who have to be excluded to achieve reasonably homogeneous treatment groups. On the other hand, all treatment benefits are relative. Randomization seems the best way to sufficiently minimize the effects of chance.

Box 15.2   Economic constraints on the design of trials of manual therapy

- Number of subjects
- Number of treatments
- Length of follow-up

This trade-off between 'generalizability' and 'representativeness' is a continuing conundrum in the field. To some extent the problem can be minimized by using a 'pragmatic' trial design, which evaluates the overall management approach, in contrast to a more 'fastidious' or 'explanatory' method, which tries to identify which method's key element is more effective. Both methods have inherent strengths and dangers.

The first pragmatic trial of a manual therapy profession addressed British chiropractic (Meade et al 1990, 1995). This was explicitly a trial of a profession's approach to a defined condition (low back pain of mechanical origins and of all durations) against conventional hospital outpatient management. As a starting point, the trial designers chose to be 'pragmatic' and sacrifice a more explanatory design in order to obtain information which would be immediately applicable in health care. The result was a methodologically strong trial which showed a clear but modest result in favour of chiropractic over 3 years.

Subsequent discussion about the significance of this trial's results was a cameo of contemporary issues in complementary medicine research. Surrounding this trial, in a window of time of some 20 years, were some 36 other, more fastidious trials of manipulation (Shekelle et al 1992). These compared manipulation with a variety of other treatments, from corsets to analgesics and bed rest. Such was the interest in their results that some 53 reviews of them were published (Waddell et al 1999). These attempted, often in highly individual ways, to clarify the nature of the evidence provided and point out where doubt remained.

Much of the remaining doubt surrounded the optimal timing for manipulation and the type of patient who might benefit best from it – questions which remain unanswered. There is also disagreement about how manipulation is itself best defined and how other procedures, such as exercise programs and cognitive behavioral therapy, might be combined with it. For this type of problem, more powerful statistical methods have been developed. These allow a variety of 'factors' to be evaluated in a single trial (Altman 1991). It remains to be seen to what extent this can help to alleviate the methodological difficulties of trials in the manual therapy area.

This procession of trials is expensive, yet the expense is insignificant compared to the suffering and costs associated with the complaints. The results should ultimately suggest what to emphasize in treatment and for whom.

Table 15.1 Pragmatic and fastidious trial designs

	Pragmatic	Fastidious
Strengths	Represents treatment applied in practice	Specific method tested
	Eligible subjects readily available	Specific conditions identified
	Immediate applicability	Identifies effective components
Weaknesses	Effective components not identified	Numbers of eligible subjects small
	Specific conditions not known	Limited applicability (likely to miss effective components)

Adverse effects

Any suggestion in the press that there may be a significant risk in a therapy, however small, highlights the risk and undermines public trust (Bennett & Calman 1999). It is therefore essential that alleged risk is substantiated by evidence because, once lost, reestablishing trust is a long and uphill task. The public, however, has a right to expect best practice, hence the importance of research into risks and adverse effects.

Reports of serious adverse effects from manual therapies are extremely rare but also apparently unpredictable (Haldeman et al 1999). They may also go unreported. It is, however, also important to distinguish between adverse effects which are serious and treatment reactions which are not. Events which merit the term 'serious' are normally those which require admission to hospital, whereas a treatment reaction usually amounts to a temporary increase in the severity of the presenting complaint following treatment.

Serious adverse effects The most notorious serious adverse effect of manual therapy is probably stroke, resulting from dissection of one of the cerebrobasilar arteries following neck manipulation. The incidence of this has been estimated at between 1:400 000 and 1:1 300 000 (Haldeman et al 1999). The other main serious event is loss of power or sensation in a limb following spinal manipulation. This is reported to be even more rare at 1:100 000 000 (Haldeman & Rubenstein 1992).

Since the incidence is so low, such events are all but impossible to study prospectively. Moreover, it is important to distinguish 'risk' from 'incidence following', for the latter does not discriminate between events which happen 'because of' from 'after' the intervention. To calculate true risk, therefore, it is necessary to compare untreated subjects with treated ones over some years.

The ideal vehicle for doing this is a clinical trial in which subjects are randomly allocated to groups exposed and unexposed to the treatment. The relative risk is determined from a count of those in each group who suffer adverse events. When such events are rare, however, this level of rigor is impossible to achieve and therefore doubt must always remain about the exact level of risk.

This does not mean that research in this area is fruitless. Retrospective reviews of emergency hospital admissions for cerebrovascular accidents are in progress and will investigate any cases which followed manipulative treatment. Over many years there have been attempts to pool these statistics in order to come closer to a reasonable estimate of population risk, plus a closer description of the treatment components concerned (Assendelft et al 1996). Progress is incremental and, if kept abreast of, should lead to better treatment optimization and diminished risk.

Table 15.2 Estimation of relative risks for exposed and unexposed subjects (from Levine et al 1994)

Patient	Adverse event (case)	No adverse event (control)
Exposed	a	b
Not exposed	c	d

Relative risk = [a/(a+b)]/[c(c+d)]

> **Box 15.3**   Suggested methodological criteria for studies of treatment reactions
>
> - Prospective design
> - Blinded outcome evaluation
> - Exclusion of subjects whose conditions are unstable

Treatment reactions Transient increases in pain following manipulation are, unlike serious events, quite common, occurring after 25–50% of all manipulations (Barrett & Breen 2000, Leboeuf-Yde et al 1997, Senstadt et al 1996) and usually subsiding within 24 hours. This does not, however, necessarily mean that they are acceptable, especially if avoidable.

Research into reactions using questionnaires or patient interviews can represent a worst-case scenario if done blind to the practitioner or potentially underrepresent the intensity of the reaction if administered by the practice which gave the treatment. An additional (and somewhat obvious) consideration is that manual treatments are usually used for patients who are already in pain, with the intention of reducing disability in order to facilitate return to normal activities. This increased activity is usually essential but can in itself cause some additional pain.

Future studies aimed at distinguishing 'acceptable' from 'unacceptable' reactions should therefore also take into account which reactions are followed by overall improvement and which are not, as well as the patient's own perception of their acceptability or otherwise.

SYSTEMATIC REVIEWS OF MANUAL THERAPIES

As noted at the beginning of this chapter, the whole topic of manual therapy is a very heterogeneous one. This makes clear interpretation of context essential if clinical policies and decisions are to avoid continual argument without agreement. The literature holds many answers, all of them imperfect, hence the need for extreme clarity in attempting to use it to improve knowledge.

One way to achieve this is to insist on a systematic approach to arriving at conclusions based on evidence, whether these are to be used to drive clinical decisions or to start new research. We can experience this for ourselves in the following exercise of a limited systematic review.

An exercise in evidence appraisal

This exercise can be as brief or as ambitious as the reader desires. It is hoped that, for the majority of practitioners or researchers who are setting out in this field, it will be at least a moderately rewarding experience and be found relevant to practice and helpful in professional development. It can be conducted either as an individual or a group project. The exercise involves seeking an evidence-based view of a specific clinical topic. The steps are:

1. selecting the topic
2. finding the evidence
3. appraising the evidence
4. formulating (an) evidence-linked statement(s).

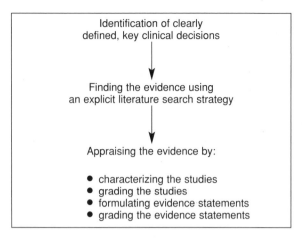

Figure 15.1 The systematic review process.

The first three of these steps are expanded upon in Figure 15.1 where the topic is, in fact, a key clinical decision for practice, where finding the evidence follows an explicit process and appraisal goes through some defined stages. After this process is completed, the exercise ends with an attempt to formulate one or two evidence-linked statements.

Selecting the topic (the key clinical decision)

A key clinical decision usually relates to diagnosis (i.e. which methods are valid and when should they be used) or to treatment or advice (i.e. which kinds and when to use them). The scope is endless and a brief excursion into the literature may result in the topic being dropped because of a lack of acceptable studies. An example might be the effectiveness of a treatment (or a group of treatments) for a specific problem, such as shoulder pain. As clear a definition as possible should be formulated before a literature search is started.

Finding the evidence

For this exercise, a MEDLINE search is all that is recommended. This takes little time and it is rewarding, although not essential, to do it with the help of a medical librarian.

The initial search strategy might be a computer search of all papers published in the past 10 years under a few search terms, for example *'shoulder'*, *'clinical trials'* and *'review'*. The latter term will ensure that the full benefits of any reviews already published are not missed.

The follow-up search strategy would then be to perform a second MEDLINE search using revised search terms in the light of information gained from reading the review paper, but leaving out the term *'review'*. For example, *'rotator cuff tear'*, *'adhesive capsulitis'*, *'clinical trials'*, *'treatments'*.

Table 15.3 Evidence table for randomized controlled trials

Authors/date	N	Patients	Setting	Treatment (t)
(Example) Philips et al 1996	117	Acute LBP 1st episode < 15 days	Family pract. or emergency dept	Graded reactivation +/– counseling

Controls (c)	Outcomes	Results
'Let pain be your guide' until return to normal	Pain at 6/12 (no rating of severity or disability) exercise level	NS dif pain at 6/12 begin exer by 3 days: t86% c 55% P < 0.01

Table 15.4 Methodological quality grading for clinical trials

CRITERIA				TOTAL	
Authors /date	Randomization	Blinding outcome assessment	Intention to treat analysis	Drop-outs and withdrawals	(Out of 6)
(maximum)	2	2	1	1	6

Appraising the evidence

This begins with **characterizing the studies** by summarizing their content in an evidence table (Table 15.3) (for example, randomized controlled trials of reactivation exercises for back pain). This allows the reviewer to make informed choices about what studies to include by considering clearly to what extent they address the key clinical decision.

The next step is **grading the studies for methodological quality**. There are some key criteria for this which fit well with manual therapy topics. They are shown in Box 15.4. This results in a score out of 6 for each paper and enables the reviewer to see clearly whether the evidence is based on high- or low-quality studies. This is an important and often revealing part of the exercise, which illustrates the truth in the statement 'The best evidence may not necessarily be good evidence.' The results of grading can be summarized in a table, as shown in Table 15.4.

Formulating graded evidence statements is an exercise in qualitative judgment. It is helpful to consider what kind of statements current evidence will actually support and there are a number of ways of grading this. The suggested method for this exercise is as used in the RCGP guidelines evidence review (Waddell et al 1999) and is on three levels, as shown in Box 15.5.

If this exercise is being done in a group, it can be a valuable experience to try to agree on graded evidence statements with specific reference to the search criteria, evidence tables and methodological grading.

Box 15.4 Methodological Quality Grading for Clinical Trials (adapted from Moher et al 1998 and Schulz et al 1995)

Criterion	Points
RANDOMIZATION	
Randomized	+1
Method described and appropriate[1]	+1
Method inappropriate[1]	−1
BLINDING OF OUTCOME ASSESSMENT[2]	
Double blind	+1
Masking described and appropriate	+1
Method inappropriate	−1
INTENTION TO TREAT ANALYSIS[3]	+1
DROP-OUTS AND WITHDRAWALS	
Numbers and reasons for withdrawal reported	+1
MAXIMUM TOTAL POINTS	6

[1] Random numbers generated by computer, random numbers table, shuffled cards or tossed coins and minimization. Randomization clearly (authors explicitly state method) and adequately concealed from treatment and assessment.
[2] Outcome evaluators shielded from knowledge of treatment assignments.
[3] No exclusions from analysis regardless of whether they: (a) deviated from protocol; (b) withdrew; (c) dropped out; (d) were lost to follow-up.

Box 15.5   Grading criteria for evidence statements

Strong evidence
Generally consistent finding in a majority of multiple acceptable studies

Moderate evidence
Either based on a single acceptable study or a weak or inconsistent finding in some multiple acceptable studies

Weak evidence
Limited scientific evidence, which does not meet all the criteria of acceptable studies

---

Formulating recommendations for clinical practice is the final step in this exercise. For many key clinical decisions, it may become clear that the research evidence, as obtained in the review, will not support any recommendations for practice but does suggest how further work or a more rigorous review might fill the gaps. If it is thought possible to formulate recommendations, these should be:

- clearly linked to the evidence statements
- unambiguous
- related to a key clinical decision
- agreed by a consensus
- graded as strong, medium or weak (optional).

CLINICAL PRACTICE GUIDELINES

The purpose of clinical guidelines is to help practitioners and their patients to make informed decisions about care. The process is very much like the exercise described above, but with a much more comprehensive search strategy (Breen & Feder 1999). Guidelines are 'tools, not rules' and are meant to be neither slavishly followed nor studiously ignored. The best of them are the result of multidisciplinary consensus, based on a substantial body of evidence that is sufficiently well organized and explicit to make it possible to accommodate different professional perspectives.

The RCGP Back Pain Guidelines

For back pain, major evidence reviews carried out in the United States (AHCPR 1994) and Great Britain (CSAG 1994) sought to bring together best evidence about the condition and its treatment in the acute and subacute phases (i.e. up to 6 weeks from onset). This was because of the need to prevent chronicity and because most of the evidence related to the acute phase.

The question 'How good is the evidence?' was crucial to making recommendations for this guideline. As in our exercise (above), research evidence was graded for methodological quality before summary statements were made. These statements were then themselves given a score to indicate the quality of the evidence behind them. Then, recommendations based on the evidence statements were added to constitute the guideline. In the example below, the evidence statements are based on the clinical trials of manipulation which met the criteria at the time of the review.

Box 15.6   Manipulation evidence statements and recommendations (from Waddell et al 1999)

Evidence

There is strong evidence that: In acute and subacute back pain manipulation provides better short-term improvement in pain and activity levels and higher patient satisfaction than the treatments to which it has been compared.

There is moderate evidence that: the risks of manipulation are very low, provided patients are selected and assessed properly and it is carried out by a trained therapist or practitioner. Manipulation should not be used in patients with severe or progressive neurological deficit in view of the rare but serious risk of neurological complication.

There is limited evidence that: it is possible to select which patients will respond or what kind of manipulation is most effective. The optimum timing for this intervention is unclear.

Recommendation

Consider manipulative treatment for patients who need additional help with pain relief or who are failing to return to normal activities

---

Not all of them were of high quality and not all related to exactly the same kind of manipulation.

CONCLUSION

Research is seldom conducive to sweeping statements. When made without qualification, these can lead to unhelpful hermeneutical discussion. Research into evocative topics also tends to be misquoted. If there are antidotes to these conflicts, they probably lie in explicit context and systematic review, where the criteria for evaluation are a part of the assessments themselves. Hopefully, more collaborative efforts will deal with the topics more equitably.

The ability and preparedness of practitioners across disciplines to accept the need to make changes to practice is also essential to progress. We are influenced to change by convincing evidence of a better approach and not to change by disruption of already complex health-care practices (Grol et al 1998). Evidence-based recommendations about manual therapies, which are feasible and about issues that matter, should have a chance, even if they introduce a context which seems foreign.

Manual therapy is currently among the most researched areas of complementary medicine. This chapter highlights the areas and methodologies which are prominent at time of writing as well as those which have helped to shape the status of these treatments. They mainly address the natural history and diagnosis of commonly treated complaints and the potential benefits and harms of the treatments themselves. The focus is mainly on issues related to cohort studies and clinical trials.

Methods for investigating these issues are challenging, partly because of the conflict between the need to generalize while at the same time representing the therapies as they are offered to patients. The criteria for successful studies have been put forward as benchmarks for those who may be contemplating involvement in such studies or using existing ones as evidence for change. An exercise in critical appraisal is also offered which, it is hoped, will be useful to practitioners as an introduction to the various methodologies, particularly that of randomized trials.

The chapter concludes with a brief reference to evidence-based clinical practice guidelines. Like summarized research evidence, these are subject to revision in the light of further research and its critical appraisal. That this evidence can be both helpful and limited is the nature of research. Hopefully, any discomfort resulting from this conflict will be made more tolerable by this discussion.

Acknowledgments

This chapter owes much to exposure to the groups which participated in the preparation of the Clinical Standards Advisory Group's Back Pain report and the RCGP Acute Back Pain Guidelines. Its construction owes even more to the help of my secretary Mrs Jane Baker.

REFERENCES

Agency for Health Care Policy Research 1994 Clinical practice guidelines for acute low back pain problems in adults. US Department of Health and Human Services, Washington DC

Altman DG 1991 Practical statistics for medical research. Chapman and Hall, London

Assendelft WJ, Bouter LM, Knipschild PG 1996 Complications of spinal manipulation: a comprehensive review of the literature. Journal of Family Practice 42(5): 475–480

Barrett A, Breen AC 2000 Adverse effects of spinal manipulation. Journal of the Royal Society of Medicine (in press)

Bennett P, Calman K 1999 Risk communication and public health. Oxford University Press, Oxford

Breen A, Feder G 1999 Where does the evidence come from? In: Hutchinson A, Baker R (eds) Making use of guidelines in clinical practice. Radcliffe Medical Press, Oxford, pp 15–28

Burton AK 1981 Back pain in osteopathic practice. Rheumatology and Rehabilitation 20: 239–246

Clinical Standards Advisory Group, Department of Health 1994 Epidemiology review: the epidemiology and cost of back pain. HMSO, London

Cochrane AL 1979 A Working Group on Back Pain report to Secretary of State of Social Services, Department of Health and Social Security. HMSO, London

Coxhead CE, Meade TW, Inskip H, North WRS, Troup JDG 1981 Multicentre trial of physiotherapy in the management of sciatic symptoms. Lancet 1: 1065–1068

Foster NE, Thompson KA, Baxter GD, Allen JM 1999 Management of nonspecific low back pain by physiotherapists in Britain and Ireland. Spine 24(13): 1332–1342

Grol R, Dalhuijsen J, Thomas S, Int Veld C, Rutten G, Mokkink H 1998 Attributes of clinical guidelines that influence use of guidelines in general practice: observational study. British Medical Journal 317: 858–861

Haldeman S, Rubinstein SM 1992 Cauda equina syndrome in patients undergoing manipulation of the lumbar spine. Spine 17(12): 1469–1473

Haldeman S, Kohlbeck FJ, McGregor M 1999 Risk factors and precipitating neck movements causing vertebrobasilar artery dissection after cervical trauma and spinal manipulation. Spine 24(8): 785–794

Jaeschke R, Singler J, Guyatt GH 1989 Measurement of health status: ascertaining the minimal clinically important difference. Controlled Clinical Trials 10: 407–415

Leboeuf-Yde C, Hennius B, Rudberg E, Leufvenmark P 1997 Side effects of chiropractic treatment: a prospective study. Journal of Manipulative and Physiological Therapeutics 20(8): 511–515

Levine L, Walter S, Lee H, Haines T, Holbrook A, Moyer V 1994 Users' guides to the medical literature: IV. How to use an article about harm. Journal of the American Medical Association 271(20): 1615–1619

Meade TW, Dyer S, Browne W, Townsend J, Frank AO 1990 Low back pain of mechanical origin: randomised comparison of chiropractic and hospital outpatient treatment. British Medical Journal 300: 1431–1437

Meade TW, Dyer S, Browne W, Frank AO 1995 Randomised comparison of chiropractic and hospital outpatient management for low back pain: results from extended follow-up. British Medical Journal 311: 349–351

Moher D, Pham B, Jones A 1998 Does quality of reports of randomised trials affect estimates of intervention efficacy reported in meta-analyses? Lancet 352: 609–613

National Institute of Neurological and Communicative Disorders and Stroke 1976 The research status of spinal manipulative therapy. Monograph no. 5. NINCDS, Bethesda, MD

Pedersen P 1994 A survey of chiropractic practice in Europe. European Journal of Chiropractic 42(S): 3–28

Schulz KF, Chalmers I, Hayes RJ, Altman DG 1995 Review: empirical evidence of bias. Journal of the American Medical Association 273(5): 408–412

Senstad O, Leboeuf-Yde C, Borchgrevink CF 1996 Side effects of chiropractic spinal manipulation: types, frequency, discomfort and course. Scandinavian Journal of Primary Health Care 14: 50–53

Shekelle PG, Adams AJ, Chassin MR, Hurwitz EL, Brook RH 1992 Review: spinal manipulation for low-back pain. Annals of Internal Medicine 117(7): 590–597

Spitzer WO 1995 Scientific monograph of the Quebec Task Force on whiplash-associated disorders: redefining 'whiplash' and its management. Spine 20(8S)

Staquet MJ, Hays RD, Fayers PM 1998 Quality of life assessment in clinical trials: methods and practice. Oxford University Press, Oxford

Thomas E, Silman AJ, Croft PR, Papageorgiou AC, Jayson MIV 1999 Predicting who develops chronic low back pain in primary care: a prospective study. British Medical Journal 318: 1662–1667

Waddell G, McIntosh A, Hutchinson A, Feder G, Lewis M 1999 Low back pain evidence review. Royal College of General Practitioners, London

---

FURTHER READING

Bennett P, Calman K 1999 Risk communication and public health. Oxford University Press, Oxford

Senior figures from within government departments, the NHS, the Consumers' Association, the King's Fund and other prominent institutions have contributed to this useful book which is a great help in building confidence in what constitutes 'good practice' in risk communication. Manual therapy practitioners and researchers alike can learn much from the wisdom contained here.

Bronfort G 1997 Efficacy of manual therapies of the spine. Institute for Research in Extramural Medicine, Vrije Universiteit, Amsterdam, Van der Boechorststraat 7, 1081 BT Amsterdam, The Netherlands

This PhD thesis is at the same time a good coverage of the evidence of effectiveness of manual therapies from the indexed literature and an expanded illustration of how systematic reviews might be used. Its methodology is as was current in 1997 and although there has been some progress since then, the approach is well worth digesting.

Chalmers I, Altman DG 1995 Systematic reviews. BMJ Publishing, London

This seminal work on systematic reviews is only 119 pages long. It conceptualizes admirably and in unembellished language the rationale for this ground-breaking innovation.

Daly J, Kellehear A, Gliksman M 1997 The public health researcher: a methodological guide. Oxford University Press, Melbourne

Written for students with no background in public health, this paperback volume provides the pragmatic view of research. Based on the viewpoint of policymakers, its perspective is one which practitioners and even researchers may encounter seldom but without which an understanding of the implementation of research can be elusive.

Hulley SB, Cummings SR 1988 Designing clinical research – an epidemiological approach. Williams and Wilkins, Baltimore

This is a helpful reference text for anyone wishing to select, or understand, a research design related to manual therapies. This is an inexpensive, paperback book by a group of epidemiologists in America which informs, without intimidating, in this complex subject.

Hutchinson A, Baker B 1999 Making use of guidelines in clinical practice. Radcliffe Medical Press, Oxford

This is a very current work of 18 contributors whose task was to bridge the gap between research and clinical decision making. It is particularly recommended for those who are concerned about possible prescriptive handling of research results by standard-setters in the future. It demystifies guidelines by describing their nature, from development to implementation.

Institute for Alternative Futures 1998 The future of complementary and alternative approaches (CAAs) in US health care. NCMIC Insurance Company, Virginia

This is a report which presents the view of insurers, having consulted both medical and chiropractic experts in the US. It is a pragmatic treatment of the sociological possibilities emanating from research, especially in manual therapy.

Kraemer HC, Thiermann S 1987 How many subjects? Statistical power analysis in research. Sage Publications, London

This is a small (120 pages) but authoritative book, which provides the rationale and method necessary for determining the sample size in clinical trials. Complete with power tables, this book is a concise solution for hands-on researchers of clinical effectiveness.

Lederman E 1997 Fundamentals of manual therapy: physiology, neurology and psychology. Churchill Livingstone, New York

For readers who have an interest in manual therapy but wish to gain understanding of how it works on patients, this book provides a useful source of physiological and psychophysiological information. Written by a practicing osteopath undertaking doctoral research in the neurophysiological basis of manual therapy, this is one of the best reference sources about mechanisms available.

Murray DM 1998 Design and analysis of group-randomized trials. Monographs in Epidemiology and Biostatistics Vol 27. Oxford University Press, New York

This book is recommended because the issue that it addresses is a growing one in trials of manual therapy, that of identifying the patients who will benefit. By randomizing groups, as opposed to individuals, it becomes possible to further allocate to subgroups without compromising the randomization process. This means greater ability to discover subgroups who respond best – an important and outstanding question for manual therapy. Unfortunately, despite its potential, this method is full of pitfalls dealt with admirably in this substantial monograph.

Peckham M, Smith R 1996 Scientific basis of health services. BMJ Publishing, London

A product of 27 expert contributors, this paperback volume takes on the problems of organizing evidence-based services in the presence of shifting evidence. The authors suggest innovative ways of dealing with this through continuous appraisal methods, which researchers should be aware of.

Pynsent P, Fairbank J, Carr A 1993 Outcome measures in orthopaedics. Butterworth Heinemann, Oxford

Manual therapies are used principally for musculoskeletal complaints and any measurement of outcomes requires some form of device, be it a goniometer or questionnaire. This book catalogues a number of such instruments in a useful reference volume which is relevant to the whole body.

Waddell G 1998 The back pain revolution. Churchill Livingstone, Edinburgh

This is a highly authoritative monograph on the current status of back pain research. Fully referenced, it puts into words the radical change which research has brought to the subject and sets the scene for a very different future for manual therapies and those who practice them.

16

Massage therapy research methods

Tiffany Field

AN EVOLVING RESEARCH PROCESS

Historical background

Massage therapy dates to prerecorded time and was epitomized by Hippocrates in 400 BC as 'medicine being the art of rubbing'. Research in the field of massage therapy also goes back many years. The first academic journal publications date back to the 1930s when massage therapy research on humans and animals was fairly popular. Many of those research projects focused on documenting the increased blood flow associated with massage therapy as well as reducing muscle atrophy. Although many of the questions then are the same questions now, the approach to research was limited by the measurement technology and the studies often featured either single cases or very small sample sizes which were typically self-selected samples of clinical patients being treated for one condition. Measurement technology, for example, was limited to physiological measures such as heart rate, blood pressure and temperature and was basically a biomechanical model. The advent of biochemical assay technology has enabled more expansive models. Even in the last few years the ability to assay neurohormonal activity in non-invasive procedures has advanced the field significantly in terms of looking at underlying mechanisms.

Additional methodological problems included a lack of control groups which meant the effects being measured could be placebo effects or effects of simply receiving attention from a human being. Later came the use of control groups but they were non-treatment groups that did not control for attention from the therapist. Even more recently, massage therapy has been compared to other treatments such as relaxation therapy. However, these group comparisons are confounded by compliance problems as relaxation therapy is often viewed as requiring work and concentration.

The research question

Typically the research question for massage therapy studies is whether massage therapy is an effective and cost-effective treatment for a given condition. Much of research is 'me-search', the questions often derived from the investigator's personal interest, such as somebody close having experienced that condition or because that is a condition seen in one's practice or research setting or because the condition is a recent funding priority and the research is intended to provide pilot data for seeking funding in that area. Determining how effective the massage therapy is means finding meaningful variables such as the gold standard variables for that particular condition, designing the most effective massage therapy technique for that condition and selecting the most appropriate treatment comparison group and attention control group. To address these questions typically leads first to a literature search.

Literature search

MEDLINE and Psychology Abstracts are the biggest sources of current literature abstracts. Although it is fascinating to read the older literature, which often serves as a source of good ideas for replication studies using more sophisticated approaches to problems, the typical published paper features references from the last decade. Thus, literature searches are typically confined to the last decade. In searching through the abstracts yielded by the computer literature search, researchers look to see if the question has already been addressed, if the condition has been treated by massage therapy and if the literature suggests the next steps. Entering a term for the condition along with massage therapy is likely to yield the most specific information needed. However, starting with a more global approach using simply the terms 'treatment' or 'therapy' and the name of the condition would yield significantly more abstracts and more general information about:

- the condition
- the hypothesized underlying etiology
- the gold standard and other measures that have been used in research on other treatments of the condition
- ideas for treatment comparisons that might serve as an attention control group.

The literature search can serve as the background for the first part of the paper, the introduction. To be sure one knows the problem being addressed and the methods used to study that problem, it is always a good idea to write the first half of the paper before starting the study. The literature search will provide background on the incidence of the problem, the symptoms, possibly the etiology or hypothesized etiology, previous treatments both allopathic and alternative, and the efficacy of those treatments. Once the background and methods sections are drafted, the paper can serve as a proposal that can go to potential collaborators who will facilitate the research.

Selection of collaborators

Selecting a clinic or a hospital setting or a school setting for non-clinical problems is always advantageous given their provision of participants for the research. Another advantage is that clinical settings are often the places where potential collaborators work, such as allopathic or alternative physicians in osteopathic medicine. Having a medical collaborator is important in terms of being able to keep abreast of the most important clinical measures for the condition being studied, having a referral source and someone who can administer the clinical measures and having clinically relevant research that is considered credible by potential journals for publication and by potential reviewers for grant funding. Important scientific collaborators include a neuroscientist for assays of biochemical measures or for interpretation of physiological, e.g. EEG, data and a statistician or PhD researcher to assist with designing and conducting the statistical analyses for the project. Massage therapy collaborators are also needed, particularly if the researcher is not a massage therapist, for the design of the massage therapy procedure to be used and to help identify measures that can directly assess the effects of that procedure. Another important collaboration consideration is locating a source of volunteer massage therapists for the actual treatments or for demonstration of the treatments if parents or significant others are going to be the therapists.

Selecting treatment and attention control comparison groups

Traditionally, the alternative treatment group has been compared to a standard treatment control group, for comparison assessments made on the first and last days of treatment. However, a potential placebo effect or an effect of the therapist simply providing attention to the subject has highlighted the need for using treatment comparison and/or attention control groups. In much of our early work we used relaxation therapy as a comparison treatment group because relaxation therapy has been shown to be effective particularly in alleviating stress and anxiety, which often exacerbate the medical conditions we are studying. Also, we considered it important to establish a greater efficacy of massage therapy (versus relaxation therapy) in order to justify the greater expense of massage therapy treatment. The problem we found was that it may be a biased comparison inasmuch as people view relaxation therapy as hard work, requiring significant concentration and self-discipline. Thus, we may be experiencing compliance problems when we use relaxation therapy as a control. In addition, because relaxation therapy requires a certain amount of cognitive sophistication along with a reasonable attention span, it may be too difficult for young children. Therefore, we have used attention controls such as rocking the child, holding the child or playing with toys and holding and reading to the child as comparison groups in massage therapy research with children.

More recently, since we discovered the critical importance of stimulating pressure receptors for the massage to be effective, we have elected to use a sham massage therapy procedure comparison group which receives exactly the same massage as the treatment group, but with no pressure. This also enables the subjects to be 'naïve' or 'blind' to expecting a unique effect of their particular treatment condition. The subjects or participants in each group would expect to receive some benefit from massage whether it was deep pressure (in the case of the real treatment group) or light pressure as applied in the sham group. Double blinding is also possible insofar as the physicians who are providing the standard treatment and the massage therapists providing the experimental treatment do not necessarily have expectations that one or the other massage style is going to be more effective. This is the closest we can come to a double-blinded situation in massage therapy research. This way neither the participant nor the therapists are biased towards the treatment.

Selection of sample parameters and random assignment to groups

Demographic variables including age, gender, ethnicity and socioeconomic status are considered the most basic sampling parameters that need to be equivalent across groups. Generally, by virtue of the location and demographics of the clinical setting, the age, ethnicity and socioeconomic status of the participants are somewhat homogeneous. The ethnicity is often predominantly one ethnic group or another and the socioeconomic status is limited in range. This helps prevent the research design from being confounded by variability as a function of varying ethnicity or socioeconomic status and the random assignment to groups would be expected to result in a roughly equivalent distribution in each group. Clinics are also generally separated by pediatrics, adulthood and sometimes even by aging, by function of the condition and by the specialty of the physician, so they are also typically homogeneous on age and condition.

Another critical background variable, particularly in medical research, is the severity of the condition. This variable is more likely to result in a heterogeneous grouping and therefore would need careful matching or stratification. Typically, participants are randomly assigned to groups by a table of random numbers or by flipping a coin and it is intended that the randomization would yield roughly equivalent groups on background variables. The most conservative way to ensure equivalent groups is to match subjects across groups. For example, in studies on premature babies, the subjects are frequently matched on birthweight and gestational age and then randomly assigned to treatment and control groups. The less conservative way is a random stratification procedure whereby cells would be made so that if there were two birthweight groups (low birthweight and very low birthweight) and two gestational age groups (short gestation and very short gestation), there would be four cells (a very short gestation and very low birthweight group, a very short gestation and low birthweight group, a short gestation and very low birthweight group, and a short gestation and low birthweight group). Subjects would then be randomly assigned to these cells and there would be a roughly equal number of subjects assigned to each cell in each group by the end of the study.

The selection of the sample size involves several considerations, including economic considerations. The typical first step for determining sample size is to conduct a power analysis to determine whether there will be enough statistical power for the data analysis given the sample size. Power can be determined by taking the difference of the two group means from a previous study and dividing that by the larger of the two standard deviations for the same means.

Despite the sample size determined by the power analysis, economic consideration constrain the sample size to a minimum. One way to remain economical is by conducting data analyses at intervals of 10 subjects per group to determine whether groups are significantly different on the key variables. If there is simply a trend for statistical significance for those variables, then the absence of significance may mean that the sample is still too small and more subjects are needed. This can be done at intervals of two subjects per group.

Selection of variables

The most important variable is the gold standard clinical variable that is typically viewed as a criterion for clinical improvement in any condition. For example, in diabetes the gold standard variable is typically the glucose level and in asthma it is typically the peak air flow measure. The clinical gold standard measure can be designated by a collaborating physician or can be found in the literature. Often there is more than one clinical gold standard measure. If there are multiple variables that would be considered redundant, some selection needs to be made. For statistical analysis reasons, researchers try to keep in mind a five-subjects-to-one-variable ratio, attempting not to be variable heavy.

The second important set of variables are stress variables as they are thought to exacerbate any clinical condition. Because of the subjective nature of stress, it is good to have not only self-report stress variables such as the State Anxiety Index and the Profile of Mood State measures (to be elaborated later) but also a converging physiological measure, e.g. vagal tone or a chemical measure, e.g. salivary cortisol, to provide validation of the subject's self-report on stress.

Typically, treatment research involves assessing the immediate effects of the therapy session and the longer term effects at the end of the treatment period. Occasionally effects are also assessed after some interval of time after the end of therapy as a follow-up assessment. The immediate effects of the session are often measured by self-reports of how the subject feels, the anxiety level and the mood state, and saliva samples are taken for assaying stress hormone (cortisol). Sometimes a heart rate or a blood pressure measure would also be taken as a physiological index of stress. In the clinical condition of itching, as in burn during healing, some kind of temperature gauge of the itchiness immediately following the treatment would be made. Similarly, if the pain condition of juvenile rheumatoid arthritis was the subject of study, the immediate effects might be the response to a dolorimeter which is a pressure gauge that determines the threshold beyond which the subject could no longer tolerate the pressure of the rod-like dolorimeter. Longer term measures are, of course, the gold standard or criteria for the success of the therapy. Typically the longer term measures include a clinical index such as the number of back pain-free days or number of migraine-free days, the glucose levels or the pulmonary measures taken in children with asthma. Those might also include a change in the level of depression and a change in the level of urinary stress hormones (norepinephrine, epinephrine).

The importance of having converging variables from several levels (behavioral, physiological and biochemical) cannot be overstated. Almost invariably, self-report measures are taken on pencil and paper forms. Recently, manual physiologic assessments have been popular such as heart rate and blood pressure. More sophisticated measures such as vagal tone, which needs to be derived from the respiratory sinus arrhythmia of heart rate, are more difficult to collect because of the sophisticated equipment required and the data reduction that not only requires technical expertise but is also considered labor intensive. Serious consideration needs to be given to biochemical assays and the significance of those to the research because assaying salivary and urinary cortisol levels requires expensive assay kits or neuroscientists in an expensively equipped laboratory. For example, a salivary cortisol assay costs $25.00. If you consider that at least two (one pre- and one post-therapy session) would need to be taken at each of the two assessment periods (first day, last day), the salivary cortisol protocol for each subject would cost approximately $100.00.

Other measures include sleep/wake behavior observations which typically are valuable as they indicate how sleep and wake behavior can be significantly affected across treatment and as the clinical condition changes. Because sleep and wake behavior are the best index of the subject's functioning, these are important measures. They do, however, require training of observers either to conduct live observations by using time sample unit coding systems or laptop computers or to code videotapes of the behavior if it has been videotaped. This then requires assessing interobserver reliability or the process whereby observers come to agree on the behaviors that they are observing and to code them similarly. The standard for interobserver reliability is 90%; that is, that the two observers agree on 90% of the time sample intervals on the behaviors being observed. This requires significant amounts of practice time on the part of the observers and interobserver reliability assessment time. Interobserver reliability needs to be calculated using what is called a kappa coefficient, a statistical calculation that corrects for chance disagreement.

Other important variables have already been mentioned, including the gold standard clinical measure that is typically performed by the physician. Sometimes when children are involved, it is important to tap measures of parental stress and mood state to determine whether their stress may be affecting the child's clinical course and whether the child's clinical course is, in turn, affecting them.

Procedures

The treatment and research procedures need considerable attention and careful thought prior to the beginning of the study. In a sense, it is good to have completed the first half of the paper (the introduction and the methods) prior to the study so that they can be critiqued by colleagues and collaborators and so that every person in the treatment and research process is 'on the same page'.

One of the most important aspects of the research procedure is that the observers be blind to the hypotheses of the study and to the subject's group assignment. Otherwise their treatment of the subject and their observations would be biased by knowing the intent of the study and the subject's group assignment. Having multiple assessors and multiple observers often prevents this biasing process but training each of the individuals and then working to achieve interobserver reliability is a costly process.

Similarly, the treatment procedure requires careful thought. On the one hand, the procedures need to be extremely detailed and in most cases need to cover many muscle groups and different parts of the body to be effective. However, there are also cost considerations like the length of the session both for the cost of the study but also for the cost of transporting the treatment once it is determined to be effective. Most individuals are unable to afford more than one half-hour session of a professional massage therapist per week and even if their significant other is trained in the procedure, that person is not likely to conduct massages more than a couple of times a week at 20–30 minutes per session. Thus, these are important time and cost-effectiveness considerations. Volunteer massage therapists can often be found for research studies given that they appreciate the research experience, particularly when that involves children, whom they are rarely able to see otherwise. The research can end up being fairly inexpensive in that way. But, at the termination of the study the subjects are less likely to continue their treatment if the procedure that has proven effective is too costly. Thus, in our studies we try to limit the therapy sessions to once or twice a week at approximately 20 minutes a session and have a built-in period for training a significant other to conduct the massage following the end of the study and we provide that individual with a video demonstration of the therapy procedure. In the case of children, parents are often the therapists for the massage studies and this becomes part of their ritual (typically bedtime ritual) that helps not only the children but themselves as well. We have documented that the therapist benefits from providing the massage in the same way that the recipient benefits. Massage therapy by parents, of course, is a very cost-effective procedure and one that not only helps the child's clinical condition but also helps make the parent feel empowered as part of the treatment process and helps the relationship between parent and child.

In the next section, special considerations are reviewed for specific research protocols, including growth and development prenatally and in early infancy, attention deficit disorders, psychiatric conditions and addictions, pain syndromes, autoimmune conditions including asthma, diabetes and dermatitis, and immune conditions including HIV and breast cancer.

SPECIFIC CONSIDERATIONS FOR SPECIFIC CONDITIONS

Growth and development

Prenatal development

A very large literature documents the effects of stress and, more recently, of depression on the developing fetus. Some data suggest that the cortisol levels of the pregnant woman at 28 weeks gestation can predict premature delivery with a reliability of 0.98 (Wadwha et al 1998). The babies born prematurely in turn had significantly higher cortisol levels than those who went to term. In another study conducted by our group, the mothers' prenatal catecholamines (norepinephrine and epinephrine) and stress neurohormones (cortisol) during the last trimester of gestation were mimicked by their newborns, suggesting that the mothers' hormones were crossing the placenta (Lundy et al 1998). This is consistent with data showing that in a study 40% of the mothers' cortisol crossed the placenta (Glover et al 1999). Fetuses of depressed mothers in our study were more active from the fifth to the seventh gestational month, at which point they become more like fetuses of non-depressed women (Dieter et al 2000).

These data highlight the importance of conducting stress and depression-reducing interventions during pregnancy. In one of our recent studies we documented that pregnancy massage conducted twice a week over the last trimester of pregnancy did in fact reduce perinatal complications, the most important one being a reduction in prematurity (Field et al 1998c). In addition, the mothers' leg and back pains were reduced and, in turn, they were able to sleep better. In a current study we are looking at the effects of pregnancy massage specifically on depressed mothers with the expectation that massage will not only reduce depression and anxiety but also the neurotransmitters and hormones associated with stress (norepinephrine and cortisol) will increase the antidepressant hormone serotonin, will reduce fetal activity and finally will improve the newborn outcome, including a reduction in neonatal stress hormones and complications such as prematurity and an increase in birthweight. We have added a significant number of variables to this current study because of the greater involvement of the depressed mothers and because we expect to impact on a greater number of variables than the previous study.

Labor massage

We have piloted a labor massage study with women with normal deliveries (Field et al 1998c) and, following the positive effects, we are now replicating that procedure for depressed women. In that study we were able to reduce labor pain simply by the significant other being taught the labor massage and giving the massage for the first 15 minutes of every hour of labor. The labors were shorter, the need for labor medication was less and the mothers were hospitalized for a shorter period of time and experienced less postpartum depression. In the replication study, we will add more measures that might better inform us as to the underlying mechanism. In the current labor study we will also record fetal activity and fetal heart rate as well as the periodicity and intensity of the mother's contractions and obstetric interventions, including medication.

Preterm growth and development

Unfortunately for some infants, preterm deliveries are unavoidable and those infants are hospitalized in neonatal intensive care units for sometimes 2–5 months. Prematurity-related stress is accompanied by the iatrogenic stresses of the nursery, including loud sounds and bright lights. At some point when the newborn is no longer in medical jeopardy, the only reason for the infant remaining in the intensive care unit is to gain sufficient weight to be discharged. At this time we conduct massage. Typically we have conducted the massages for three 15-minute periods a day for a 10-day period, although, in our most recent study, we were able to establish a 47% weight gain (same weight gain achieved in the 10-day study) in a 5-day study (Dieter et al 2001). Therefore, we have converted to using the more cost-effective 5-day treatment period. We are also trying to teach the parents to continue the massage following discharge.

In our early studies, the most important measure was, of course, weight gain. We also learned a significant amount about the infant's state by recording 45-minute sleep/wake sessions. We were able to document that indeterminate sleep (a sleep state that is very difficult to code because it is disorganized and does not look like deep sleep or active sleep) was a very important variable. In fact, the only neonatal variable that was noted to relate to childhood IQ was the amount of indeterminate sleep (which was negatively related). The other critical measures, of course, were the number of days in the hospital and the cost associated with that. We were able to document that we could save $4.7 billion in hospital costs if we were to provide 10 days of massage to the approximately 470 000 infants born prematurely in the US each year (saving $10 000 in hospital costs per infant). NICU costs have increased significantly since that time period, so the cost savings would now be even greater. One of the other important variables was conducting the Brazelton newborn assessments with these infants (see Appendix A for the sleep/wake behavior codes and the list of Brazelton behaviors). Had we not known how much more responsive the baby was to social stimulation following the massage therapy, we never would have been able to hypothesize why these infants go on to have a weight and developmental advantage at 8 months post-discharge (Scafidi et al 1993). Knowing that their newborn behavior was more responsive, we argued that their interactions with their parents were better and thus, the infants were able to 'pull' better stimulation from their parents and eventually show better growth and development.

In our current study we have added growth hormone (IGF1) and oxytocin measurements. These variables are considered important for growth and have been shown to increase with additional stimulation in the rat model (Uvnas-Moberg 1994). In our earlier study we speculated that the underlying mechanism for the weight gain in the preterm babies following massage was that their vagal activity (activity of the 10th cranial nerve, the vagus) was increased and thereby there were more hormones being released for more efficient food absorption since that is the function of the vegetative branch of the vagus nerve. Vagal activity was measured and shown to increase and plasma samples of insulin increased (one of the more active growth hormones). This may be one of the underlying mechanisms, along with several others including the fact that gastric motility (which is also stimulated by the vegetative branch of the vagus) may also increase. That, too, could contribute to more efficient food absorption.

Having the additional measure of IGF1 and oxytocin will enable us to further determine the underlying mechanism. Knowing underlying mechanisms is the most effective way to ensure that the massage gets put into practice in NICUs. Some investigators' use of the functional MRI method may also show that there is significant brain development that accompanies the massage therapy, most particularly the development of the hippocampus (the region that involves memory functions). In the rat model, which often serves as a model for the human with respect to growth and brain development, the rat has been noted to have significantly increased dendritic arborization in the hippocampal region following extra pressure stimulation. The experimenter can use a paintbrush to simulate the mother's deep pressure tongue licking. The stimulated rat pups were saved from senility during the aging process because their cortisol levels were lower and thereby more brain cells were saved.

Unfortunately, in the human, measures such as functional MRI and the additional growth measures (IGF1 and oxytocin) are extremely expensive. For example, the growth measures cannot be assayed until dozens of samples are collected because of the expense involved. Functional MRI is even more prohibitively expensive with respect to the equipment that is often unavailable to investigators and the technical expertise that is needed to read the functional MRI scans. Although what happens inside the brain is often very compelling evidence for the medical field, the clinical measure, in this case weight gain, is often the more important variable and it is also the easiest and least expensive to measure.

Attention and attention disorders

Two of the most reliable indicators of attention are vagal activity and EEG patterns. The stimulation of the 10th cranial nerve, the vagus, is critical for attention. Attention is accompanied by slower heart rate and increased vagal activity. Vagal activity is the heart rate that accompanies sinus arrhythmia, so it can be easily transferred from heart rate recordings by a computer program. The very expensive $6000 vagal tone monitor is not necessary, although it more readily yields vagal activity than using the computer package. EEG also requires sophisticated equipment and technical expertise for reducing the data. EEG patterns that accompany attentiveness include decreased alpha, decreased beta and increased theta. In a recent study we documented this pattern of heightened alertness/attentiveness following 15-minute chair massages in the subjects' offices (Field et al 1997a). The heightened alertness/attentiveness EEG pattern was accompanied by improved performance on math computation tasks, including being able to perform them in less time with greater accuracy following the massage sessions. We have also documented enhanced performance by infants on habituation tasks (primitive learning tasks involving learning that a repeated stimulus like the sound of a bell, used in the Brazelton scale, becomes irrelevant because it does not signal anything else happening and is therefore no longer responded to) (Cigales et al 1997). Finally, in a study on preschoolers we were able to show that following a brief massage the children were able to perform IQ tasks in less time and more accurately (Hart et al 1998).

Children with attentional disorders

Children with autism (Field et al 1997b) and children with attention deficit hyperactivity disorder (ADHD) (Field et al 1998a) are also able to perform better and stay on task for longer periods of time following massage therapy sessions. In the study on children with autism, we recorded their classroom behavior including how much time they were on task, how little attention they paid to irrelevant stimuli, how much stereotypic behavior they showed and how much social relatedness was observed toward the teacher (Field et al 1997b). Following massage therapy (two sessions per week by a massage therapist) these children were able to stay on task longer and relate more to their teachers. In a subsequent study we used parents as the therapists and we were able to show that the children not only spent more time being attentive and on-task in the classroom but they also showed fewer sleep problems. Since sleep problems are prevalent in children with autism, the sleep diaries recording the onset of sleep, duration of sleep and number of sleep wakings were a critical measure and one that surprisingly improved over this brief period of time.

Because parents of children with autism may be biased toward seeing any signs of improvement, it is particularly important to have converging measures. Since sleep behavior is likely to affect classroom behavior, classroom behavior is worth observing. In addition, in some studies we have used time lapse video equipment to record nighttime sleep by simply turning on a nightlight and running the time lapse video camera. Subsequently, eight hours of sleep can be coded in one hour. The movements on the tape look like Charlie Chaplin moving about, so they are very easy to record if you are interested in a gross rating of activity. Gross activity can differentiate deep sleep from active sleep and, of course, nightwakings and moving out of the bed are easy to code from videotapes.

A measure somewhere between the use of videotaping, which can be somewhat intrusive and requires compliance of the subject, and the more subjective sleep diaries is a device called an actometer. The actometer is a Timex watch with the spring removed such that every time the subject moves his or her arm, the time hand on the watch moves so that the time elapsed from nighttime to daytime is a total amount of activity that has occurred during nighttime sleep. These are easy to use with all age groups.

Similar measures were used with ADHD children and in a subsequent study, with adolescents with ADHD (Field et al 1998a). Here again the most meaningful measures are those taken in the classroom where the children express and perhaps experience their worst problems. In these studies, we also used teacher and parent rating scales (the Conners Scale because it is shorter than the Child Behavior Checklist, which is another measure of the same type that is frequently used by parents and teachers). In many studies, the parents' and teachers' ratings are highly correlated, although because parents and teachers observe different behaviors in the two different settings, some behaviors are difficult for the parents to rate, for example classroom attentiveness, and some are difficult for the teachers to rate, for example sleep behavior. Teachers' and parents' ratings have been criticized because of their suspected subjectivity. However, because they have been highly correlated with independent observer ratings, they have been subject to less criticism recently.

Optimally, for ratings of attentiveness we would have some kind of device that would be mounted on the head and record eye movements or free field recording of heart rate that would be unaffected by movement artefact. However, when sophisticated devices are ultimately designed for recordings of this nature, they are often shown to be highly correlated with behavioral ratings. For example, the EEG recording of sleep is highly correlated with the actometer readings of sleep activity and the time lapse video recordings of activity.

Psychiatric conditions

Most psychiatric conditions are accompanied by depression or at least depressed mood state and anxiety. Thus, in all psychiatric conditions we have studied, we have used the following self-report scales.

- The Profile of Mood States (McNair et al 1971) which taps depressed mood state, anxiety, anger and confusion.

- The Center for Epidemiological Studies Depression Scale (Radloff 1977) or the Beck Depression Inventory (Beck et al 1961), both of which measure depressive symptoms. We have found that the CESD is more sensitive (detects more individuals with depressive symptoms) and is also more user friendly or simpler such that adolescents and less educated people are more able to complete this instrument.
- The State Trait Anxiety Inventory (Spielberger et al 1970) (which also has a children's version called the STAIC), assesses state anxiety (current, short-term anxiety) and trait anxiety (closer to being a personality trait). The authors of these scales have now created two new instruments that measure depression and anger. These 20-item Likert-type scales are extremely easy to complete and have good psychometric properties, including good test-retest reliability.

In the psychiatric conditions we also try to have a converging measure of behavior, including the symptoms that are reported in the self-report scales such as depressed affect, behavioral agitation and angry behavior. For behavioral observations we designed the Behavior Observation Scale (see Appendix B). These behaviors, along with others, are rated on a five-point scale following a brief observation. Typically, like the mood scales which are completed by the subject before and after the therapy session, the behavioral observations are also made before the massage therapy session and after.

The third set of measures we have invariably collected in psychiatric conditions are saliva (for an assay of the stress hormone cortisol before and after the first and last massage therapy session) and urine (for assays of the stress neurotransmitters norepinephrine and epinephrine and the body's natural antidepressants, dopamine and serotonin). The salivary measure of cortisol is taken as an immediate index of the reduction of stress during the therapy session (see Appendix C for the assay procedure) and the urinary assays are made to assess the longer term effects of massage therapy over the course of the study (see Appendix C for assays).

We have recorded the above self-help, behavioral observation and biochemical samples in all of our studies on depressed children, adolescents and depressed mothers, as well as the studies we have conducted on eating disorders (anorexia, bulimia) to assess the longer term effects of the massage therapy treatment. While depression, eating disorders and addictions are considered to have an underlying depression base, which suggests the use of depression measures across studies, there are also, of course, measures that are unique to each of the conditions. Measures that were unique to the different studies include the following.

- Having time lapse videotaped sleep during the child and adolescent psychiatry study as well as a set of nurses' ratings of the children's and adolescents' behavior on the psychiatric unit.
- Additional measures for the eating disorder study included the Eating Disorders Inventory (Garner et al 1983).
- For a smoking addiction study, the number of cravings and cigarettes smoked.
- For the depressed adult studies we have also recorded EEG. Depressed individuals typically have relative right frontal EEG during the expression or reception of emotional expressions. The right frontal area of the brain is an area

for processing negative emotions. Activation of this area has been noted to shift to symmetry following massage therapy. Thus, in the depression studies we have employed the use of EEG (see Appendix D for an elaboration of these methods).

- For the posttraumatic stress disorder group of children (following Hurricane Andrew), we also employed the children's self-drawings using magic markers as an index of the children's change in depression. The drawings are simply scored on seven points including: (1) small self-figure on page; (2) use of dark colors; (3) missing facial features; (4) sad face; (5) distorted figure; (6) displaced body parts; and (7) agitated lines. Typically, depressed children have made drawings that feature very few facial features, distorted body parts and a small figure on the page. Self-drawings are a very reliable index of the children's mood state.

Pain syndromes

For pain alleviation, we have studied a number of pain syndromes including migraine headaches, lower back pain, premenstrual syndrome, pain from burns, fibromyalgia and juvenile rheumatoid arthritis. In these conditions we have used very similar self-report scales on pain including the McGill Pain Questionnaire, the Pain Intensity Scale and a visual analog scale which is generally in the form of a ruler with ratings along its scale or a thermometer with similar ratings or a series of sad to happy faces in the case of children's ratings of pain. In the case of adults these self-report scales are completed by themselves alone and in the case of children, we often have parents rating the amount of pain existing as well as the physician making a rating. For each of the syndromes we have also used measures unique to that syndrome for assessing functioning of the individual. So, for example, for the burn subjects who we hoped would have higher pain thresholds following the massage therapy sessions, we assessed their affective reaction to debridement (skin brushing). For juvenile rheumatoid arthritis, we had a parent's assessment of the child's ability to continue activities of daily living. For lower back pain we had functional assessments of range of motion, ability to touch toes, etc. For fibromyalgia we used a dolorimeter (a rod that exerts pressure until the patient winces which represents the pain threshold) and for migraine headaches, we had a measure of headache-free days.

Because anxiety exacerbates pain syndromes, we also used anxiety scales (State Trait Anxiety Inventory) to assess the pre-post massage therapy session anxiety levels. In addition, we used salivary cortisol as the secondary index of anxiety/stress levels pre and post massage therapy sessions. In addition, because sleep is considered disturbed in most pain syndromes, either because of the pain or because the sleep syndrome is contributing to the pain (the direction of effects is not certain here), we have used sleep recordings (typically sleep diaries). More recently, because we have come to notice that in all of the pain syndrome studies sleep improved following massage therapy and pain in turn was reduced, we are now trying to get better measures of sleep, including actometer readings during sleep. One current theory about the origins of pain syndromes is that there is insufficient quiet or restorative sleep and when that happens, there are increased levels of substance P which causes pain. Because substance P can be measured in salivary samples, we are assaying substance P at the beginning and end of the massage therapy treatment periods.

Autoimmune disorders

Once again, because stress and particularly stress hormones such as cortisol are known to interact and affect autoimmune and immune conditions, we measure cortisol in saliva before and after the massage therapy sessions and in urine at the beginning and end of the study period. In all of the autoimmune diseases we have studied to date (asthma, diabetes and dermatitis) we have studied children and used the parents as the massage therapists. We know that the parents are also likely to benefit from the therapy because grandparent volunteer massage therapists who massaged infants became less depressed and had lower cortisol levels (Field et al 1998b). We also know that parents' stress levels impact on children's stress levels and, in turn, may affect their autoimmune condition. Thus, we also assess stress in the parents using self-report measures. Otherwise, the measures for the autoimmune diseases have been as different as the diseases themselves.

For asthma, the gold standard clinical measure is the peak air flow monitor value recorded by the child and parent. Typically these are done on a daily basis and a diary-like recording is made. The pulmonologist also has the four standard pulmonary measures that are recorded at the beginning and the end of the study. These include the forced vital flow capacity, forced expiratory volume, average flow rate and peak expiratory flow.

In the case of diabetes, a self-report measure was completed by the parents, in this case on the child's glucose regulation, insulin and food regulation and exercise. In addition, glucose levels were measured by the children and their parents using a calibrated glucometer which we provided. Here it was important for the readings to be taken at the same time of day by the parents. The use of confirmatory measures such as fructosamine and glycosylated hemoglobin would provide confirmatory data in a future study.

For the clinical assessment of changes in dermatitis following the massage therapy treatment period, the physician assessed the following in both the focal area and the global area of the dermatitis:

- redness
- lichenification (thickening and hardening of the skin, often resulting from the irritation caused by repeated scratching of a pruritic lesion)
- scaling
- excoriation (an abrasion typically from scratching)
- pruritus (the symptom of itching).
  These were rated on a scale from 0–3 by the dermatologist and a dermatology fellow, who were blind to the child's group assignment.

Immune disorders

One of the immune measures that seems to be invariably improved following massage therapy across all of our immune studies, including HIV in adults (Ironson et al 1996), HIV in adolescents (Diego et al 2001) and breast cancer (Hernandez-Reif et al 2001), is the increased production of natural killer cells. Natural killer cells are considered the front line of the immune system and they ward off viral and cancer cells. A current theory suggests that they may even substitute for the destroyed CD4 cells in HIV. Therefore, we have invariably assayed natural killer cell number and natural killer cell cytotoxicity (activity). Of course, a number of other CD cells are related and those too have been measured (see Appendix E for the immune measures we typically assay). In more immune-compromised conditions such as the study on HIV men, the CD4 cell number was so low that it was not possible to reverse those numbers, whereas in the less immune-compromised adolescent HIV study, we were able not only to increase natural killer cells but also reverse the CD4 cell number and improve the CD4:CD8 ratio (the HIV disease marker). Again, like all the other conditions we have studied, these immune conditions are highly affected by stress hormones so we have also assayed cortisol levels (cortisol being known to kill immune cells).

STATISTICAL ANALYSES

The statistical analyses should be left to a statistician or a PhD trained researcher on the project. While the actual use of the statistical analysis software is like following a recipe, it is important to know the appropriate statistics to use and how to interpret the results. A brief description of the basics will be given here.

In any group treatment comparison research, the scores or values of the variables are averaged across the group to obtain a mean score/rating/value. The distribution of the individuals around the mean performance is called variability and a typical distribution would have a mean in the middle of a line with most of the individuals falling in a hill around the mean but as individuals depart from the group value, they become farther out on 'downward slopes of the hill' either to the left or to the right of the peak of the hill. To give an example, the mean IQ score for the population at large is 100. However, there are many individuals who perform higher and many that perform lower. One standard deviation from the mean would be 16 points higher, or a score of 116, or 16 points lower, or a score of 84. Two standard deviations would be twice 16 or 132 or 100 minus 32, and very few people would be out beyond the two standard deviations. The standard deviation is the term for variability.

A simple statistical comparison between groups can be made by a t-test where the group means and the group standard deviations are taken into consideration to arrive at a t-value which is then indicated as being significant if this value could only happen five times out of 100 times or significantly more often than chance (which would be five in 100 times) (at the $P =$ or > 0.05 level). Typically t values greater than 2.00 are significant. After performing a t-test by hand on the calculator or computer, the t-values can be looked for in a table of t-values and the P-value or significance level also checked. The significance level only indicates whether the test result was statistically significant, suggesting that the groups were significantly different on that value.

Another group comparison test is called the F test which is basically the same as a t-test but is performed when there are more than two groups being compared. The test for yielding an F-value is called the analysis of variance (ANOVA). Once again, an F test would be checked in a statistics book table to determine the P-level (significance level). Typically F-values greater than 4.00 are significant. More complex ANOVAs can be performed when there are more than two groups and more than three variables. These are called MANOVAs which is an abbreviation for multivariate analyses of variance. Whenever there are multiple variables and multiple groups, a MANOVA is performed on the group of variables followed by post-hoc ANOVAs on each of the variables. The MANOVA indicates whether the groups are significantly different on the group of variables as a whole. Subsequently, the ANOVAs are conducted to determine whether the groups are different on each of the individual variables. If there is more than one independent measure describing the group, for example age and gender, and the MANOVAs and ANOVAs yield significant differences, it is then necessary to conduct post-hoc t-tests to test all the possible comparisons.

Another way of looking at the data is to determine the relationships between the variables. For example, does gender relate to anxiety scores such that higher anxiety scores are noted for males versus females? The entire group of variables can be entered into a correlation analysis and the relationships between variables can be determined. The computer program prints out a matrix of correlation coefficients that range from 0 to 0.99. If gender and anxiety are correlated 0.83, this is an extremely high correlation or a strong relationship. If anxiety levels run from low to high with higher values reflecting higher anxiety and males are classified as a 1 and females as a 2, then the relationship between gender and anxiety would be a negative 0.83 (−0.83) relationship with males having higher anxiety. If females had higher anxiety, the correlation coefficient would be a positive 0.83. Again, the table of numbers is checked for the P-level (if the computer output does not provide that).

Further analyses can be conducted, for example stepwise regression analyses. In this analysis it is possible to determine the relative importance of the predictor variables or the independent variables. Again, if we are talking about gender and anxiety we would enter into the stepwise regression analysis the anxiety score as the dependent measure (or the outcome measure) and gender along with age would be entered as the predictor variables. If gender has a high correlation (0.83), as was already noted, the computer program will enter gender as a predictor variable into the equation. This would be interpreted as explaining 64% of the outcome variance or variability. If you multiply 0.83 (which is the R or the correlation coefficient by itself to get the R square or variance), this would tell you how much the variable gender is contributing to the outcome variable anxiety (64%). If then age came into the equation at the second step and the correlation coefficient was 0.91 with an R square of 0.81 or 81%, that would have added 17% to the variance (64% plus 17% equaling 81%).

These, then, are some of the simplest analyses performed in treatment research. Many things are considered in selecting the types of data analysis, including whether the data are normally distributed or skewed, for example. It may be necessary to use non-parametric statistics (instead of the parametric statistics just described) because the database fails to meet the required assumptions to perform the parametric analyses. These considerations are complex and understanding them as well as using them appropriately requires considerable coursework in statistics.

CONCLUSION

In summary, the methodology for massage therapy research is similar to methodology for many kinds of research in psychology and medicine. Designing the study, including the treatments and the measures, is the most important aspect of conducting the research. Careful attention to detail at all stages of the process is critical. Finally, being careful not to overinterpret or overgeneralize from the data is very important. Collaboration between therapists and scientists throughout the scientific process is critical for improving and advancing the research methodology and for addressing the important questions in the field.

Acknowledgments

We would like to thank the subjects who participated in our research and the researchers who collected and analyzed data. This research was supported by an NIMH Senior Research Scientist Award (MH#00331) and by a merit award from NIMH to Tiffany Field (MH#46586) and by funding from Johnson & Johnson.

REFERENCES

Beck A, Ward C, Mendelson M, Mach J, Erbaugh J 1961 An inventory for measuring depression. Archives of General Psychiatry 4: 561–571

Cigales M, Field T, Lundy B, Cuadra A, Hart S 1997 Massage enhances recovery from habituation in normal infants. Infant Behavior and Development 20: 29–34

Diego MA, Hernandez-Reif M, Field T, Friedman L, Shaw K 2001 Massage therapy effects on immune function in adolescents with HIV. International Journal of Neuroscience 106: 35–45

Dieter JNI, Field T, Hernandez-Reif M et al 2000 Fetal activity in fetuses of depressed mothers. Journal of Pediatrics (in press)

Field T, Quintino O, Henteleff T, Wells-Keife L, Delvecchio-Feinberg G 1997a Job stress reduction therapies. Alternative Therapies 3: 54–56

Field T, Lasko D, Mundy P et al 1997b Brief report: autistic children's attentiveness and responsivity improved after touch therapy. Journal of Autism and Developmental Disorder 27(3): 333–338

Field T, Quintino O, Hernandez-Reif M, Koslovsky G 1998a Adolescents with attention deficit hyperactivity disorder benefit from massage therapy. Adolescence 33: 103–108

Field T, Hernandez-Reif M, Quintino O, Schanberg S, Kuhn C 1998b Elder retired volunteers benefit from giving massage therapy to infants. Journal of Applied Gerontology 17: 229–239

Field T, Hernandez-Reif M, Taylor S, Quintino O, Burman I 1998c Labor pain is reduced by massage therapy. Journal of Psychosomatic Obstetrics and Gynecology 18:•286–291

Garner DM, Olmstead MP, Polivy J 1983 The Eating Disorders Inventory: a measure of cognitive behavioral dimensions of anorexia nervosa and bulimia. In: Darby PL, Garfinkel PR, Garner DM, Coscina DV (eds) Anorexia nervosa: recent developments in research. Alan R Liss, New York, pp 173–184

Glover V, Teixeira J, Gitau R, Fisk NM 1999 Mechanisms by which maternal mood in pregnancy may affect the fetus. Contemporary Reviews in Obstetrics and Gynecology 25: 1–6

Hart S, Field T, Hernandez-Reif M, Lundy B 1998 Preschoolers' cognitive performance improves following massage. Early Child Development and Care 143: 59–64

Hernandez-Reif M, Ironson G, Field T et al 2000 Immunological responses of breast cancer patients to massage therapy.

Ironson G, Field T, Scafidi F et al 1996 Massage therapy is associated with enhancement of the immune system's cytotoxic capacity. International Journal of Neuroscience 84: 205–218

Lundy B, Jones NA, Field T et al 1998 Prenatal depressive symptoms and neonatal outcome. Infant Behavior and Development 22: 121–137

McNair DM, Lorr M, Droppleman LF 1971 POMS – profile of mood states. Educational and Industrial Testing Services, San Diego, CA

Radloff L 1977 The CES-D Scale: a self-report depression scale for research in the general population. Applied Psychological Measures 1: 385–401

Scafidi F, Field T, Schanberg SM 1993 Factors that predict which preterm infants benefit most from massage therapy. Journal of Developmental and Behavioral Pediatrics 14(3): 176–180

Spielberger CD, Gorusch TC, Lushene RE 1970 The State Trait Anxiety Inventory. Consulting Psychologists Press, Palo Alto, CA

Uvnas-Moberg K 1994 Role of efferent and afferent vagal nerve activity during reproduction: integrating function of oxytocin on metabolism and behavior. Psychoneuroendocrinology 19: 687–695

Wadwha PD, Porto M, Garite TJ, Chicz-DeMet A, Sandman CA 1998 Maternal corticotropin releasing hormone levels in the early third trimester predict length of gestation in human pregnancy. American Journal of Obstetrics and Gynecology 179: 1079–1085

APPENDIX A   SLEEP STATES AND BRAZELTON NEONATAL BEHAVIOR ASSESSMENT SCALE

Sleep states
Deep
Light
Drowsy
Alert
Active
Crying

Brazelton items
In sleep
　Flashlight
　Rattle
　Bell

Uncover
Pin prick
Ankle clonus
Foot grasp (plantar)
Babinski

Undress
Passive movements: arms——legs——
General tone

Hold
Palmar grasp——pull-to-sit——
Standing——Walking——
Placing——Incurvation——
Body tone——Crawling——
Rooting——Sucking——
Nystagmus——Glabella——
Cuddliness——Tonic dev.——

Orientation
Inanimate visual (ball)
Inanimate aud. (rattle)
Inanimate aud. and visual (rattle)
Animate visual (face)
Animate auditory (voice)
Animate aud. and visual

Return to bassinette
Defensive (cloth on face)
Tonic neck reflex
Moro reflex

Brazelton behaviors
State changes
　Predominant states
　# of changes

Self quieting
Attempts
Brief (5 seconds)
Successful (15 seconds)

Hand to mouth
None
Swipes
Contact
Insertion
Startles

Tremulousness

Skin color

Irritable crying
Pull-to-sit
Uncover
Pin prick
Undress
TNR
Prone
Moro
Defensive

APPENDIX B BEHAVIOR RATINGS DURING MASSAGE

Date _____

Subject name _____   Evaluator _____

A.	PRE	Pulse			
1.	State	–	Drowsy	Inactive Alert	Active Alert
2.	Affect	–	Negative/Flat	Neutral	Positive
3.	Activity	–	Low	Moderate	High
4.	Vocalization	–	Low	Moderate	High
5.	Anxiety	–	Low	Moderate	High
6.	Cooperation	–	Low	Moderate	High
7.	Fidgeting/ Nerv. Behavior	–	Low	Moderate	High

B.	DURING	Pulse			
1.	State	–	Drowsy	Inactive Alert	Active Alert
2.	Affect	–	Negative/Flat	Neutral	Positive
3.	Activity	–	Low	Moderate	High
4.	Vocalization	–	Low	Moderate	High
5.	Anxiety	–	Low	Moderate	High
6.	Cooperation	–	Low	Moderate	High
7.	Fidgeting/ Nerv. Behavior	–	Low	Moderate	High

C.	POST	Pulse			
1.	State	–	Drowsy	Inactive Alert	Active Alert
2.	Affect	–	Negative/Flat	Neutral	Positive
3.	Activity	–	Low	Moderate	High
4.	Vocalization	–	Low	Moderate	High
5.	Anxiety	–	Low	Moderate	High
6.	Cooperation	–	Low	Moderate	High
7.	Fidgeting/ Nerv. Behavior	–	Low	Moderate	High

APPENDIX C   CORTISOL, CATECHOLAMINES AND SEROTONIN (5HIAA)

Cortisol assays

Cortisol is measured in plasma or urine by radioimmunoassay using an extremely specific antiserum from Radioassay Systems Laboratories (Carson City, CA). The specificity of the assay is such that biological fluids can be assayed directly following heat inactivation of CBG, eliminating the need for time-consuming extraction into organic solvents which is usually required for this assay. Only 5–10 µl of sample is needed for triplicate assay. Specially purified 3H-cortisol from the same supplier is used as the labeled hormone. Bound and free hormones are separated by the dextran-coated charcoal technique. The sensitivity of the assay is 0.025 ng/tube. The interassay and intraassay coefficients of variation are less than 10% and 5% respectively. Standards are prepared from cortisol from the same supplier and quality control samples representing low, medium and high values are run in every assay.

Catecholamine and serotonin (5HIAA) assays

Recent advances on HPLC have vastly simplified analysis of urinary catecholamines and their metabolites from a time-consuming procedure involving multiple purification steps to a single-step purification, followed by chromatographic separation and electrochemical detection. These new methodologic developments, which we have previously used to great advantage in analysis of plasma catecholamines, will greatly simplify what was previously an extremely difficult task. Analysis of urinary catecholamines (norepinephrine, epinephrine and dopamine) will be conducted in two steps. Urinary catecholamines and O-methylated metabolites will be measured by high pressure liquid chromatography (HPLC) and electrochemical detection following online purification by cation exchange chromatography using a methodology already being used in this laboratory for plasma catecholamines. Urine, VMA, HVA and MHPG will be measured similarly by HPLC following extraction into ethyl acetate.

As the goal of these studies is to measure integrated sympathetic activity rather than to identify the specific pattern of urinary metabolites, all urine will be treated with glucalase, a combination of glucuronidase and sulfatase, in order to hydrolyze conjugated metabolites before the analysis is conducted. The pH of urine is adjusted to 5.2 with acetate buffer and the urine incubated for 16 hours with the enzyme preparation. After hydrolysis, aliquots are taken for analysis of catecholamines and metabolites as described below.

The assay for the urinary catecholamines and O-methylated metabolites is the same as that used currently in this laboratory for plasma catecholamines. Urine is injected directly onto the chromatograph, which contains an on-line cation exchange column. Samples are absorbed onto this precolumn using a mobile phase of low ionic strength (0.02 M citrate, 0.2M potassium acetate, 1.5 mM EDTA, pH 3.5). Norepinephrine, epinephrine, dopamine, normetanephrine and metanephrine are eluted with a mobile phase of higher ionic strength (0.02 M citrate, 0.2 M potassium acetate and 1.5 mM octanesulfonate (as ion-pair reagent) with a final pH of 5.5). Catecholamines are separated by reverse phase chromatography using C18-bonded 5 µm microparticulate silica (Spherisorb ODS). Catecholamines are detected with a TL-5A glassy carbon working electrode maintained at +600 mV vs an Ag/AgCl reference electrode in conjunction with a LC-4A controller (Bioanalytical Systems). An internal standard (3.4 dihydroxybenzylamine) is added at the beginning of the procedure. Standard curves are generated from catecholamine-free urine to which known amounts of standard have been added. Sensitivity of the assay is 25–50 pg.

An analogous method for measurement of acidic catecholamine metabolites in urine which has been developed for use with urine from patient populations including infants will be used. Urine is acidified by addition of 6N HCl and acidic metabolites (HVA, VMA and MHPG) extracted into ethyl acetate. The ethyl acetate extract is dried under nitrogen, redissolved in distilled water for injection. Samples are chromatographed on the same reverse phase C18 column described above. HVA, MHPG and HVA are eluted by gradient elution. The low ionic strength mobile phase is 0.1 potassium phosphate, pH 2.5 and the high-strength eluent is an acetonitrile:water (3:2) mixture. A 45-minute linear gradient from 0 to 60% of the high-strength mobile phase is used at a flow rate of 1.4 ml/min. Samples are detected by electrochemical detection as described above. The optimum oxidation voltage for these compounds is +1 V. Standards are prepared and recovery determined as described above.

APPENDIX D   EEG MEASURES AND PROCEDURES

EEG for a baseline measure of relative right or left frontal EEG activation

EEG will be recorded for 10 minutes while the subject is in a quiet alert state. The subject will face a researcher who will blow bubbles in front of the subject's face to keep the subject distracted during placement of the electrodes as well as during the recording. We have reported significant 1–3 month stability of EEG ($r = 0.45$) (Jones et al 1996) as well as significant 3-month to 3-year stability (Jones et al 1997).

EEG recording

The EEG for the subjects will be recorded using Lycra stretchable caps (manufactured by Electro-Cap, Inc.) that will be positioned on the subject's head using anatomical landmarks (Bloom & Anneveldt 1982). Electrode gel will be injected into the electrodes at the following sites: F3, F4, P3, P4, T3, T4, O1, O2 and Cz (used as the reference during recording) and impedances will be brought below 5000 ohms. Additional electrodes will be positioned on the external canthus and above the supra orbit of the right eye to record the subject's EEG, which will be used to determine horizontal and vertical eye movement artefacts.

The signal will be passed through a Biopac MP100 aquisition system with amplifiers set as follows: low-frequency filter, 1 Hz; high-frequency filter, 100 Hz; amplification, 20 000. The line frequency filter is on for all channels. The output from the amplifiers will be directed to a Dell Inspiron 7000 laptop. The signal will be sampled at a rate of 512 Hz and streamed to hard disk using data acquisition software (Acq Knowledge software V.3.5, Biopac Systems Inc., 1999).

EEG analyses

EEG data will be analyzed using an EEG analysis software package (EEG Analysis System v. 5.3, James M. Long, 1987–1990). The first step of this process involves computing EEG off-line to derive a computer-averaged reference, followed by the manual elimination of sections of data that are unusable due to artefact (eye movements, muscle activity or technical difficulties). The remaining artefact-free data will be spectrally analyzed using discrete Fourier transforms to yield power data for specific frequency bands. The subject EEG data will be analyzed from 1 to 12 Hz in 1 Hz bins. Data analyses will be conducted on the natural log power data for both hemispheres in frontal and parietal regions. Frontal alpha laterality ratios (FLR) will be computed by obtaining the difference of mean log power density scores of a right hemisphere site and its homologous left hemisphere site (LnRight-LnLeft). A score of zero represents hemispheric symmetry, a negative score represents relative right frontal activation and a positive score represents relative left frontal activation.

APPENDIX E   IMMUNE MEASURES

Immunoassays

1. Preparation of PBMC

Samples of venous blood collected in Vacutainer tubes with heparin (green-top) from the volunteers, who had willingly signed the informed consent form prior to blood collection. Peripheral blood mononuclear cells were isolated by the Ficoll-Hypaque method, washed twice in RPMI-1640 medium (Sigma Chem, St Louis, MO) and adjusted to 1×10/ml.

2. Purification of lymphocyte subsets

To examine the function of CD8+, CD14+ and CD19+ subsets, the isolated PBMC will be treated with either Dynabeads CD8 only or the combination of CD8, CD14 and CD19 (Dynal, Great Neck, NY). The cells which bind to the beads will be isolated by the use of a magnetic particle concentrator (Dynal), washed twice in RPMI-1640 medium (Sigma) and adjusted to 1×10/ml. To study isolated subpopulations (CD4 or CD8 cells), PBMC will stained with 20 of anti-CD4 monoclonal antibody (Mab) conjugated with peridinin chlorophyll protein (PerCP: emission peak at 670 nm) and anti-CD8 Mab conjugated with fluoresceine isothiocyanate (FITC: emission peak at 530 nm) (Beckton Dickinson Immunocytometry Systems, San Jose, CA) for 20 min. Cells will be washed in RPMI-1640 medium and adjusted to 1×10/ml. The washed cells will be sorted by using a FACS-Calibur (Beckton Dickinson). Briefly, region one (R1) was drawn to identify lymphocytes on forward scatter (FSC) and side scatter (SSC) dot plots. Region two (R2) will be drawn on CD4+ cells using the FL3 channel and region three (R3) on CD8+ cells using the FL1 channel. Logical gate 8 (LG8 = R1 and R2) will be used to sort CD4+ cells and logical gate 7 (LG7 = R1 and 113) will be used to sort CD8+ cells. The sorted cells will be collected in sterile tubes precoated for one hour with fetal calf serum (FCS) to prevent T-cell adhesion. The cells will be counted and the purity verified. It is expected that the purity of the sorted CD4 or CD8 cells would exceed 99%.

3. Activation of T-lymphocytes

Approximately 1×10 cells/ml will be cultured in RPMI-1640 medium containing 10% serum at 37°C under humidified air containing 5% CO_2. Phorbol 12-myristate 13-acetate (PMA) (Sigma) (50 ng/ml), murine anti-CD28 and anti-CD3 Mab (1 μg/ml each) (Research Diagnostics, Flanders, NJ) will be added to the culture and the cultures will be incubated for 10 hr. In the last 6 hr of incubation 2 μM Monensin (Sigma) will be added. In Monensin-treated cells, newly synthesized proteins accumulate in intracellular vacuoles and some of the post-translational modifications such as glycosylation and proteolytic cleavage are blocked.

4. Flow cytometric assessment of intracytoplasmic cytokines

Cells will be washed twice in phosphate-buffered saline (PBS) containing 1% bovine serum and 0.1% sodium azide at pH 7.4–7.6 (staining buffer). Cells will be fixed with 0.5% paraformaldehyde (PFA) (Sigma) for 30 min (or overnight) at 4°C, followed by the addition of a second fixation in 4% paraformaldehyde (PFA) for additional 30 min at 4°C. They will be washed with PBS containing 1% fetal bovine serum supplemented with 0.1% sodium azide and 0.1% saponin (Sigma) (permeabilization buffer) and stained with 3 of phycoerythrin-conjugated (PE: emission peak at 570 nm) anti-cytokine Mab (PharMingen, San Diego, CA) for 30 min at 4°C. Cells will be washed twice with staining buffer and then treated with FITC-conjugated anti-CD8 Mab and PerCP-conjugated anti-CD3 Mab (Beckton Dickinson) for 20 min, washed twice and resuspended in 0.5% PFA for flow cytometric analysis. To analyze cytokine production by certain T-cell subset, FL2 (cytokine) profiles of CD8 (FL1 positive) or CD4 (FL1 negative) T-cells will be plotted as contour graphs of the logically gated population. Both the percentage of cytokine-producing cells and the average amount of cytokine produced, i.e. Y geometric mean (gm), will be obtained. The relative quantity of cytokine produced by each T-cell subset will be calculated as (% gated events) × (Y gm).

5. Detection of interleukins

Culture supernatants will be assayed for the following interleukins: IL-4, IL-5, IL-8 and IL-12. The assay will be conducted according to the vendor's specifications (Genzyme Diagnostics, Cambridge, MA and R&D Systems, Minneapolis, MN).

CAM laboratory of immunology

The laboratory will be fully equipped to run all of the immune assays. The major equipment that will be available includes: cell analyzer and sorter, laminar flow sterile hood, refrigerated centrifuge, cell counter, kinetic ELISA reader, deep freezer, refrigerator, fluorescence reader, gamma counter, electrophoresis.

17

Research aspects of environmental medicine

Honor M Anthony

INTRODUCTION

Clinical environmental medicine shares problems of acceptance and of research methodology with complementary medicine but is not itself complementary: rather, it is the common-sense central strand of all medical practice, putting into clinical practice the widely accepted adage 'prevention is better than cure'. As interest in positive health and in the environment increases and the dangers of medication become clearer, this type of practice will undoubtedly come into its own.

The most controversial aspect of clinical environmental medicine is the demonstration that hidden reactions to foods and pollutants are responsible for much chronic illness. For centuries there have been sporadic reports that idiosyncratic adverse reactions to foods cause exacerbations of chronic illnesses. These started with the Ancient Greeks and particularly clear descriptions in asthma remain from the 12th and 17th centuries and in migraine from the 19th century (Anthony et al 1997). The symptoms provoked by foods and environmental factors (and therefore prevented by avoiding those incitants) which Hare listed in 1905 were virtually identical to those listed independently by Rowe in 1928 and by Hearn in 1978 (Anthony et al 1997), and the symptoms that had improved in an environmental medicine outcome audit in 1996 (Maberly et al 1996). The symptoms involve many systems. Some of these symptoms are readily recognized as allergic or as having an allergic component but many others are not; some are common illnesses whose origin remains largely unrecognized and others are still regarded as 'medically-unexplained' (Mayou 1991). This term is usually used as a synonym for 'psychologically-induced' but for these illnesses there is no convincing evidence that psychological factors are a primary cause and much evidence for an environmental cause.

In the last 50 years, there have been increases in the prevalence, not only of allergic reactivity (Sibbald et al 1990) and explicit allergic illnesses (Aberg et al 1995, Foucard 1991) but also of those other groups. Asthma, for instance (which occupies an intermediate status), has increased not only in prevalence but also in severity and epidemiologists regard the changes as being of environmental origin, probably due to foods or pollutants (Burney 1988), although mainstream clinical management regularly considers a few of the latter only. In spite of medical advances, by 1990 'medically-unexplained' conditions were so common that they represented 52% and 45% respectively of two series of 191 and 229 new referrals to general medical outpatients (Speckens et al 1995, Van Hemert et al 1993); three-quarters still had symptoms 10 weeks later in spite of investigations and reassurance.

The role of the environment in these conditions has been largely neglected and, at the beginning of the 21st century, the usual medical treatment is palliative – symptom suppression mainly using medication – usually without any attempt to find out what the provoking factors are or whether the symptoms can be prevented. Managed in a palliative fashion, these symptoms present a very substantial problem which is a drain on the NHS in terms of money, labor and morale. It is, sadly, not unusual for patients who have recognized that a food makes their symptoms worse to be told that this cannot be so, or even ridiculed.

The provocation of a symptom by a different range of foods in different individuals does not fit into the systems view which currently characterizes medicine. Causes common to the condition fit into this thinking but causes which are individual to each of the patients who suffer from it do not. So doctors do not have difficulty with the possibility that high-amine foods provoke migraine (although few cases are solved entirely by avoiding these foods alone) but most of them disbelieve the evidence that patients who have suffered from migraine for years become migraine free if they avoid a range of foods identified by doing an elimination diet (Egger et al 1983, Grant 1979).

WHAT MECHANISM IS INVOLVED?

Some adverse reactions to foods are clearly allergic in nature, others have an idiosyncratic biochemical mechanism but the largest group are often referred to as 'hidden food allergy' because of the hidden nature of the symptom provocation and the circumstantial evidence that they are caused by non-IgE mediated allergic mechanisms. The need to use an elimination diet to detect such triggers arises from the curious natural history of hidden food allergy, which is another bar to recognition of the environmental nature of these illnesses. In hidden food allergy, it is usual for multiple trigger foods to be involved, mainly foods eaten frequently: the reaction is often delayed and the link between consumption of the food and the symptoms is obscured. The patient is ill but does not recognize the common foods that are responsible, although they may have noticed that they are worse after a food they only eat occasionally or when they have missed a meal. Excluding a single food and then challenging with it may not expose the cause of the symptoms but excluding all, or nearly all, the incitants will do so. So, during the first stage of an elimination diet, the patient excludes all the most commonly incriminated foods. If they have successfully avoided their main incitants, symptoms often get worse for 2 or 3 days and then clear; by days 5–10 many patients are symptom free. The initial worsening (known as withdrawal) may be very marked and the uninitiated often draw quite the wrong conclusions. After symptoms have cleared on the elimination diet, the patient performs structured challenges with the excluded foods: food incitants provoke symptoms and signs whereas other foods ('safe' foods) will provoke neither. If the diet is subsequently restricted to these safe foods, the patient may succeed in remaining virtually symptom-free for years and in time some of the incitant foods may again be tolerated in moderation.

The natural history of hidden food allergy, its role in chronic illness and the role of allergic reactions to biological aeroallergens in chronic illnesses were clearly described in the first half of the 20th century (see Rowe & Rowe 1972); the contribution of chemical additives and pollutants was only recognized later. During the 1950s Dr Theron Randolph admitted patients with multiple symptoms to a hospital side ward for elimination diets; he noticed that chemical pollutants seemed to interfere with the results, so he progressively cleaned up the environment into which he admitted them, lining the walls and ceilings with impermeable natural materials, fitting double doors and good ventilation with air filtration, filtering the water, using organic produce and banning smoking, perfumes and any products or materials which gave off volatile chemicals. As the environment improved the proportion of patients he could help increased (Randolph 1987) and it became clear that some of the patients' symptoms were caused by reactions to volatile chemicals at everyday concentrations, to medications and to contaminants in food and water. This chemical sensitivity shows much the same natural history as hidden food allergy and a period of complete avoidance of the chemical mixture or compound is often essential before sensitivity can be demonstrated. Dr Randolph's findings led to the development of comprehensive environmentally-controlled inpatient units (Randolph 1965), now seen as essential for the investigation of severe cases of environmental illness. I had the good fortune to be associated with the first purpose-built unit in the world, the Airedale Allergy Centre, for over 10 years.

It has recently been suggested that this group of conditions represents a previously unrecognized patho-etiology which is likely in time to prove to be at least as important for the understanding of disease causation as the germ theory was at the end of the 19th century. Miller (1997) has named this 'toxicant-induced loss of tolerance' (TILT) and proposed the following postulates.

- When a subject simultaneously avoids all chemical, food, inhalant and drug incitants, remission of symptoms occurs (unmasking).
- A specific constellation of symptoms occurs with reintroduction of a particular incitant.
- Symptoms resolve when the incitant is again avoided.
- With reexposure to the same incitant, the same constellation of symptoms reoccurs, provided that the challenge is conducted within an appropriate window of time. Clinical observations suggest that an ideal window is 4–7 days following the last exposure to the test incitant.

Clinically, one of the characteristics of this condition is that the patients' histories tend to show a strong link with the amount of exposure to foods eaten repetitively, to synthetic and pollutant chemicals, to biological aeroallergens and particularly with exposures to them during periods of stress, and with a high total load of such exposures. If it is possible to reduce the overall level of exposure substantially, the patient's progress is usually much better than if this is not possible; some may then keep well for years.

RESEARCH

Clinical environmental medicine is the medical discipline which involves the management of patients with environmental illness with the aim of enabling them to keep well with little or no medication. To date there has been little public funding of research into clinical environmental medicine, and what has been funded has not always been undertaken by researchers who are familiar with the natural history of the condition. This has had serious consequences for the planning and ultimate validity of the studies. One study (Young et al 1994), examining the prevalence of food intolerance, used double-blind testing after a week's avoidance to confirm that reported reactions to foods were genuine, but only patients who were already aware of adverse reactions to foods were tested. Moreover, patients were excluded from the challenge if they had intercurrent illness during the investigation, thereby excluding just those patients who were most likely to show positive reactions (Anthony et al 1994, Finn 1994, Moneret-Vautrin & Kanny 1994).

There are six main areas in which research is needed:

- evidence of efficacy
- the prevalence of the conditions which respond well to these methods
- the mechanisms involved
- potential savings in health costs and in sickness-related benefits
- improving methods of diagnosis and treatment
- investigating the interactions of TILT with deficiencies of minerals, vitamins and essential fatty acids and with abnormalities of gut flora.

I shall discuss the first and touch on the others, concentrating on the importance of careful planning which takes account of the natural history of the condition if studies are to be valid.

EVIDENCE OF EFFICACY

It is generally considered that research into efficacy is the most needed, both in complementary medicine and in environmental allergy and nutrition, but in the case of the latter there is more need for a change in attitude so that the research which has been done is interpreted without bias. A bias against the publication of a trial of homeopathy has recently been reported (Resch et al 2000) in a blinded study where peer reviewers were supplied with identical imaginary trial data. They were more likely to recommend publication if the data referred to drug treatments than if it referred to homeopathy. The bias was significant in spite of the fact that homeopathy is relatively well accepted and has been part of NHS medicine since its inception. It seems likely that the results would have shown even more bias had the data been attributed to a less accepted therapeutic modality.

Even when good trials have been published they tend to be disregarded, especially if the results do not fit easily into the framework of systematic medicine that has become entrenched in the last 40 years. The judgment of whether a trial is good or not does not always consider whether the trial plan was appropriate, taking into account the nature and natural history of the condition treated and the nature of the therapies investigated. A good trial must test the therapy applied in a form which would be chosen as optimal by good therapists engaged in that discipline and must use relevant investigation, timescale and recording. Bias must be avoided as far as possible but it is also important that the trial does not distort either the therapy given or the confidence of the patients in it. For much of complementary and clinical environmental medicine, the usual patterns of trial design are not consistent with these principles.

'EVIDENCE-BASED' MEDICINE

There are profound questions about what should be considered to be 'evidence-based' medicine. Trial design aims to produce two groups of patients differing only in the treatment used and unaware of how they have been treated, so that statistical evaluation can be applied to compare outcomes or, if there are no carry-over effects, to randomize the order of application of the active and placebo treatments to single patients or randomize patients to a crossover design so that the patients can be their own controls. Statistical evaluation is essential to draw conclusions from what would otherwise be doubtful data. But when a treatment can immediately be seen to be highly beneficial on logic alone, the only source of doubt is about the reliability of the assessments and the honesty of the report; neither of these is solved by using statistics to check a comparison. When the patients have had chronic illness for years and a high proportion of them report marked and sustained improvement with the new treatment, the differences revealed by the comparison with their previous state are not doubtful and confirmation by statistical analysis is inappropriate. Statistics may be essential in validating the assessment systems and demonstrating the characteristics of the patients who responded (helping to establish the genuine nature of the improvements reported) but this can equally well be applied to well-disciplined uncontrolled or unblinded studies (Anthony 1987). Studies subject to statistical analysis may be falsely relied on, forgetting their limitations. They are no less subject to assessment errors or fraud and they introduce other sources of error.

Many of the studies in clinical environmental medicine were in patients with a long history of failed mainstream management which must be regarded as a natural control period. In order to apply the therapeutic strategy appropriately, most were not double-blind placebo-controlled trials throughout, and some were conceived only as observational studies or audits; most involved long follow-up periods in which a majority of patients claimed to be very much better. Are they then acceptable or not acceptable as evidence?

The double-blind placebo-controlled trial (DBPCT) was introduced for drug trials to reduce bias arising from the allocation of patients between the two arms and from the placebo and the 'please the doctor' effects, but this format is not applicable to all circumstances and is less reliable for evaluating longer term outcomes. Over longer terms it is difficult to maintain the blinding and difficult to keep the co-operation of the required high proportion of the patients. Patients who are doing less well are particularly likely to look round for some other treatment to give them some relief. This problem can be accentuated by asking for informed consent (essential for trials) and by contact between patients on different arms of the trial. The longer the trial, the more likely patients are to withdraw, break the protocol or have intercurrent illnesses; it is difficult to manage the data about these patients without introducing some kind of bias to the overall results. The numbers of protocol breakers may be large enough to destroy the validity of the trial entirely.

As usually employed, DBPCTs test one treatment against another, for instance a new drug against the current drug of choice. They test uniform treatments, giving each member of the group the same treatment at the same or a weight-related dose. It is this uniformity which is largely responsible for the unpopularity of trials among doctors because doctors like to feel free to consider each patient in choosing the drug and the dose to prescribe and to modify this if necessary. Moreover, uniform treatments are not always either possible or desirable. Some therapeutic strategies have to be individually designed: this is particularly true for patients in whom there is a need to identify and correct individual nutrient deficiencies or identify individual intolerances so that the incitants can be avoided. Trials which test supplementation with, for instance, zinc or magnesium in pregnancy would only have satisfactory sensitivity when deficiency was common or when only those with low values were included. Any treatment plan which is inappropriate for a proportion of the patients will not provide a valid estimate of what the treatment could do if applied in an individually appropriate manner.

For these therapies, if there is doubt about therapeutic efficacy, the trial plan of choice either involves using the patient as his own control or randomization between two therapeutic strategies before referral. Formal use of a patient as their own control uses randomization of the order of treatments, double blind if possible, with appropriate wash-out periods between (usually referred to as $N=1$ studies) or a randomized group crossover design. These are only satisfactory for those treatments which do not have long-term effects which may be carried over; they cannot be applied if advice is given, nutrition improved or lifestyle changes recommended, although a one-sided crossover design (randomizing to immediate or delayed treatment) may be used in these circumstances. For randomization between treatment strategies, the patients must be identified and assessed by a third party before randomization determines referral to one or other strategy; treatment can then be applied individually to each patient within that strategy as required, preferably with independent outcome assessment of the patients in each arm and without contact between the two groups of patients. This trial plan was used most effectively in a trial which compared doctors and chiropractors in their management of back pain (Meade et al 1995).

The most serious worry about the pre-eminence of the DBPCT is that it imparts an active bias to the types of therapy that are accepted as 'evidence based'. Hands-on therapies cannot be used double blind and the appropriateness of the placebo arm in single-blind studies may be questionable. Randomized studies which were not performed in a blinded fashion are often disregarded. No treatment which requires active cooperation from the patient (such as in doing an elimination diet or reducing exposure to house dust mite allergen or making observations about the circumstances when their symptoms are better or worse) can be carried out blind, although in some circumstances challenge may be blinded. Challenges in the elucidation of hidden food allergy are a special case. False-negative results are common unless foods are excluded for an appropriate period before challenge testing. Since there is no universally safe food, before double-blind challenge it is essential not only to relieve the patient's symptoms but also to test foods openly in order to identify foods that can be used as placebos for that patient. Only then can double-blind testing be used. A corn placebo caused difficulties in one double-blind study (Atkins et al 1985a) where a reaction to corn was disregarded in a patient because she also reacted to the placebo (glucose), the authors being apparently unaware that most glucose is made from corn. There is also a report that the gelatine capsules used to blind food challenge may cause migraine in some patients (Strong 2000). However, there are other circumstances under which double-blind testing may give rise to false-negative reactions – if too little is given (Atkins et al 1985b) (and not all foods can be given blind in sufficient quantities) and, in some patients, if the food does not make contact with the mouth (Kaplan 1994). In one case, it was reported that reliance on the results of double-blind food challenge endangered the life of a child with immediate allergy (Kaplan 1994). Positive responses to double-blind food challenge therefore reliably confirm food reactions, but negative results cannot exclude them. Relying only on double-blind food challenges in patients with TILT (if it were practicable in adults, which it is not) would risk getting inferior clinical results.

With chronic illness, the aim of therapy is to get the patient better and keep them more or less well long term and it is this that studies must establish. When the therapy cannot be used blind, a number of different approaches may be needed. All studies must be well planned and performed with discipline, preferably with the initial and outcome assessments undertaken by an independent observer, measuring any measurable features as in studies, for instance, in asthma (peak expiratory flow rate, Hoj et al 1981) and rheumatoid arthritis (clinical and laboratory indices, Darlington & Mansfield 1986, Kjeldsen-Krach et al 1991) or supported by questionnaire responses. For symptoms which cannot be measured, it is important to use a questionnaire which is appropriate to the patients concerned, to get as high a response rate as possible and to make it clear that the patients should answer even if they are disappointed with the outcome of treatment. Data about degree of cooperation, rescue medication required and ability to work or pursue a normal life are useful confirmation. The collection of data should be as impersonal as possible so as to keep 'please the doctor' effects to a minimum. The patients must always be a defined cohort of patients because otherwise there is a risk that those who have done well will be overrepresented: patients should ideally be followed prospectively.

At the present time it seems that, however good the methodology, results of underregarded management methods are likely to be received with disbelief, particularly if the results are substantially better than those achieved with orthodox management. This is a problem which needs to be faced by the medical profession and some solution found. Disbelief is damaging to the development of medicine as a scientific clinical discipline whether it affects acceptance for publication or acceptance of the findings by reviewers and by teaching staff. Clearly, the records (and if studies are likely to be received with disbelief, the patients themselves) should be available for checking if required, but such checks are dependent on others since the profession is unlikely to pay attention to an independent check arranged by the researcher. There is a need for some unbiased, truly independent group of medical scientists of high status to whom requests for such checks could be addressed, either by the journals or by the researchers, and rigid standards about who they appoint to perform such checks and how they should be done. Some years ago one of our colleagues was apparently subjected to something akin to a witch hunt by academics determined to disprove his findings, and an earlier investigation by the journal *Nature* attempted to debunk a French study of the mechanisms of homeo-pathy (Anthony 1988, Davenas et al 1988, Maddox et al 1988), using scientists unfamiliar with the laboratory techniques used, helped by a magician. These are not reputable scientific ways of proceeding. But equally, waiting for a study to be replicated is ineffective since even findings confirmed by two further studies have been disregarded.

EVIDENCE IN CLINICAL ENVIRONMENTAL MEDICINE

Half the patients involved in the outcome audit of polysymptomatic patients treat-ed by environmental methods (Maberly et al 1996) (see Figure 17.1) had been having symptoms for 10 years or more before referral, without much relief from mainstream treatments; this is in line with the general experience of environmental physicians. The pre-referral period represents a natural 'control' period during which most patients get worse, with increasing numbers of symptoms of increasing severity. If treatment is followed by substantial and sustained relief in a high pro-portion of patients, the cause and effect relationship cannot logically be doubted, particularly if the patients report that symptoms recur when they are unable to fol-low the regime recommended (Maberly & Anthony 1992, Maberly et al 1996). It is true that the severity of the symptoms of the conditions which are caused by TILT characteristically fluctuate from day to day or week to week, but sudden, sponta-neous, lasting improvements are rare and if they occur, they can usually be traced to a change in exposures and reversed temporarily by challenge testing. Under these circumstances, establishing efficacy primarily involves establishing the hon-esty of the reports and the genuine nature of the improvements reported; many doctors think that these are too good to be true.

Table 17.1 shows a list of symptoms which have been provoked by double-blind food challenge after an elimination diet in a number of different studies: the list is not exhaustive because most chose to study symptoms which could be confirmed by observation or measurement. Table 17.2 shows the high percentage of patients in such studies whose symptoms were prevented long term while the patient remained on a safe diet.

These reports of symptom provocation by double-blind challenge, from many different sources and predominantly published in mainline medical journals, clear-ly prove that a wide variety of symptoms can be provoked by food challenge in appropriate circumstances in sensitive patients. The avoidance/challenge regimes used by the studies were also similar and the common description of the circum-stances under which food challenge could be confirmed strongly supports the con-cept of 'hidden food allergy' as an entity and supports the claims about its curious natural history, although the evidence that allergy is involved is only circumstan-tial. In many of these studies the patients had persistent and disabling symptoms that had failed to improve with standard treatments; other studies included con-secutive referrals. In view of the consistency with which studies have shown long-term advantage following the avoidance of the recognized food triggers in high proportions of the patients, the conclusion must be that either the management is highly effective or it is the subject of multiple hoaxes: having done an outcome audit myself, I know the latter view to be untenable.

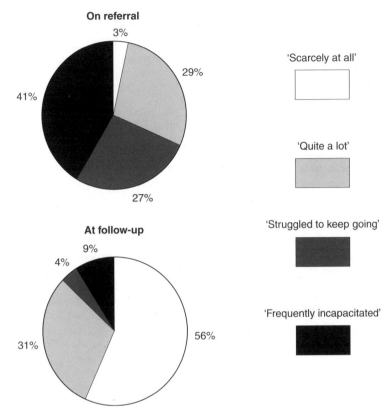

Figure 17.1   Degree of life disruption on admission to the Airedale Allergy Centre and on follow-up 6 months to $2\frac{1}{2}$ years later. The pie chart shows responses from the patients at follow-up to the following questions:

1. *How much was your life disrupted before admission? Scarcely at all/Quite a lot/Struggled to keep going/Frequently incapacitated/Kept needing hospital admission*
2. *How much is your life disrupted now (same categories)?*
Similar questions were answered by the patients on admission and independently by a relative or close friend of the patient on follow-up: these agreed closely with the above responses (after Maberly et al 1996).

Outcome audit, if properly and honestly performed, reflects the normal clinical situation, without the restrictions, selections and stresses involved in clinical trials, for the patients as well as the organizers, and may be a more accurate reflection of the potentialities of the treatment. Audit does not carry the same limitations on length of follow-up. It depends on scrupulous application of inclusion criteria and accounting for all failures to follow-up. Care must be taken in applying statistics when comparing the patients' condition during the natural inbuilt control period with the post-treatment period but it can be applied if data about a baseline period are collected and compared to a similar period or periods during follow-up (Kjeldsen-Krach et al 1991) or if condition at referral is compared to that at the point of follow-up (Maberly et al 1996).

Table 17.1 Symptoms provoked by double-blind food challenge

Symptoms	Author
Adults	
Supraventricular tachycardia, vomiting, sore throat	Finn & Cohen 1978
Rhinorrhea, stomatitis, urticaria, conjunctivitis, pruritus, abdominal pain, dypsnea, nausea, diarrhea, headache	Bernstein et al 1982
Asthma	Wraith 1982
Rhinitis, flushing, urticaria, laryngeal edema, pruritus, cramps, eczema	Atkins et al 1985b
Asthma	Burr et al 1985
Headache, lethargy	Mills 1986
Asthma	Pelikan et al 1987
Asthma, rhinitis, urticaria, angio-edema, diarrhea, vomiting	Pastorello et al 1989
IBS	Alun-Jones et al 1982
Mixed ages	
Asthma, atopic dermatitis, nausea, abdominal pain, diarrhea	Onorato et al 1986
Children	
Eczema	Atherton et al 1978
Puffy eyes, nasal congestion, irritability	Rapp 1978a
Weeping eyes	Rapp 1978b
Migraine, epilepsy, abdominal pain and distension	Egger et al 1983
Hyperactivity	Egger et al 1985
Enuresis	Egger et al 1992
Sleeplessness, agitation, vomiting, diarrhea	Kahn et al 1989
Hyperactivity	Carter et al 1993
Hyperactivity	Boris & Mandel 1994
Under 1 year	
Anaphylaxis, atopic dermatitis, urticaria, angio-edema, rhinorrhea, conjunctivitis, wheezing, cough, vomiting, diarrhea, bloody stools, growth retardation	Bock & Sampson 1994 (review)

We performed an outcome audit doing our utmost to avoid bias. It was an audit of long-term outcome in severely affected polysymptomatic TILT patients using the same questionnaires at two centers. The patients were from defined cohorts and represented, in each case, approximately a fifth of the patients referred, the most

Table 17.2 Percentage improvement in follow-up studies

Illness	Age group	Better (%)	Some DB food challenges	Author
Hyperactivity	Children	82	Yes	Egger et al 1985
		76	Yes	Carter et al 1993
		73	Yes	Boris & Mandel 1994
Irritable bowel	Adults	67	Yes	Hunter et al 1985
		48[x]	Yes	Nanda et al 1989
Migraine	Children	88[*]	Yes	Egger et al 1983
	Adults	85[*]	No	Grant 1979
Asthma	Adults	66	No	Lindahl et al 1985
Eczema (refractory)	Children	73	Yes	Devlin et al 1991
Polysymptomatic	Adults	77	No	Maberly et al 1996

[x] One diet regime only used, permitting consumption of some foods provoking IBS
[*] Headache free without medication

severely affected. One series included those patients referred to Keighley who had been admitted for a full investigation in the Airedale Allergy Centre (AAC), a purpose-built comprehensive environmentally-controlled unit. Figure 17.1 shows the AAC patients' assessment of their condition on admission and at follow-up 6 months to $2\frac{1}{2}$ years later in terms of life disruption. The questionnaire responses were validated statistically in two ways: by comparing the retrospective reports of condition on admission with the responses to a similar question answered at the time of admission, and by comparing the patients' responses at follow-up with those sent independently by a relative or close friend. There was a very close match in each case and no differences approaching significance. The second series were patients referred to Dr Birtwistle in Cambridge and treated as outpatients and were included retrospectively only if they had had three or more enzyme-potentiated desensitization treatments.

The referral patterns and inclusion and exclusion criteria in the two series were not identical and the timescales of treatment and therefore of follow-up were different, outpatient responses being slower and follow-up later. The effectiveness of the two management regimes cannot therefore be compared. However, the *philosophy* of the management was the same and the outcomes almost identical (Maberly et al 1996). Figure 17.2 shows the prevalence, and the frequency and severity (reported separately and then combined) of each of 64 symptoms in each series, with the upper bars representing percentages having symptoms on referral and the lower bars on follow-up; the darker the shading, the more frequent and severe the symptoms. The two series show strikingly similar patterns of the prevalence and frequency/severity of symptoms on referral and of changes at follow-up. The detailed patterns of improvement in the symptoms varied somewhat, both between patients and between symptoms: patients reported that symptoms had become less severe or less frequent or both, often reporting different patterns of change for different symptoms, an additional validation of the questionnaire. By questionnaire

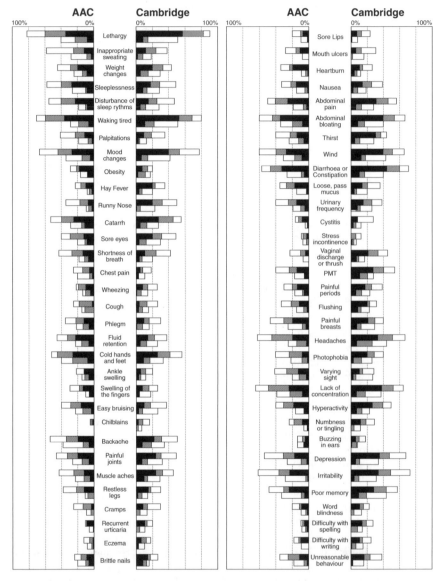

Figure 17.2 Percentage of patients in the AAC series (left) and the Cambridge series (right) reporting each symptom on presentation (upper bars) and at FU (lower bars) at symptom scores above the trivial. Most patients were polysymptomatic (after Maberly et al 1996).

Key   ■   F/S = 4 (severe and frequent/constant)
       ■   F/S = 3 (severe and occasional *or* moderate and frequent/constant)
       □   F/S = 2 (moderate and occasional *or* slight and frequent/constant)

standards, the response in both arms of this study was good and non-responders in an AAC asthma subgroup did not have a worse outcome than responders (Maberly & Anthony 1992).

When considering sustained improvements of this magnitude in patients with a long natural control period before referral, occurring in such a high proportion of patients with severe and disabling problems, statistics are irrelevant. If others disbelieve this audit we would be happy to go through the data with them or put them in touch with the patients, or both. This is, probably, the only way of further validating the results of such a study.

Unfortunately, even studies with double-blind elements tend to be disregarded. In 1998 and 1999 there were three reviews published in top mainline journals on attention deficit hyperactivity disorder (ADHD) (Hill 1998, Swanson et al, 1998, Zametkin & Ernst 1999). They all concentrated on the management of these children with drugs and psychotherapy although the three trials shown in Table 17.2 (Boris & Mandel 1994, Carter et al 1993, Egger et al 1985) had all found marked (and highly significant) reductions of Conners' short scores after an elimination diet. For instance, scores reduced from means of 24 to 12 (Egger et al 1985) and from 25 to 9.6 (Boris & Mandel 1994) during the initial diet and rose on challenge with some foods and not others, whether they were given as open or as double-blind challenges. In the double-blind challenges the pretest mean of 8.1 rose to 13.9 with active challenge (8.8 placebo) in one study (Carter et al 1993) and from 8.4 to 18.1 with active challenge (8.2 placebo) in another (Boris & Mandel 1994), with similar results, displayed differently, in the third. There was long-term improvement when incitant foods were avoided. One of the reviews (Zametkin & Ernst 1999) went so far as to comment that there were claims that excluding foods could help in a small number of patients but implied that it was difficult and not worth trying. In fact, each of the three published studies found substantial improvement in over 70% of the children. Doctors who use environmental methods in these children get similar results using simpler dietary regimes and find that most of the children are unexpectedly co-operative once they have found what it is like to feel well and to get on better with their friends and family.

The same applies to irritable bowel syndrome (IBS) which mainstream gastroenterologists regard as a difficult condition to treat. In the study which used a strict elimination diet (Alun-Jones et al 1982, Hunter et al 1985) the symptoms of most patients were relieved (Table 17.2), confirmed by double-blind challenge with foods which had been found to trigger symptoms; the second of these studies (Nanda et al 1989) had good results in about half the patients in spite of using a single diet which did not exclude some of the likely incitant foods. In Crohn's disease, management by hypoallergenic diet, challenges and long-term exclusion of incitant foods has been found to be as effective as the standard steroid regimes (Alun-Jones & Hunter 1985, Hunter 1985, Riordan et al 1993). Neither of these conditions is routinely managed in this way except by a small group of environmental physicians.

There has been a similar trial in children who had had severe migraine at least once a week for at least 6 months, some for as long as 11 years (Egger et al 1983). An elimination diet followed by challenges and the avoidance of incitant foods relieved migraine entirely in 88% of the children, confirmed by double-blind challenge with some of the incitant foods. A study in migrainous adults (Grant 1979) reported that 80% became symptom free after doing an elimination diet, stopping smoking and withdrawal of the contraceptive pill, although this trial did not have double-blind confirmation. However, 15 out of 60 had raised blood pressure on referral and all became normotensive while they avoided the environmental factors and foods which provoked symptoms.

There have been rather similar studies in serous otitis media, epilepsy in patients with migraine, enuresis, asthma, eczema and other conditions (Anthony et al 1997).

PROBLEMS IN OTHER RESEARCH ENDEAVORS

Other types of research into TILT also present difficulties.

It would be a great benefit if a laboratory test (or small battery of tests) could be developed which would effectively diagnose TILT, but such a test would need to be at least as sensitive and specific as prick tests or the variants of RAST are at diagnosing atopy. Poor specificity leads to false positives, poor sensitivity to false negatives, both equally undesirable. Successful development of such tests might contribute substantially to the understanding of the mechanisms of TILT, but might well have to await the elucidation of such mechanisms.

Characteristically, before the condition is recognized, patients suffering from TILT develop increasing numbers of symptoms with time and react to increasing numbers of incitants – foods and biological and chemical pollutants. Effective diagnostic tests might be of two kinds. One kind might establish the diagnosis of TILT as a patho-etiological mechanism, establishing that the patient suffered from TILT; the other would identify all the environmental factors to which the patient was sensitive. The sensitivity and specificity of diagnostic tests can only be established by comparing the results with a 'gold standard'. However, no gold standard is available, even for TILT as a patho-etiological entity, let alone for the details of all the incitants: the nearest at present is optimal clinical improvement following the detection of all relevant triggers. For less severely affected patients a return to full health is probably a satisfactory criterion but for the more severe cases, this may not be possible and the best alternative would require admission to a comprehensive environmentally controlled inpatient facility. There can be no certainty that chronic or recurrent symptoms are not of environmental origin unless this has been tried.

Patients who show adverse responses to foods and environmental factors often also have symptoms due to chronic toxicity or to anomalies of the internal environment – deficient production of digestive enzymes, disturbance of gut organisms or deficiencies of vitamins, minerals and essential fatty acids. They may not improve unless these are addressed. Research to elucidate these interactions is much needed. At present it is not clear whether poor nutrition and gut flora anomalies are predisposing factors for intolerance or whether allergies and dysbioses cause deficiencies by increasing the utilization or excretion of such nutrients and reducing absorption. Functional tests have been developed for a few nutrients only and further development of tests and clinical studies using them is much needed.

Valid estimates of the numbers of the population who suffer from TILT, and could be helped by these methods, would require the prevalence of chronic symptoms to be investigated in a random population sample and for a subsample to be treated to see what percentage responded. This raises the problem of making a firm diagnosis of TILT. As patients become more severely affected it becomes increasingly difficult to get them well, which would be the best marker. Most epidemiological studies to date which have attempted to confirm adverse reactions to foods have used double-blind challenges and sacrificed sensitivity for specificity: both are needed if the estimates are to be valid. Even if the subgroup were subjected to the best clinical environmental management, the result might still be an underestimate since the management methods in use at present are not necessarily optimally effective, particularly if an environmentally controlled inpatient facility is not available. Such a facility is regarded as essential for research into multiple chemical sensitivity, which is another element of TILT (Miller 1997); no such facility is available in the UK at present.

Similarly, accurate costing of potential savings cannot be achieved until the scale of the problem has been assessed and the costs of mainstream managements are more accurately defined; this area is currently muddied by the confusion between overall costs and add-on costs and by the inclusion or exclusion of the costs of training health service personnel. The personal costs of long-term chronic illness are even more difficult to calculate.

CONCLUSION

It is important that medical treatments are properly assessed, but equally important that the methods of assessment do not dictate the types of therapy that are seen to be effective. The most pressing problem is to set up a fair and equitable means by which all studies which report markedly good results can be scrutinized on the ground by fair-minded independent assessors to make sure that effective therapies are not penalized because they are not suitable for standard statistical evaluation. In view of the increasing pressures on doctors to produce publications for career advancement, it would not be out of place for a random sample of DBPCT to be regularly subjected to the same sort of detailed examination.

REFERENCES

Aberg N, Hesselmar B, Aberg B et al 1995 Increase of asthma, allergic rhinitis and eczema in Swedish schoolchildren between 1979 and 1991. Clinical and Experimental Allergy 25: 815–819

Alun-Jones V, Shorthouse M, McLoughlan P et al 1982 Food intolerance, a major factor in the pathogenesis of the irritable bowel syndrome. Lancet 2: 1117–1120

Alun-Jones VA, Hunter JO 1985 Crohn's disease: maintenance of remission by diet. Lancet 2: 177

Anthony H, Birtwistle S, Eaton K, Maberly J 1997 Environmental Medicine in Clinical Practice. BSAENM Publications (Tel: 02380 812124), Southampton

Anthony HM 1987 Some methodological problems in the assessment of complementary therapy. Statistics in Medicine 6: 761–771 (reprinted with permission in the 1st edition of the book pp 108–121)

Anthony HM 1988 Homoeopathy: the controversy in Nature. Complementary Medical Research 3: 79–86; reply pp 86–87

Anthony HM, Birtwistle S, Brostoff J et al 1994 Letters: food intolerance. Lancet 344: 136–137

Atherton DJ, Sewell M, Soothill JF et al 1978 A double-blind crossover trial of an antigen avoidance diet in atopic eczema. Lancet 1: 401–403

Atkins FM, Steinberg SS, Metcalfe DD 1985a Evaluation of immediate adverse reactions to food in adult patients. 2. A detailed analysis of reaction patterns during challenge. Journal of Allergy and Clinical Immunology 75: 356–363

Atkins FM, Steinberg SS, Metcalfe DD 1985b Evaluation of immediate adverse reactions to foods in adult patients. 1. Correlation of laboratory & prick test data with controlled oral challenge. Journal of Allergy and Clinical Immunology 75: 348–355

Bernstein M, Day JH, Welsh A 1982 Double-blind food challenge in a diagnosis of food sensitivity in the adult. Journal of Allergy and Clinical Immunology 70: 205

Bock SA, Sampson HA 1994 Food allergy in infancy. Pediatric Clinics of America 14(5): 1047–1067

Boris M, Mandel FS 1994 Foods and additives are common causes of the attention deficit hyperactive disorder in children. Annals of Allergy 72: 462–468

Burney PGJ 1988 Why study the epidemiology of asthma? Thorax 43: 425–428

Burr ML, Fehily AM, Stott NC, Merrett TG 1985 Food-allergic asthma in general practice. Human Nutrition–Applied Nutrition 39: 349–355

Carter CM, Urbanowicz M, Hemsley R et al 1993 Effects of few food diet in attention deficit disorder. Archives of Diseases in Childhood 69: 564–568

Darlington LG, Mansfield JR 1986 Placebo-controlled blind study of dietary manipulation in rheumatoid arthritis. Lancet 1: 236–238

Davenas E, Beauvais F, Amara J et al 1988 Human basophil degranulation triggered by very dilute antiserum against IgE. Nature 333: 816–818

Devlin J, David TJ, Stanton RHJ 1991 Elemental diet for refractory atopic eczema. Archives of Diseases in Childhood 66: 93–99

Egger J, Carter CH, Soothill JF et al 1992 Effect of diet treatment on enuresis in children with migraine or hyperkinetic behaviour. Clinical Pediatrics 31: 302–307

Egger J, Carter CM, Wilson J et al 1983 Is migraine food allergy? A double blind controlled trial of oligo-antigenic diet treatment. Lancet 2: 865–869

Egger J, Graham PJ, Carter CM et al 1985 Controlled trial of oligoantigenic treatment in the hyperkinetic syndrome. Lancet 1: 540–545

Finn R 1994 Letters: food intolerance. Lancet 344: 137

Finn R, Cohen HN 1978 Food allergy: fact or fiction? Lancet 1: 426–428

Foucard T 1991 Allergy and allergy-like symptoms in 1050 medical students. Allergy 46: 20–26

Grant ECG 1979 Food allergies and migraine. Lancet i: 966–968

Hill P 1998 Attention deficit hyperactivity disorder. Archives of Diseases in Childhood 79: 381–385

Hoj L, Osterballe A, Bundgaard A et al 1981 A double-blind controlled trial of elemental diet in severe perennial asthma. Allergy (Copenhagen) 36: 257–262

Hunter JO 1985 The dietary management of Crohn's disease. In: Alun-Jones VA, Hunter JO (eds) Food and the Gut. Baillière Tindall, Eastbourne, 221–237

Hunter JO, Workman EM, Alun-Jones V 1985 Dietary studies. Topics in Gastroenterology 12: 305–313

Kahn A, Mozin MJ, Rebuffat E et al 1989 Milk intolerance in children with persistent sleeplessness: a prospective double-blind crossover evaluation. Pediatrics 84: 595–603

Kaplan MS 1994 The importance of appropriate challenges in diagnosing food sensitivity. Clinical Experimental Allergy 24: 291–293

Kjeldsen-Krach J, Haughen M, Borchgrevink CF et al 1991 Controlled trial of fasting and 1-yr vegetarian diet in rheumatoid arthritis. Lancet 338: 899–902

Lindahl O, Lindwall L, Spangberg A et al 1985 Vegan regimen with reduced medication in the treatment of bronchial asthma. Journal of Asthma 22: 45–55

Maberly DJ, Anthony HM 1992 Asthma management in a 'clean' environment: 2. Progress and outcome in a cohort of patients. Journal of Nutritional Medicine 3: 231–248

Maberly DJ, Anthony HM, Birtwistle S 1996 Polysymptomatic patients: a two-centre outcome audit study. Journal of Nutrition and Environmental Medicine 6: 7–32

Maddox J, Rand J, Stewart WW 1988 'High dilution' experiments a delusion. Nature 334: 287–290; reply p 291

Mayou R 1991 Medically unexplained physical symptoms. British Medical Journal 303: 534–535

Meade TW, Dyer S, Browne W et al 1995 Randomised comparison of chiropractic and hospital outpatient management for low back pain: results from extended follow-up. British Medical Journal 311: 349–351

Miller C, Ashford N, Doty R et al 1997 Working Group Report. Empirical approaches for the investigation of toxicant-induced lack of tolerance. Environmental Health Perspectives 105 (suppl 2): 515–520

Miller CS 1997 Toxicant-induced loss of tolerance - an emerging theory of disease? Environmental Health Perspectives 105 (suppl 2): 445–454

Mills N 1986 Depression and food intolerance. Human Nutrition–Applied Nutrition 40A: 141–145

Moneret-Vautrin DA, Kanny G 1994 Letters: food intolerance. Lancet 344: 137

Nanda R, James R, Smith H et al 1989 Food intolerance and the irritable bowel syndrome. Gut 30: 1099–1104

Onorato J, Merland N, Terral C et al 1986 Placebo-controlled double-blind food challenge in asthma. Journal of Allergy and Clinical Immunology 78: 1139–1146

Pastorello EA, Stocchi L, Pravettoni V et al 1989 Role of the elimination diet in adults with food allergy. Journal of Allergy-Clinical Immunology 84: 475–483

Pelikan Z, Pelikan-Filipek M 1987 Bronchial response to food ingestion challenge. Annals of Allergy 58: 164–172

Randolph TG 1965 Ecologic orientation in medicine: comprehensive environmental control in diagnosis and therapy. Annals of Allergy 23: 7–22

Randolph TG 1987 Environmental Medicine - beginnings and biographies of clinical ecology. Clinical Ecology Publishers, Colorado

Rapp DJ 1978a Double blind confirmation and treatment of milk sensitivity. Medical Journal of Australia 1: 571–572

Rapp DJ 1978b Weeping eyes in wheat allergy. Transactions of the American Society of Ophthalmology and Otolaryngology 18: 149

Resch KI, Ernst E, Garrow J 2000 A randomised controlled study of reviewer bias against unconventional therapy. Journal of the Royal Society of Medicine 93: 164–167

Riordan AM, Hunter JO, Cowan RE et al 1993 Treatment of active Crohn's disease by exclusion diet: East Anglian Multicentre Controlled Trial. Lancet 342; 1131–1134

Rowe AH, Rowe A Jr 1972 Food Allergy: its manifestations and control and the elimination diets. A compendium. Charles C Thomas, Springfield, IL

Sibbald B, Rink E, De Souza M 1990 Is the prevalence of atopy increasing? British Journal of General Practice 40: 338–340

Speckens AEM, Van Hemert AM, Spinhoven P et al 1995 Cognitive behavioural therapy for medically unexplained physical symptoms: a randomised controlled trial. British Medical Journal 311: 1328–1332

Strong FC 2000 Why do some dietary migraine patients claim they get headaches from placebos? Clinical and Experimental Allergy 30: 739–743

Swanson JM, Sergeant JA, Taylor E et al 1998 Attention-deficit hyperactivity disorder and hyperkinetic disorder. Lancet 351: 429–433

Van Hemert AM, Hengeveld MW, Bolk JH et al 1993 Psychiatric disorders in relation to medical illness among patients of a general medical outpatient clinic. Psychological Medicine 23: 167–173

Wraith DG 1982 Asthma and rhinitis. Clinical Immunology and Allergy 2: 101–112

Young E, Stoneham MD, Petruckevitch A et al 1994 A population study of food intolerance. Lancet 343: 1127–1130

Zametkin AJ, Ernst M 1999 Problems in the management of attention-deficit-hyperactivity disorder. New England Journal of Medicine 340: 780–788

18

Acupuncture research methodology

Adrian R White

INTRODUCTION

The aim of this chapter is to describe the methods of clinical research into acupuncture and to identify promising areas for future investigation. It starts from the basic premises that:

- sick patients should have access to whatever is the most effective health care
- RCTs are unsurpassed in determining clinical effectiveness
- the highest level of evidence of effectiveness is a well-performed systematic review that considers appropriate, high-quality RCTs
- the basic 'mindset' needed for this research is to *test whether acupuncture works* rather than to *prove that acupuncture does work*. This attitude may seem incomprehensible to practitioners because they are surrounded by grateful patients every day.

It is important to distinguish between *explanatory* (or *causal*) and *pragmatic* trials of acupuncture, which address different questions. Explanatory studies use groups of highly selected, homogenous subjects, with all variables tightly controlled and data analyzed in terms of statistical significance; they address rather esoteric questions such as whether one form of acupuncture is superior to another or to placebo. In contrast, pragmatic trials recruit patients under real-life conditions without tight selection criteria, allow much more leeway in treatment protocols, give results in terms of the clinical significance and address practical questions such as whether acupuncture is effective enough to be used in the health service.

Because acupuncture has not been shown beyond doubt to be more efficacious than a placebo, which is seen as a crucial step before any intervention can be recommended to patients, explanatory studies are the main concern of this chapter. The main difficulties relating to the design of acupuncture trials are:

- selecting the condition to be studied
- optimizing the acupuncture
- choosing an appropriate control.

Some rather fundamental questions about acupuncture practice are still unanswered, such as: How valid are the diagnostic methods of traditional acupuncture? What does each part of the acupuncture consultation contribute to the overall benefit? Where should we insert the needles and what should we do with them then? Opinions on these matters vary enormously and until they have been answered by rigorous research, acupuncture will have difficulty in being taken seriously. Many people have problems in accepting the fundamental concept of traditional Chinese acupuncture, viz. that energy circulates in meridians and can be controlled by needling certain points. In an effort to make acupuncture comprehensible, some authors have reinterpreted it in Western, biomedical terms (Baldry 1993, Filshie & Cummings 1999, Mann 1992). However, it is argued that this ignores important parts of acupuncture and perhaps even loses its essence. This chapter is not concerned with such issues and hopes to be relevant for all types or schools of acupuncture.

EXPLANATORY STUDIES

Explanatory studies address questions of statistical significance. One such question (but by no means the only one) is whether acupuncture has 'specific' efficacy, i.e. has more than a placebo effect. Acupuncture has features which are likely to evoke a powerful placebo response (Ernst 1994) which may even reach 100% (Taub et al 1979). Placebo effects depend on context and environment; public attitudes at the beginning of the 21st century are clearly positive towards ancient therapies and natural treatments in general, and acupuncture in particular. Thus, its placebo effect appears to be powerful. However, public attitudes change. Therefore it is important to know what the 'specific' effect is, beyond placebo; this gives us a kind of irreducible minimum effectiveness of acupuncture that will remain truly independent of context.

Clinical efficacy: current evidence

Chronic pain systematic reviews

The first 'modern' systematic review of acupuncture that used an assessment of trial quality included 32 sham-controlled studies of acupuncture for chronic pain (Ter Riet et al 1990). Overall, 15 studies were positive and 17 negative. This result is compatible with a modest efficacy of acupuncture, particularly considering that chronic pain is difficult to treat. Combining studies in different conditions can be criticized as there is a risk of not identifying an effect in one particular condition or subgroup. The major conclusion of ter Riet and colleagues was that 'The efficacy of acupuncture in the treatment of chronic pain remains doubtful'. This use of the word 'doubtful' was seen as seriously undermining by the acupuncture profession, who failed to recognize that, in the scientific context, the author simply meant that the efficacy of acupuncture is in doubt through insufficient good-quality evidence:

'absence of evidence of an effect, not evidence of absence of an effect'. Clinicians have different needs and must treat the patient in front of them by applying the available evidence in the light of their own clinical judgment.

The second important finding of this review was the poor quality of the studies. The reviewers made the following general suggestions for improvement:

- larger sample sizes
- subject groups that are more homogeneous
- fewer drop-outs
- longer follow-up periods
- more reliable and sophisticated measures of outcome.

The third result of the review was that the better the quality of the study, the more likely it was to be negative. The same conclusion was reached in two later reviews, one in chronic pain (Ezzo et al 2000), using the method of Jadad for assessing quality (Jadad et al 1996), and one in back and neck pain studies only (Smith et al 2000), using a newly developed method to assess quality. Interestingly, the latter review did not find the same inverse relationship between quality and result when they used the original authors' own conclusions but only when the reviewers reinterpreted the data. This association between higher trial quality and smaller effect size is seen in all clinical research, because removing bias inevitably leads to a smaller observed effect (Schulz et al 1995). What we need to know is whether there is any effect left when all bias has been minimized.

Nausea and vomiting systematic reviews

Another quality-based systematic review considered acupuncture for the treatment of nausea and vomiting (N&V) (Vickers 1996). This review included 33 studies (12 of high quality) of PC6 stimulation for N&V from three causes: surgery, early pregnancy or chemotherapy. Excluding four studies in which acupuncture stimulation was applied under anesthesia, 27 out of 29 (and 11 out of 12 high quality) trials were positive. This result has been confirmed for early postoperative N&V in a meta-analysis of five studies with 392 patients (Lee & Done 1999). A later review of acupressure for early morning sickness (Murphy 1998) questioned the success of blinding and included a fresh, negative study. It reached a more cautious conclusion, that it was clear that women benefit from acupressure but it was not possible to say if the effect was superior to placebo.

Headache and dental pain systematic reviews

Eight sham-controlled studies of acupuncture for dental pain (experimental or clinical) were included in a review (Ernst & Pittler 1998). Seven were positive, although their poor quality limits the strength of the conclusion. A similar result was found for acupuncture for migraine (Melchart et al 1999) but the overall quality of the studies was poor, with a median score of only 2 points out of a possible 5 (Jadad et al 1996). The authors combined the results in an exploratory quantitative analysis using 'global response', i.e. at least 33% improvement. Out of 14 sham-controlled studies, six showed acupuncture superior to sham, three showed trends in favor of acupuncture, in two there was no difference and three were uninterpretable and could not be included. Results for treatment of tension headache were not conclusive. These reviewers commented that the outcome measures used in these trials were not uniform or appropriate and did not adhere to international guidelines (International Headache Society 1995). It is an important principle that anyone undertaking research must become familiar with the literature on the conventional management of the condition, including the best outcome measures, and not just with the acupuncture literature. The authors conclude that, because of heterogeneity, poor methodology, small sample sizes and difference in treatment strategies, 'no clear recommendation can be made of the use of acupuncture for headache'.

Other systematic reviews

Acupuncture for back pain has been systematically reviewed twice (Ernst & White 1998, Tulder et al 2000). Neither found any evidence that acupuncture was superior to placebo, but one combined studies in a metaanalysis and found acupuncture overall superior to all control interventions (Ernst & White 1998). The second reviewers (Tulder et al 2000) argued that the trials were too heterogeneous to combine. Similar conclusions, i.e. no evidence that acupuncture was superior to placebo, were reached for treatment of asthma (Linde et al 2000), neck pain (White & Ernst 1999) and tinnitus (Park et al 1999) as well as in smoking cessation (White et al 1999) and weight loss (Ernst 1997).

Individual randomized controlled trials

There are several instances where there is insufficient evidence for formal review, but a single good-quality study has shown acupuncture to be superior to placebo. For example, Deluze and colleagues recruited 70 patients with fibromyalgia and found real acupuncture to be superior to sham on five out of eight outcome measures, including blinded physician's assessment (Deluze 1992). Kleinhenz and colleagues showed that real acupuncture was better than a non-penetrating sham needle in helping recovery from sports injury (rotator cuff tendinitis) in sportsmen (Kleinhenz et al 1999). Aune and colleagues found acupuncture to be superior to sham acupuncture in preventing recurrent urinary tract infection in women (Aune et al 1998). All these studies are promising but need independent replication.

In other cases, early studies suggested that acupuncture was promising but later sham-controlled studies failed to reveal any specific effect. For example, a review of controlled trials concluded that acupuncture looked promising for stroke recovery when it was compared to no additional therapy (Ernst & White 1996). However, a subsequent sham-controlled study found no effect (Gosman-Hedstroem et al 1998). In fact, in the latter study, a control group with no additional treatment was included for comparison and neither real nor sham acupuncture proved to have an effect. It is noteworthy that the therapeutic interaction between therapist and subjects was carefully minimized, which suggests that the earlier positive effects might have been due to placebo effects such as the practitioner's enthusiasm.

A similar story may be unfolding for acupuncture for osteoarthritis of the knee: acupuncture has been shown to be clearly better than waiting list (Berman et al 1999, Christensen et al 1992), but a later trial found acupuncture no better than sham control (Takeda & Wessel 1994). The latter study seems generally well designed and conducted, although one weakness is that the sample size calculation was based on pain threshold, whereas the primary outcome was pain score. The sample may have been too small to be definitive (type II error). The question of acupuncture's specific efficacy for osteoarthritis of the knee is now being addressed again in a large multicenter study (Berman, personal communication).

In conclusion, with the possible exception of early postoperative nausea and vomiting in adults, acupuncture has not been convincingly established to have an effect beyond placebo. However, it is fair to say that acupuncture still has considerable promise and further research is certainly justified.

Clinical efficacy: design of explanatory trials

Rigorous RCTs of acupuncture are clearly feasible in principle. In contrast to the results in daily clinical practice, the formal evidence from trials shows a strongly negative trend. Some will argue that this is because acupuncture is no more than a good placebo. However, it is also possible that the acupuncture in these trials has been constrained in some way, so that its effect size was reduced and failed to show up in relation to a large placebo effect. It is therefore crucial that every possible attempt must be made to optimize the design of future trials in order to answer this crucial question. Three particular aspects of design are discussed here.

Appropriate condition

Laboratory studies provide information on the mechanisms of acupuncture. Their aim is to inform both research and practice, for example by guiding the selection or exclusion of particular patients for physiological reasons such as changing neurological response with age.

It is tempting to measure a physiologic response in humans, to provide evidence for the effect of acupuncture. Physiologic effects that have been described in controlled trials include changes in skin temperature (Dyrehag et al 1997), blood flow (Blom et al 1993) and heart rate variability (Haker et al 2000). However, none of this evidence demonstrates that acupuncture has a clinically relevant effect. The most convincing research must involve patients with clinical conditions.

Experimental pain can be tested in a laboratory but the findings can be extended to the clinical situation of acute (e.g. postoperative) pain. A recent review found a number of laboratory studies testing the analgesic effect of acupuncture on experimental pain (White 1999). The balance of the evidence was positive, more convincingly for electroacupuncture than manual stimulation. Acupuncture may have an effect size not very different from that of some analgesics. Pain has the advantage that it can be assessed reliably by validated measures. Postoperative pain can be tested with some precision, reliability and relevance by measuring patient-controlled analgesia (Christensen et al 1993). This use of acupuncture under general anesthetic provides a perfect opportunity for subject blinding.

Nausea and vomiting (N&V) also provides an appropriate model (Vickers 1996). It is commonly induced by particular circumstances, so that homogeneous groups can be identified. Assessment of nausea seems to be reliable and measurement of vomiting is objective. The outcome can be measured over a short timeframe, so drop-outs and confounding factors are not likely to be a problem. Treatment with acupuncture is by a simple formula which is agreed by most acupuncturists. On the other hand, N&V responds strongly to placebo, so large sample sizes are likely to be needed, and the incidence rate for postoperative nausea has been found to vary from 10% to 96% in different trials, which makes both sample size calculation and the assessment of effects unreliable (Tramèr et al 1998).

Functional conditions, such as asthma, irritable colon or tension-type headache, would be considered by some to be less suitable for demonstrating a physical effect of acupuncture, because they have a large psychological component. This is unnecessarily reductionist. Some of acupuncture's clinical effect may be due to influence on brain centers such as the limbic system (Campbell 1999); laboratory research provides supporting evidence (White 1999). Effects on attitude, motivation and the stress response are quite feasible, so conditions in which these factors are important should not be excluded.

Recovery from injury has rarely been used for testing acupuncture but appears promising (Kleinhenz et al 1999). Outcomes must be measured at appropriate times so that differences between the groups are not overlooked. Back pain is probably not a suitable condition for efficacy studies: acute back pain recovers quickly so treatment effects may be difficult to demonstrate and chronic pain involves many confounding factors, such as stress at work, which confound the effects of acupuncture. Pragmatic studies are more appropriate.

It may be necessary to choose particular subgroups for trials, i.e. those who have best likelihood of response. For example, Blom and colleagues (1996) showed that acupuncture was superior to sham acupuncture at increasing salivary secretion overall in patients with dry mouth syndrome. However, the best response was seen in those who showed a good short-term change after stimulation by pilocarpine, i.e. had some residual gland function (Blom et al 1999).

Optimal therapy

The acupuncture technique used in the study should be optimal. In some published studies the treatment has been less than optimal, such as using only three treatment sessions to treat cervical spondylosis (Emery & Lythgoe 1986) or using oversimplified regimes for chronic conditions (Biernacki & Peake 1998). However, there is no general agreement on what constitutes the optimal technique. For example, when six experienced acupuncturists were asked to evaluate the treatment regimes used in 15 controlled trials of acupuncture for back pain, there was a remarkable divergence of opinion (White & Ernst 1998).

There have been various attempts to establish the optimal treatment. Birch used classic and widely accepted texts to produce a description of 'best practice' by amalgamating the various protocols (Birch 1997). Another method is to survey clinicians to form a consensus (Foster et al 1999). Another approach is to arrange for every subject to be examined by a committee of recognized experienced practitioners, who form a consensus diagnosis and treatment strategy: this procedure has been described for studies of homeopathy (Walach et al 1997). Treatment guidelines may already exist, as is the case for auricular acupuncture for cocaine addiction (Margolin et al 1998).

Aspects of the optimal use of acupuncture that need to be considered are the diagnosis, therapeutic approach and treatment protocol.

Diagnosis Subjects may be diagnosed by Western methods, by traditional methods (for example, Wind-Cold) or by both (Vincent & Furnham 1997). For a trial to be meaningful, the method of diagnosis must be valid. Interrater reliability involves two or more acupuncturists making independent diagnoses on a series of subjects. Subjects could be rated for categories (such as Wind, Cold, Heat and Damp) on a scale of 0–5 and the results compared using the kappa statistic or preferably weighted kappa (Altman 1991). The simpler method of testing for correlation is likely to produce false-positive results (Altman 1991). Birch found that interrater reliability of practitioners using Japanese diagnostic methods was poor for pulse and abdominal diagnosis but good for overall diagnosis when information from the history was included (Birch, personal communication). One alternative approach is to develop and validate a patient questionnaire that can distinguish syndromes by different combinations of symptoms (Alraek et al 2000).

Therapeutic approach A variety of therapeutic approaches is available.

• A 'formula' approach in which points predefined for the condition are used. Some flexibility can be introduced to make treatment more realistic, by selecting points from a list either according to symptoms (Thomas & Lundeberg 1994) or according to tenderness (Kleinhenz et al 1999, Vincent 1989, White et al 1996).

• Selection may be made from predefined points according to patient type, which could be called 'tailored' treatment (Park et al 1999).

• Treatment may be individualized according to energy diagnosis. In order to make such a study reproducible, treatment must be according to a particular known style or the teaching of a specified school. It is by no means impossible to individualize treatment in clinical trials (see below).

Treatment protocol It is essential that the acupuncture protocol for a proposed trial should be accepted as valid by at least one reputable acupuncture authority. Two aspects of treatment protocol are discussed here: point selection and needling technique.

Acupuncture students traditionally spend considerable time and effort learning the locations of more than 300 points. The challenge is to show that this is time well spent, i.e. that these points are more effective than random points. So far, there is little evidence: some studies have not been able to show that standard acupuncture is more successful than similar needling performed at off-point, off-meridian sites (Gaw et al 1975, Ghia et al 1976, Mao et al 1980). The hypothesis has been stated that some conditions such as nausea should be treated accurately at a correct point, whereas treatment of other conditions, such as smoking cessation, requires opioid peptide release that might be achieved by placing needles anywhere (Lewith & Vincent 1998).

Acupuncture students also learn how to select particular points that are believed to be appropriate for each patient. However, it is not established whether this is important. The present evidence suggests that it makes little difference: appropriate and inappropriate points were compared in 193 patients with chronic pain and no difference was found in the outcome (Godfrey & Morgan 1978). However, acupuncturists cannot agree what are inappropriate points. Treatments chosen as ineffective by one practitioner were considered effective by another (Jobst 1995). This represents a serious challenge to the integrity of acupuncture.

Several fundamental questions about needling technique still need to be answered.

- *Is it necessary to penetrate the skin?* The findings of Kleinhenz suggest that penetration itself is the critical process in successful treatment (Kleinhenz et al 1999, Streitberger & Kleinhenz 1998).
- *Is the sensation of deqi necessary for a good outcome?* This has rarely been investigated. One study found that 48% of patients who responded to treatment experienced deqi, but only 23% of those who failed to respond (Chen, personal communication). In another study, subjects who experienced deqi had a better response than those who did not, whether the needles were in the appropriate points or not; however, the sample size was small and this analysis was post hoc, so no firm conclusions can be drawn (Takeda & Wessel 1994). The precise characteristics of deqi have not yet been firmly determined. Vincent established which components of the McGill Pain Questionnaire are significantly associated with acupuncture treatment, using factor analysis of patient questionnaires (Vincent et al 1989). One group of four adjectives seems similar to classic descriptions of deqi and further studies to validate questionnaires for deqi are under way.
- *What is the optimum duration of needling?* One study found little difference in the outcome after 20 and after 5 minutes' needling, though baseline differences between the groups prevented firm conclusions (Hansen 1997).
- *What is the appropriate depth of needling?* One study found that children with migraine were more likely to respond to subcutaneous needling than when the needles were inserted only as far as the stratum corneum (Pintov et al 1997).
- *What is the optimum regimen for treatment?* There is evidence that the body's response to needling changes over time; after a course of treatment, there was a significant change detected in the circulatory effects of acupuncture (Dyrehag et al 1997).

Controls and subject blinding

Choice of control procedure An explanatory investigation into the efficacy of acupuncture requires a 'placebo' control. A placebo should be indistinguishable from the real intervention in all respects (appearance, sensation, etc.) but devoid of therapeutic or physiological action. However, in the case of acupuncture, it seems necessary for a placebo to touch the skin. This is perceived as a problem because it involves physiological stimulation which, it has been argued, excites diffuse noxious inhibitory control (Bing et al 1991) and may have clinical effects on pain (Lewith & Vincent 1995). The duration of diffuse noxious inhibitory control may be too short to have clinical effects (Bing et al 1991). However, Ezzo and colleagues (2000) noted, in a systematic review of acupuncture for chronic pain, that control groups who received shallow 'placebo' needling had a higher response rate than control groups who received non-needle placebos, such as sham tablets or dummy TENS. These authors comment that this finding is comptabile with shallow needling being an active treatment. But it is also compatible with sham needling being a more power-ful placebo than the other procedures. This question of whether superficial needling has a clinical effect is still open.

There is some confusion over the terminology used for acupuncture controls. Lewith and Machin used the term 'sham' acupuncture to mean needling the wrong points (Hammerschlag 1998, Lewith & Vincent 1998, Lewith et al 1983) and 'mini-mal' acupuncture to mean superficial needling. Others have argued that since noth-ing that touches the skin can be guaranteed to be inactive, the word 'placebo' is altogether inappropriate and the term 'sham' places emphasis on the psychological impact on the subject (Park et al 1999). The term 'sham' is used here for any procedure (see below) that is a pretence of acupuncture but to avoid confusion the procedure should always be described in full.

The essential features of the ideal acupuncture sham are (1) that it should match what the subject (or at least an acupuncture-naïve one) expects to see and experi-ence with needling, but (2) that it should not produce the specific needle sensation, deqi. Margolin suggests an additional test: that it should have the same likelihood of adverse events leading to drop-out as the real intervention (Margolin et al 1998), but this applies only to its appearance and acceptability and not to its physiological effects.

Several sham acupuncture procedures have been devised, in five main categories with varying degrees of appropriateness. A list and discussion of possible control interventions are available (Filshie & Cummings 1999).

1. Standard needles inserted in inappropriate sites and/or superficially.

2. Standard needles used in an abnormal way, either pressing with the handle (Hesse et al 1994) or just pricking the surface of the skin (Moore & Berk 1976).

3. Other devices used to touch or press the skin, such as the finger-nail (Junnila 1982), an empty guide tube (Lao et al 1994) or a cocktail stick (White et al 1996). Ingeniously, Lao and Berman attached leads from inactive electrostimulation apparatus to both groups in order to reduce the perceived differences between the procedures (Lao et al 1995).

4. Sham forms of other treatments, such as inactivated TENS or laser apparatus (Dowson et al 1985, Macdonald et al 1983). This is problematic because the placebo effects of inactivated electrical devices are likely to be different from those of needles. Therefore, any differences in the outcomes of the two groups cannot be attributed solely to the specific effect of acupuncture. This control has been described as a 'fatal flaw' by Ter Riet and colleagues (1990).

5. Needles modified in some way, e.g. by placing an adhesive plug on the tip so that the needle does not penetrate (Gallacchi et al 1981). A major advance was to develop a sham needle that is blunt and in which the shaft of the needle is free to move inside the handle (Streitberger & Kleinhenz 1998). When pressed on the skin, the needle appears to penetrate but the handle simply telescopes over the shaft. The needle is supported vertically on the skin by an adhesive dressing applied over an O-ring around the point. In a validation study, 22% of volunteers could feel 'a dull sensation' with the sham needle, compared with 57% with a real needle. This 'dull sensation' was called deqi by the authors, though it may not accurately reflect true needle sensation. This sham needle needs to be tested in a variety of locations, with different methods of manual stimulation and with variation in direction of needle

insertion (Kaptchuk 1998). An RCT using the sham needle showed a significant difference in treatment effect between real needle and sham needle in treatment of rotator cuff lesions in sportsmen (Kleinhenz et al 1999). The credibility of the intervention was not different between the groups. A different method of supporting the needle was developed by Park, consisting of an oversize guide tube with a silicon flange which adheres to the skin by means of double-sided tape (Park et al 1999). The standard guide tube makes a sliding fit within the Park tube. More experience of these procedures is awaited and validation in different types of subject.

Selection of sham points Although the new sham needle may prove a satisfactory control for use at genuine points, it may still have physiological activity. Until this is established, it is better to use it on sham points. Choice of sham points involves several considerations. A sufficient number and variety of sham points should be defined before the study to give the user some choice (Zaslawski et al 1997). The practical process of locating them (for example, measuring from landmarks) should be comparable to using real points and practitioners must become as familiar with using them as with real points. It is not known how close sham points should be to the site of the complaint in order to be credible. Some studies have placed needles in the knee (Jobst et al 1986, Waite & Clough 1998, Williamson et al 1996), but the credibility was not tested. The points should not be in the affected anatomical segment: a metaanalysis of 90 sham-controlled studies found that real acupuncture was much more likely to be superior when controls were not in the relevant segment than when they were close to it (Araujo 1998). Finally, sham points should be properly validated, as exemplified by Margolin and colleagues in preparation for a definitive study of auricular acupuncture for cocaine dependency (Margolin et al 1998).

Testing the success of blinding The success of blinding should be tested, either indirectly by comparing the credibility of real and sham interventions, to show that they have the same psychological impact, or directly by asking subjects which intervention they believe they received. Neither method is straightforward.

A common approach (Vincent & Lewith 1995) to credibility testing involves four questions:

- How confident do you feel that this treatment can alleviate your complaint?
- How confident would you be in recommending this treatment to a friend who suffered from similar complaints?
- How logical does this treatment seem to you?
- How successful do you think this treatment would be in alleviating other complaints?

The responses can be recorded on a 6-point scale or VAS (Petrie & Hazleman 1985). Two additional questions, about how severe current symptoms are and willingness to receive the treatment, were used by these authors (Petrie & Hazleman 1985). The original questionnaire was developed as an exercise to rate the credibility of novel therapies and control procedures that had just been described to (though not experienced by) a class of healthy psychology students (Borkovec & Nau 1972). Although the original context was very different from a clinical trial, the questionnaire was shown to have test-retest validity and internal consistency in the context of a clinical trial (Vincent 1990) and has been used in several subsequent studies

(Kleinhenz et al 1999, White et al 1996, Wood & Lewith 1998). However, the subjects' response could vary according to information they received on recruitment; for example, whether they were told 'You will receive one of two forms of acupuncture' or 'You will receive either acupuncture or a placebo'. The subjects must be judging the intervention they have actually experienced and not just giving answers about acupuncture in general; for example, Kleinhenz reports that, even after treatment had failed, 'acupuncture was continued to be judged as effective'. The questionnaire wording must be both precise and fully understood.

Other investigators (Moore & Berk 1976, White et al 1996, Zaslawski et al 1997) have used a direct question such as: 'You were told you would receive either acupuncture or another treatment very similar to it. Which do you believe you have received?'. We found this method less than ideal: subjects may try to give the answer which they think the researcher wants (interviewer bias) and the question focuses their attention on the details of therapy which may cause doubt and confound the outcome. Also, we observed that it is quite stressful for subjects who do not want to 'lose face' by not recognizing the fact that they had false treatment. Zaslawski analyzed the responses in some detail and found that the subjects' decision depended on four factors: layout of the needles, needle sensation, general responses such as drowsiness, and alteration of symptoms (Zaslawski et al 1997).

It seems, then, that there is no entirely satisfactory method of testing subject blinding and it is provisionally recommended to use the credibility questions as they are less stressful for subjects, taking great care in setting the correct context.

Practitioner blinding The influence of the therapist can be powerful, possibly more powerful than many interventions (Balint 1957), and is best minimized by masking (blinding) the practitioner. However, it is difficult or impossible to mask an acupuncturist and still offer technically optimal treatment. In one attempt, a doctor with no special knowledge of acupuncture was trained specifically for the study, learning two sets of points without knowing which were the correct ones (Lagrue et al 1977). In another attempt, the practitioner was given either the true or false diagnosis, made by another physician (Godfrey & Morgan 1978). This method has been adapted for rigorous, truly 'double-blind' studies of individualized acupuncture (Allen et al 1998): the diagnosing practitioner (or preferably team) would write down both appropriate and inappropriate selections of points, place them in different envelopes marked A and B, and leave the room. An independent practitioner would then enter, select one envelope according to a code and treat the subject. This way, all acupuncture practitioners would remain blinded as well as the subject, so it only remains to arrange a blinded assessor. This method is, however, still not acceptable by practitioners who use immediate feedback from the patient, e.g. by feeling the pulse, as a guide for further treatment.

The closest substitute for practitioner blinding is standardized, minimal interaction (Hansen & Hansen 1985) in which the acupuncturist must avoid discussing the therapy or the response with the patient. A modification involves answering questions about acupuncture using prepared responses (Kleinhenz et al 1999). Social discussion should also be forbidden, even though this creates a rather stilted atmosphere. Care must be taken that the actual performance of the intervention is identical in both groups. If subjects might see different practitioners on subsequent attendances, the approaches must be standardized. In a study in the UK, it was found that interventions were more credible when they were given by a male practitioner than a female and working in a holistic manner rather than sympto-matically (Choi & Tweed 1996).

PRAGMATIC STUDIES

Pragmatic studies investigate the effectiveness of acupuncture in real life, often comparing it with an existing treatment for conditions in which acupuncture is already in use and (ideally) after explanatory studies have shown a statistically sig-nificant effect in the same or similar conditions. Pragmatic studies have the attrac-tion of offering all participants a treatment which is believed to be active; in addition, they allow an assessment of the time course of response and duration of effect and an assessment of comparative costs (Hammerschlag 1998). Since neither subject nor practitioner is blinded, it is crucially important that the assessor is blinded. Rather few explicitly pragmatic studies have been performed for acupuncture though one study in progress compares acupuncture for chronic headache with standard general practitioner care (Vickers et al 1999).

Subjects

Inclusion criteria are usually broad and exclusion criteria few, in order to represent the patients seen in normal practice. Large sample sizes are required because effect sizes may be smaller than in efficacy studies, as some patients will not respond optimally, e.g. because of other medical conditions. Larger sample sizes are also required to answer questions of clinical effectiveness compared with questions of statistical significance alone. Moore and colleagues explored the group size required for studies of analgesic drugs for acute pain (Moore et al 1998). A group size of 40 in an explanatory study provides 90% confidence of obtaining a statistically significant result in the correct direction; a group size of 320 would be required in a pragmatic study to calculate number needed to treat (NNT) within ±0.5 of the true value, with 90% confidence.

Preference arm

How much the patient's preference for a particular treatment contributes towards the outcome is unknown and may be considerable. Pragmatic trials offer the chance to investigate this question systematically, using a preference arm. Subjects who express a preference for either therapy are given that therapy and only those who had no preference are randomized to the treatment arms (Melchart et al 2000, Thomas & Fitter 1997).

Intervention and control

Practitioners have much greater flexibility of treatment in pragmatic than in explanatory studies and may use co-interventions (for example, dietary advice) if they would offer them in normal practice. In order to minimize the impact of the individual advice of a single therapist, several practitioners should be used in each arm of the trial. This will improve the generalizability of the study.

The control procedure is likely to be standard clinical practice. However, there may be doubt about the effectiveness of standard practice. If standard practice is not already regarded as gold standard (i.e. supported by at least one good-quality RCT) then the design should include a third arm, either an untreated control group or a sham acupuncture control group, in order to provide a meaningful result. For example, acupuncture was shown to be no different from physiotherapy in treatment of neck pain (David et al 1998, Kisiel & Lindh 1996) and no different from TENS in treatment of back pain in elderly subjects (Grant et al 1999). Since neither of the control interventions meets the criteria for a gold-standard therapy, we can only conclude that the treatments are either equally effective or equally ineffective.

Outcomes

Pragmatic studies need pragmatic outcome measures, usually focused on what is important for the patient, such as quality of life or disease-specific quality of life. These studies also provide a good opportunity to measure costs (Van Haselen et al 1999, White 1996). Reports on the costs and cost consequences of acupuncture have been published (Downey 1995, Lindall 1999, Myers 1991) and reviewed (White & Ernst 2000) but more experience is required to provide rigorous evidence of cost benefit and comparison with other therapies.

CONCLUSION

Ideally, all patients should be offered the most effective, safe and cost-effective treatment within the available resources. Acupuncture is promoted by its practitioners as meeting these criteria but the evidence for this is by no means conclusive. Because the underlying principles of traditional acupuncture are not understood according to current scientific knowledge, good-quality studies are required to demonstrate its specific efficacy beyond placebo. Subsequently it will be necessary to compare its effectiveness in practice with other available treatments in pragmatic designs. Recent advances in the design of a sham control procedure will facilitate research. Meanwhile, considerable research effort is called for in establishing the optimal approach to acupuncture diagnosis and treatment.

REFERENCES

Allen JJB, Schnyer RN, Hitt SK 1998 The efficacy of acupuncture in the treatment of major depression in women. Psychological Science 9: 397–401
Alraek T, Aune A, Baerheim A 2000 Traditional Chinese medicine syndromes in women with frequently recurring cystitis: frequencies of syndromes and symptoms. Complementary Therapies and Medicine
Altman DG 1991 Practical statistics for medical research. Chapman and Hall, London
Araujo MS 1998 Does the choice of placebo determine the results of clinical studies on acupuncture: Forschende Komplementärmedizin 5(suppl): 8–11
Aune A, Alraek T, LiHua H, Baerheim A 1998 Acupuncture in the prophylaxis of recurrent lower urinary tract infection in adult women. Scandinavian Journal of Primary Health Care 16: 37–39
Baldry PE 1993 Acupuncture, trigger points and musculoskeletal pain, 2nd edn. Churchill Livingstone, Edinburgh

Balint M 1957 The doctor, the patient and the illness. Pitman Medical, London

Berman BM, Singh BB, Lao L et al 1999 A randomized trial of acupuncture as an adjunctive therapy in osteoarthritis of the knee. Rheumatology (Oxford) 38: 346–354

Biernacki W, Peake M 1998 Acupuncture in treatment of stable asthma. Respiratory Medicine 92: 1143–1145

Bing Z, Cesselin F, Bourgoin S, Clot AM, Hamon M, LeBars D 1991 Acupuncture-like stimulation induces a heterosegmental release of Met-enkephalin-like material in the rat spinal cord. Pain 47: 71–77

Birch S 1997 Issues to consider in determining an adequate treatment in a clinical trial of acupuncture. Complementary Therapies in Medicine 5: 8–12

Blom M, Lundeberg T, Dawidson I, Angmar-Mansson B 1993 Effects on local blood flux of acupuncture stimulation used to treat xerostomia in patients suffering from Sjögren's syndrome. Journal of Oral Rehabilitation 20: 541–548

Blom M, Dawidson I, Fernberg JO, Johnson G, Angmar-Mansson B 1996 Acupuncture treatment of patients with radiation-induced xerostomia. European Journal of Cancer 32B: 182–190

Blom M, Kopp S, Lundeberg T 1999 Prognostic value of the pilocarpine test to identify patients who may obtain long-term relief from xerostomia by acupuncture treatment. Archives of Otolaryngology – Head and Neck Surgery 125: 561–566

Borkovec TD, Nau SD 1972 Credibility of analogue therapy rationales. Journal of Behavioural and Experimental Psychiatry 3: 257–260

Campbell A 1999 The limbic system and emotion in relation to acupuncture. Acupuncture in Medicine 17: 124–130

Choi PYL, Tweed A 1996 The holistic approach in acupuncture treatment: implications for clinical trials. Journal of Psychosomatic Research 41: 349–356

Christensen BV, Iuhl IU, Vilbek H, Bulow HH, Dreijer NC, Rasmussen HF 1992 Acupuncture treatment of severe knee osteoarthrosis: a long-term study. Acta Anaesthesiologica Scandinavica 36: 519–525

Christensen PA, Rotne M, Vedelsdal R, Jensen RH, Jacobsen K, Husted C 1993 Electroacupuncture in anaesthesia for hysterectomy. British Journal of Anaesthesia 71: 835–838

David J, Modi S, Aluko AA, Robertshaw C, Farebrother J 1998 Chronic neck pain: a comparison of acupuncture treatment and physiotherapy. British Journal of Rheumatology 37: 1118–1122

Deluze C 1992 Electroacupuncture in fibromyalgia: results of a controlled trial. British Medical Journal 305: 1249–1252

Downey PO 1995 Acupuncture in the normal general practice consultation: an assessment of clinical and cost effectiveness. Acupuncture in Medicine 13: 45–47

Dowson DI, Lewith G, Machin D 1985 The effects of acupuncture versus placebo in the treatment of headache. Pain 21: 35

Dyrehag LE, Widerstroem-Noga EG, Carlsson SG, Andersson SA 1997 Effects of repeated sensory stimulation sessions (electro-acupuncture) on skin temperature in chronic pain patients. Scandinavian Journal of Rehabilitation Medicine 29: 243–250

Emery P, Lythgoe S 1986 The effect of acupuncture on ankylosing spondylitis. British Journal of Rheumatology 25: 132–133

Ernst E 1994 Acupuncture research: where are the problems? Acupuncture in Medicine 12: 93–97

Ernst E 1997 Acupuncture/acupressure for weight reduction? A systematic review. Wiener Klinische Wochenschrift 109: 60–62

Ernst E, Pittler MH 1998 The effectiveness of acupuncture in treating acute dental pain: a systematic review. British Dental Journal 184: 443–447

Ernst E, White AR 1996 Acupuncture as an adjuvant therapy in stroke rehabilitation? Wiener Medizinische Wochenschrift 146: 556–558

Ernst E, White AR 1998 Acupuncture for back pain: a meta-analysis of randomized controlled trials. Archives of Internal Medicine 158: 2235–2241

Ezzo J, Berman B, Hadhazy V, Jadad AR, Lao L, Singh BB 2000 Is acupuncture effective for the treatment of chronic pain? A systematic review. Pain 86: 217–225

Filshie J, Cummings TM 1999 Western medical acupuncture. In: Ernst E, White A (eds) Acupuncture: a scientific appraisal. Butterworth Heinemann, Oxford, pp 31–59

Foster N, Barlas P, Daniels J, Dziedzic K, Gray R 1999 Use of acupuncture by physiotherapists in the treatment of osteoarthritis of the knee: current trends inform a clinical trial. Proceedings of the Chartered Society of Physiotherapy Congress, October, p 27

Gallacchi G, Mueller W, Plattner GR, Schnorrenberger CC 1981 Akupunktur- und Laserstrahlbehandlung beim Zervikal- und Lumbalsyndrom. Schweizerische Medizinische Wochenschrift 111: 1360–1366

Gaw AC, Chang LW, Shaw LC 1975 Efficacy of acupuncture on osteoarthritic pain. New England Journal of Medicine 293: 375–378

Ghia JN, Mao W, Toomey TC, Gregg JM 1976 Acupuncture and chronic pain mechanisms. Pain 2: 285–299

Godfrey CM, Morgan P 1978 A controlled trial of the theory of acupuncture in musculoskeletal pain. Journal of Rheumatology 5: 121–124

Gosman-Hedstroem G, Claesson L, Klingenstierna U et al 1998 Effects of acupuncture treatment on daily life activities and quality of life. Stroke 29: 2100–2108

Grant DJ, Bishop-Miller J, Winchester DM, Anderson M, Faulkner S 1999 A randomized comparative trial of acupuncture versus transcutaneous electrical nerve stimulation for chronic back pain in the elderly. Pain 82: 9–13

Haker E, Egekvist H, Bjerring P 2000 Effect of sensory stimulation (acupuncture) on sympathetic and parasympathetic activities in healthy subjects. Journal of the Autonomic Nervous System 79: 52–59

Hammerschlag R 1998 Methodological and ethical issues in clinical trials of acupuncture. Journal of Alternative and Complementary Medicine 4: 159–171

Hansen JA 1997 A comparative study of two methods of acupuncture treatment for neck and shoulder pain. Acupuncture in Medicine 15: 71–73

Hansen PE, Hansen JH 1985 Acupuncture treatment of chronic tension headache – a controlled cross-over trial. Cephalalgia 5: 137–142

Hesse J, Mogelvang B, Simonsen H 1994 Acupuncture versus metoprolol in migraine prophylaxis: a randomised trial of trigger point inactivation. Journal of Internal Medicine 235: 451–456

International Headache Society Committee on Clinical Trials 1995 Guidelines for trials of drug treatments in tension-type headache. Cephalalgia 15: 165–179

Jadad AR, Moore RA, Carrol D et al 1996 Assessing the quality of reports of randomised clinical trials: is blinding necessary? Controlled Clinical Trials 17: 1–12

Jobst K 1995 A critical analysis of acupuncture in pulmonary disease: efficacy and safety of the acupuncture needle. Journal of Alternative and Complementary Medicine 1: 57–86

Jobst K, Chen JH, McPherson K et al 1986 Controlled trial of acupuncture for disabling breathlessness. Lancet 328: 1416–1418

Junnila SYT 1982 Acupuncture therapy for chronic pain. American Journal of Acupuncture 10: 259–262

Kaptchuk T 1998 Placebo needle for acupuncture. Lancet 352: 992

Kisiel AC, Lindh C 1996 Smartlindring Med Fysikalisk Terapi Och Manuell Akupunktur. Sjukgymnasten 12: 24–31

Kleinhenz J, Streitberger K, Windeler J, Bacher A, Mavridis G, Martin E 1999 Randomised clinical trial comparing the effects of acupuncture and a newly designed placebo needle in rotator cuff tendinitis. Pain 83: 235–241

Lagrue G, Poupy JL, Grillot A, Ansquer JC 1977 Acupuncture anti-tabagique. La Nouvelle Presse Medicale 9: 966

Lao L, Bergman S, Anderson R, Langenberg P, Wong RH, Berman B 1994 The effect of acupuncture on post-operative pain. Acupuncture in Medicine 12: 13–17

Lao L, Bergman S, Langenberg P, Wong RH, Berman B 1995 Efficacy of Chinese acupuncture on postoperative oral surgery pain. Oral Surgery, Oral Medicine, Oral Pathology, Oral Radiology and Endodiagnosis 79: 423–428

Lee A, Done ML 1999 The use of nonpharmacologic techniques to prevent postoperative nausea and vomiting: a meta-analysis. Anesthesia and Analgesia 88: 1362–1369

Lewith G, Vincent C 1995 On the evaluation of the clinical effects of acupuncture: a problem reassessed and a framework for future research. Pain Forum 4: 29–39

Lewith GT, Vincent CA 1998 The clinical evaluation of acupuncture. In: Filshie J, White A (eds) Medical acupuncture: a Western scientific approach. Churchill Livingstone, Edinburgh, pp 205–224

Lewith G, Field J, Machin D 1983 Acupuncture compared with placebo in post-herpetic pain. Pain 17: 361–368

Lindall S 1999 Is acupuncture for pain relief in general practice cost-effective? Acupuncture in Medicine 17: 97–100

Linde K, Jobst K, Panton J 2000 Acupuncture for chronic asthma (Cochrane Review). The Cochrane Library, Issue 1. Update Software, Oxford

Macdonald AJR, Macrae KD, Master BR, Rubin A 1983 Superficial acupuncture in the relief of chronic low back pain. Annals of the Royal College of Surgeons 65: 44–46

Mann F 1992 Reinventing acupuncture. Butterworth Heinemann, Oxford

Mao W, Ghia JN, Scott DS, Duncan GH, Gregg JM 1980 High versus low intensity acupuncture analgesia for treatment of chronic pain: effects on platelet serotonin. Pain 8: 331–342

Margolin A, Avants K, Kleber H 1998 Investigating alternative medicine therapies in randomized controlled trials. Journal of the American Medical Association 280: 1626–1627

Melchart D, Linde K, Fischer P, White A, Allais G, Vickers A, Berman B 1999 Acupuncture for recurrent headaches: a systematic review of randomized controlled trials. Cephalalgia 19: 779–786

Melchart D, Steger G, Linde K, Makarian K, Hatahet Z, Brenke R, Saller R 2000 Acupuncture versus midazolam for gastroscopy – a comprehensive cohort study. Focus on Alternative and Complementary Therapies 5: 93–94

Moore ME, Berk SN 1976 Acupuncture for chronic shoulder pain. Annals of Internal Medicine 84: 381–384

Moore RA, Gavaghan D, Tramer MR, Collins SL, McQuay HJ 1998 Size is everything – large amounts of information are needed to overcome random effects in estimating direction and magnitude of treatment effects. Pain 78: 209–216

Murphy PA 1998 Alternative therapies for nausea and vomiting of pregnancy. Obstetrics and Gynaecology 91: 149–155

Myers CP 1991 Acupuncture in general practice: effect on drug expenditure. Acupuncture in Medicine 9: 71–72

Park J, White AR, Lee H, Ernst E 1999 Development of a new sham needle. Acupuncture in Medicine 17: 110–112

Petrie JP, Hazleman BL 1985 Credibility of placebo transcutaneous nerve stimulation and acupuncture. Clinical and Experimental Rheumatology 3: 151–153

Pintov S, Lahat E, Alstein M, Vogel Z, Barg J 1997 Acupuncture and the opioid system: implications in management of migraine. Paediatric Neurology 17: 129–133

Schulz KF, Chalmers I, Hayes RJ, Altman DG 1995 Empirical evidence of bias. Journal of the American Medical Association 273: 408–412

Smith LA, Oldman AD, McQuay HJ, Moore RA 2000 Teasing apart quality and validity in systematic reviews: an example from acupuncture trials in chronic neck and back pain. Pain 86: 119–132

Streitberger K, Kleinhenz J 1998 Introducing a placebo needle into acupuncture research. Lancet 352: 364–365

Takeda W, Wessel J 1994 Acupuncture for the treatment of pain of osteoarthritic knees. Arthritis Care and Research 7: 118–122

Taub HA, Mitchell JN, Stuber FE, Eisenberg L, Beard MC, McCormack RK 1979 Analgesia for operative dentistry: a comparison of acupuncture and placebo. Oral Surgery 48: 205–210

Ter Riet G, Kleijnen J, Knipschild P 1990 Acupuncture and chronic pain: a criteria-based meta-analysis. Journal of Clinical Epidemiology 43: 1191–1199

Thomas KJ, Fitter MJ 1997 Evaluating complementary therapies for use in the National Health Service: 'Horses for courses'. Part 2: alternative research strategies. Complementary Therapies in Medicine 5: 94–98

Thomas M, Lundeberg T 1994 Importance of modes of acupuncture in the treatment of chronic nociceptive low back pain. Acta Anaesthesiologica Scandinavica 38: 63–69

Tramèr MR, Reynolds DJ, Moore RA, McQuay HJ 1998 When placebo controlled trials are essential and equivalence trials are inadequate. British Medical Journal 317: 875–880

Tulder MW, Cherkin DC, Berman B, Lao L, Koes BW 2000 Acupuncture for low back pain (Cochrane Review). The Cochrane Library, Issue 1. Update Software, Oxford

Van Haselen R, Graves N, Dahiha S 1999 The costs of treating rheumatoid arthritis patients with complementary medicine: exploring the issue. Complementary Therapies in Medicine 7: 217–221

Vickers A 1996 Can acupuncture have specific effects on health? A systematic review of acupuncture antiemesis trials. Journal of the Royal Society of Medicine 89: 303–311

Vickers A, Rees R, Zollman C, Smith C, Ellis N 1999 Acupuncture for migraine and headache in primary care: a protocol for a pragmatic, randomized trial. Complementary Therapies in Medicine 7: 3–18

Vincent C 1989 A controlled trial of the treatment of migraine by acupuncture. Clinical Journal of Pain 5: 305

Vincent C 1990 Credibility assessments in trials of acupuncture. Complementary Medical Research 4(1): 8–11

Vincent C, Furnham A 1997 Complementary medicine: a research perspective. Wiley, Chichester

Vincent C, Lewith G 1995 Placebo controls for acupuncture studies. Journal of the Royal Society of Medicine 88: 199–202

Vincent CA, Richardson PH, Black JJ, Pither CE 1989 The significance of needle placement site in acupuncture. Journal of Psychosomatic Research 33: 489–496

Waite NR, Clough JB 1998 A single-blind, placebo-controlled trial of a simple acupuncture treatment in the cessation of smoking. British Journal of General Practice 48: 1487–1490

Walach H, Haeusler W, Lowes T et al 1997 Classical homeopathic treatment of cluster headaches. Cephalalgia 17: 1119–1126

White AR 1996 Economic evaluation of acupuncture. Acupuncture in Medicine 14: 109–113

White AR 1999 Neurophysiology of acupuncture analgesia. In: Ernst E, White AR (eds) Acupuncture: a scientific appraisal. Butterworth Heinemann, Oxford, pp 60–92

White AR, Ernst E 1998 A trial method for assessing the adequacy of acupuncture treatments. Alternative Therapies in Health and Medicine 4: 66–71

White AR, Ernst E 1999 A systematic review of randomized controlled trials of acupuncture for neck pain. Rheumatology (Oxford) 38: 143–147

White AR, Erust E 2000 Economic analysis of complementary medicine: a systematic review. Complementary Therapies in Medicine 8, 111–118

White AR, Eddleston C, Hardie R, Resch KL, Ernst E 1996 A pilot study of acupuncture for tension headache, using a novel placebo. Acupuncture in Medicine 14: 11–15

White AR, Rampes H, Ernst E 1999 Acupuncture for smoking cessation (Cochrane Review). The Cochrane Library, Issue 1. Update Software, Oxford

Williamson L, Yudkin P, Livingstone R, Prasad K, Fuller A, Lawrence M 1996 Hay fever treatment in general practice: a randomised controlled trial comparing standardised Western acupuncture with sham acupuncture. Acupuncture in Medicine 14(1): 6–10

Wood R, Lewith G 1998 The credibility of placebo controls in acupuncture studies. Complementary Therapies in Medicine 6: 79–82

Zaslawski C, Rogers C, Garvey M, Ryan D, Yang CX, Zhang SP 1997 Strategies to maintain the credibility of sham acupuncture used as control treatment in clinical trials. Journal of Alternative and Complementary Medicine 3: 257–266

19

Research methodology for studies of prayer and distant healing

Elisabeth Targ

INTRODUCTION

The topic of distant healing or healing intentionality brings some of the most controversial and central questions to the area of complementary medicine. Within the scientific community, the most usual explanation for any beneficial effects of prayer, energy, spiritual or 'psychic' healing efforts is that hope, expectation or the relationship with the healer mobilizes a psychogenic improvement in the patient's health. Such psychogenic effects have been well described in the psychophysiology and psychoimmunology literature and will therefore not be the focus of this chapter. Here we consider research approaches for assessing whether the intentions of one person can benefit the health of another independent of any psychological factors. The term 'distant' when applied to healing intentionality is used to emphasize the removal of ordinary channels of communication between healer and patient, but certainly the modality of healing intention could be present when a healer and patient are in proximity. More than 80% of Americans believe that their 'thoughts can cause healing for another person at a distance' (Yanklovich 1998) and this is a view shared by 75% of family practitioners. Anecdotal reports of healing in a wide variety of conditions have, however, stimulated more than 150 controlled studies dealing with human and/or biological systems. Of these, two-thirds found a statistically significant effect (for review see Benor 1992, Dossey 1993, Targ 1997). The US National Institutes of Health (NIH) now even has a category of studies entitled 'Distant Intentionality on Biological Systems' and yet the concept of distant healing implies a type of consciousness-mediated causality that has never been accepted within the medical sciences.

Few fields of research routinely raise such heartfelt opposition as research in distant healing; as one NIH reviewer wrote to this author, 'healing is intrinsically a matter of faith, and therefore cannot be studied by science'. Another reviewer from the US Department of Defense felt a study intended to determine whether distant healing could benefit breast cancer patients had 'no translational potential'. These remarks illustrate a popular belief among the scientific community that distant healing, interestingly, has also come from communities of healing practitioners and religious people as well. Some healers have voiced the concern that research cannot test or study the subtle effects of their treatments. Religionists have objected that research in distant healing may dissuade people from prayer for the purpose of strengthening faith and mistakenly focus them on a causal interaction between prayers and physical outcomes (Thomson 1996). Typical concerns are that testing healing is 'testing God' and therefore blasphemous, if not impossible (Dossey 1997).

These concerns, when removed from the heat, do reflect important issues in studying distant healing. Clearly we must consider the limits of our studies. As we interpret results, we must remember that:

- finding that a change occurs in a biological system in the context of a directed prayer or healing intention neither proves nor disproves the tenets of anyone's religion
- the spiritual, cultural and psychological contexts in which healing efforts are embedded are complex and may have many benefits (or detriments) apart from their efficacy in affecting clinical change through intention alone
- use of the double-blind randomized clinical trial has multiple inherent constraints that preclude testing of distant healing exactly as it is practiced in the community.

Researchers interested in pursuing studies in this area will take heart from a list of basic research tenets published by the NIH Panel Report on CAM Research Methodology. This report states the underlying assumptions that:

- research is always feasible – and essential, regardless of the therapy under consideration
- research rarely provides unequivocal answers
- good research aims to minimize the effects of bias, chance variation and confounding
- our priority is research that investigates whether treatments do more good than harm (Vickers et al 1997).

The methodological questions in research in distant healing necessarily rest on defining a specific intervention and evaluating its impact on a target system. This will be the main focus of this chapter. Questions of mechanisms depend on the successful negotiation of these first tasks and will be discussed more briefly at the end.

DEFINING THE INTERVENTION

There are no established protocols or practice standards for distant healing practitioners as a group. Healer inclusion criteria in published studies have ranged from novice volunteers in many studies (Braud 1989, O'Laoire 1997) to 'people who believe in God' (Harris et al 1999), to healers of international renown (Grad 1965, Rauscher & Rubik 1983) or with many years of professional experience (Sicher et al 1998, Snel & Hol 1983). Each experimenter must carefully choose and document the approach and experience level of healers in a study. The choice may have a theoretical basis, e.g. an attempt to compare one approach to another or to manipulate healing parameters. Or it may be based on a practical issue, e.g. an experimenter may wish to evaluate a method being used in a particular clinic. Documentation of healer approach or experience does not require that healers be identical on all descriptors. For example, one approach might be to require 5 years of experience or a certain score on a test of concentration but not to discriminate on the basis of philosophical approach.

Because the efficacy of distant healing as a modality has not been established, there is no test by which to choose an effective healer to participate in a particular study. In addition, unlike a pharmacological agent or a technical device, distant healing depends specifically on the consciousness of a human being. This raises the important issue that in addition to possible differing efficacy of various approaches, there may be both differing skill levels of practitioners of a particular approach or even of an individual practitioner on a day-to-day basis. In a large study, one runs the risk that certain patients might be treated by an effective healer and others by healers of no ability. One novel approach used by Sicher et al (1998) has been to have healers that meet certain inclusion criteria work on different patients on a rotating schedule, so that in case some of the healers were effective and others not, all patients would have contact with a range of practitioners. Because a healer might not always be performing at his or her maximum ability, it may also be appropriate to plan several intervention periods, rather than using a one-healer, one-session approach. Another way to think about this is that in studying intentionality as a healing modality, one has to ensure that the intentionality effort is really present and to maximize the potential effects.

Many terms have been used to describe interventions which may fall into the category of distant healing. These include: intercessory prayer, non-directed prayer, energy healing, shamanic healing, non-contact therapeutic touch, spiritual healing. Each of these describes a particular theoretical, cultural and pragmatic approach to attempts to mediate a healing or biological change through mental intentions. The following are some operational definitions of modalities which include elements of distant healing.

- *Intercessory prayer.* Any form of requesting God to bring about a specific desired outcome (O'Laoire 1997).
- *Non-directed prayer.* Intercessory prayer in which the person praying wishes only that God's will be done in the life of the subject (O'Laoire 1997). This prayer may typically be worded 'Thy will be done' (Dossey 1997).
- *Energy healing.* This large category describes attempts by a practitioner to send or direct atypical or 'subtle' energy flows either to or within the subject.

Examples include attempts to interact with the Asian concept of *chi* (or life energy) through chi gong, jin shin jyutsu or reiki or chakra (human energy centers) energetic manipulations as taught in schools influenced by Ayurvedic teaching (Brennan 1987).

- *Shamanic healing.* This approach is typical of Native American and indigenous Siberian, Tibetan, Central American, Asian and northern European cultures (Halifax 1979). These complex practices involve the healer entering a profound altered state of consciousness in which he or she experiences moving into different 'realms' and interacting with spirits whose aid may be enlisted in healing the patient.
- *Therapeutic touch.* A technique developed by nurse Dolores Krieger (1975) in which the healer uses meditative practice to induce a calm and focused state and moves his or her hands over the patient (without touching) while holding a mental intention for the patient's healing.
- *Spiritual healing.* This very general term has been used to refer to a wide range of techniques including spiritist healing seances (Krippner & Villoldo 1976), as well as meditations focused on visualizing the patient connected with God, a universal force of love or the Absolute. Such healing efforts may be performed in a religious or a non-denominational context.

In a qualitative analysis of what he termed 'transpersonal healers', Cooperstein (1992) found that whatever the cultural or religious orientation of the healer, most typically begin with a period of relaxation, followed by enhanced concentration, culminating in visualization.

Most healing efforts in the community occur within a cultural context either of interaction between the healer and the patient or expectation by the patient that healing is being performed on his or her behalf. This may or may not be the case in a study of distant healing.

What is the healer doing?

Healer strategy should be documented before any trial via interview of the healer and healers in extended studies should be asked to write daily logs describing their healing efforts. Healer selection might also involve questions as to level of experience and professional training or other issues of relevance to the study such as healer ability at concentration. At this stage, it has not yet been established whether healer experience or training are significant for outcome but based on claims that certain individuals have extraordinary healing abilities or that certain training programs increase healing ability, this will be an important variable to explore.

For how long is healing attempted?

Periods of time for healing interventions in the literature range from a few seconds in experiments attempting to arouse anesthetized mice (Watkins & Watkins 1971) to 60 hours (Sicher et al 1998). A majority of studies have required healers to perform their healing efforts serially on a daily or weekly basis for a series of treatments. Few, however, have indicated how much time the healer should spend on the healing efforts. For example, in the three major intercessory prayer studies (Byrd 1988, Harris et al 1999, Walker 1997), in which prayers continued daily for a period of weeks, no indication is given if pray-ers prayed for a few seconds at bedtime or concentrated for minutes or hours. This problem can be addressed as in Sicher et al (1998) by requiring a set amount of time for the healing effort and providing healers with a log to document the extent of their compliance. In addition, some researchers (Walker 1997, Sicher et al 1998) have pointed out that it may be important for researchers to stay in communication with and actively encourage their healers during extended studies, for the purpose of motivating their performance and ensuring that healing efforts will in fact be performed.

Individual versus group efforts

Most distant healing interventions have been organized such that one subject is treated by one healer. A variation of this approach described above involves sequential treatment of each subject by a series of different healers. Another variation is seen in the Harris study: the name of each patient was given simultaneously to a 'team of intercessors'. Thus each patient was receiving pooled prayer efforts from a group of people working individually. In the study by Byrd, prayer was performed as a group effort, by preexisting Christian prayer groups. At this point there is no evidence to suggest that individual or group healing efforts are more successful. A logistical concern is the risk that in a group setting, group members may distract one another from the task of focusing on the subject. In addition, studies using healing groups and pooled efforts have tended to use less experienced healers than those studying individual efforts. In order to comment meaningfully on the relative roles of experience versus number of interveners, it will be important that investigators considering one or another of these approaches document the experience and practice level of the healers.

Extraneous prayer

In addition to fully defining the intervention to be tested, it is also important to identify all sources from which the intervention may come. Dossey (1997) has pointed out that in clinical healing studies, especially ones in which the patient is very ill, it is quite likely that patients may be receiving prayer or healing efforts from friends and family members or may be praying for him or herself. In fact, on a daily basis, hundreds of thousands of people worldwide offer prayers 'for all the sick'.

This observation has been levied as a criticism against an important, large randomized clinical trial of intercessory prayer for patients in the coronary intensive care unit at San Francisco General Hospital (Byrd 1988). Thomson points out that the control group in this study may have been receiving intercessory prayer efforts from friends and family, thereby contaminating the study. This is an important issue to be aware of, although this scenario would suggest that both groups are being prayed for by friends and family and that the study treatment group is additionally receiving prayer from the study healers. This would be more likely to cause a false-negative result, with both groups benefiting from prayer, rather than accounting for the positive findings of the San Francisco General study.

Because of the potential for a false-negative result, or ceiling effect, with 'extraneous prayer', Dossey has suggested that target populations be ones who are less ill (and thus less likely to be receiving community prayer). Another approach would be to recruit large or variable numbers of intercessors to examine possible 'dose' (numbers) effects.

Defining the healing intention

The investigator has the responsibility to define parameters of the healing intervention engaged. This may or may not involve defining the specific mental techniques used by the healers. It does, however, require carefully defining the intentions of the treatment. Intentions may be very specifically prescribed such as having healers hold intention for 'lower blood pressure', 'reduced tumor size', 'decreased anxiety' or even 'increased emotional and physical well-being' if the investigator plans to use a broad range of measurement tools. It is *not* appropriate for healers to pray for 'religious conversion' for patients and some studies have specifically directed healers not to do this.

It is also not useful for healers to focus their intentions for change in an area which the investigator cannot measure e.g. 'change in the etheric field' or 'balancing the heart chakra'. If within a healer's theoretical orientation, such an action is believed to also be associated with changes in the target system as defined by the experimenter, this type of focus may be acceptable as part of the healer's working style but a measurable outcome intention should be defined and specified by the investigator.

Working with healers

Most healers have not worked in a laboratory or experimental setting and many are not comfortable with or sympathetic to the constraints put on their activity in the research setting. This represents a limitation of distant healing as it is performed in the community. It has been our experience that there is a great range of healing practitioners and some are eager to participate, very flexible and appreciative of research efforts. Others have been very angry about not being allowed to, for example, touch experimental Petri dishes or have felt investigators were discourteous because they were questioning the ability of the healers. As with all social and working situations, it is important that the healer–investigator team work toward mutual understanding, respect and consideration. Because of the history of scientists doubting healers, it is especially important to examine unconscious tendencies in the team to be dismissive toward healers. In addition, it is important to respect and understand cultural differences which may be present, such as whether it is important or insulting for a healer to be paid. Likewise, healers who participate in research studies should be fully appraised of the limitations they will experience and should be assessed for their motivation to participate in the study.

TARGET SYSTEMS

Distant healing studies have historically shown significant effects in trials of influence not only on human medical problems but also human physiology in the laboratory, on animals (Grad 1965, Snel & Van der Sidje 1995), bacteria (Ranscher &

Rubik 1983) and cells in vitro (Baumann et al 1986, Braud 1989). Animal and in vitro targets are often chosen for reasons including lower cost, less complexity in running a trial and ease of isolating a particular outcome measure. In addition, in animals and certainly in in vitro systems, it is much easier to eliminate psychological and placebo effects.

Population comparability

The same general rules for choosing target populations in any study apply to distant healing, with special emphasis on population homogeneity and the need for thorough baseline assessments of factors which may influence outcome such as social support, levels of depression and anxiety, meditation practice and spiritual beliefs. In smaller samples it may be appropriate to stratify or use pair matching to ensure balance between comparison groups on these and other relevant medical factors.

Pair matching

Pair matching is done to control as much as possible for variation in outcomes which might be related to major disease progression. In pair matching two or three baseline variables relevant to outcome are used to form matched subject pairs. First, a normalized z-score is computed for each subject for each variable by subtracting the mean for all subjects and dividing the result by the standard deviation for all subjects. Next all pairwise sums-of-squared differences in z-scores between subjects (over the variables) are computed. For each subject an average difference from all the other subjects is calculated. Starting with the subject with the largest average difference, the closest match is found. The two matched subjects are eliminated from the list and the procedure is iterated until all subjects are paired. A binary random number, generated by computer, is then used to randomly assign one member of each pair to the treatment group and one to control.

Healer attitude

Studies of distant healing, as with many psychosocial interventions, are studies of consciousness either directly or indirectly interacting with another living system. For this reason, it is important to consider issues pertaining to the relationship between the healer and the healing target. At the same time, we must consider the possibility of a target system contribution to the healing effect. Specifically, it may be important for the healing task to be motivating and relevant to the healer. For example, in developing studies in our own laboratory, we interview many healers who state that their preference would be to attempt to heal someone who was very ill, rather than to try and influence a minor problem. Despite staff concerns that healing someone very ill might be too hard, the healers insisted that this would bring forth their better efforts.

Another example of the importance of healer attitude toward the task and the target is a situation in which a chi gong master acting as a healer in our laboratory was asked to attempt to 'kill cancer cells in vitro'. He vehemently objected that as a healer, he was prohibited from killing anything. The situation was resolved when he agreed to 'emit harmonizing chi energy' toward the cells, holding an intention equivalent to 'Thy will be done' with regard to the cells. The cells died significantly faster than controls (Yount et al 1997). Similarly, in studies at Lawrence Berkeley Laboratories, healer Olga Worrel was not willing to attempt to kill *Salmonella bacteria* in vitro but she was willing (and able) to protect the *Salmonella* from the harmful effects of antibiotics (Rauscher & Rubik 1983).

Subject beliefs

Questions have often been raised as to the relevance of subject beliefs about healing, religious orientation and desire for healing. Studies from the literature in parapsychology, for example, have repeatedly found that subjects who believe in clairvoyance or telepathy show higher scores on tests of psychic functioning than do non-believers (Schmeidler 1998). Very few studies have examined the contribution of belief specifically to healing. In studies in our laboratory, we have not found such a correlation. However, the majority of volunteer subjects in our studies have a very high a priori belief in the power of healing such that there may not have been enough variability in our samples to see a difference. In this example, patient self-selection limits the generalizability of results. It is therefore appropriate to assess subject beliefs about healing as well as spiritual or religious issues at study admission. It may be useful to deliberately choose groups of subjects with either high or low levels of belief for the purposes of comparison.

Subject comfort with healing

In addition to differences in belief in distant healing, there may also be differences among patients in their comfort level with being the target of distant healing efforts. For example, in the Byrd study, which used 393 subjects, an additional 57 patients who were invited to participate refused. Byrd (1988) states that some of these refusals were based on religious convictions – a point of view reiterated by a commentator in the *Wall Street Journal* who stated that if any doctor tried to pray for him, 'I would sue him'. We do not know if such opposition would modify the efficacy of distant healing efforts but it emphasizes the importance of documenting patients' attitude as well as obtaining informed consent.

Subject desire for healing

A potential confounder in healing experiments became clear with the publication of a study by Walker, in which it was found that alcoholic patients remanded to an alcohol treatment facility did worse if they believed family or friends were praying for them. This emphasizes the complexity of prayer in a social context. Walker speculates that on one hand, alcoholic patients may feel criticized or worked against by the prayers of others and that in some cases their own resistance to recovery may interfere with even unknown prayer efforts by others. In designing a healing study, it would therefore be reasonable to ask subjects to indicate their own level of desire for recovery, as well as their comfort with the possibility of others praying for them.

Subject participation in healing

There has been debate among researchers doing studies in distant healing as to whether it is important for subjects to know they are receiving healing efforts. The primary objection to such trials is that telling subjects they are receiving healing eliminates the blinding and introduces possible placebo or expectation effects. Nevertheless, it would be interesting to compare blinded with open healing trials and assess the magnitude of any added benefit to patients in knowing they were receiving healing efforts.

OUTCOME MEASURES

The choice of a measurable, definable, non-confounded outcome measure is crucial to the development of a meaningful study of distant healing. Ideally, study end-points should include those that are objective, have adequate variability in the study population and are not modified by the measurement process or study participation. The outcome measurement tools should have been validated in work separate from the study.

Ceiling effects

It is important to choose an outcome measure in which there is adequate room for change. For example, if the subjects are normal healthy volunteers, it will not be appropriate to look for decreased blood pressure or improved mood scores.

Measurement effects

Avoid outcome measures that are influenced by the measurement process. For example, if the outcome measure is 'level of depression', this should not be assessed by a series of clinical interviews, as the clinical interview itself may have a thera-peutic effect and serve to mask an effect (false negative). Similarly, having patients write daily journal entries over time as a source of information about mood will risk a masking effect because journaling itself is a therapeutic tool.

Limit the number of outcome measures

As in all types of studies, hypotheses and measures must be specified before the study is begun. Appropriate statistical correction for multiple testing problems may be done using a variety of statistical methods. When outcomes are believed to be independent, which they rarely are, adjustment can be made by the Bonferroni method which simply multiplies the univariate P-values by the number of statistical tests that were used in the analysis. This is a crude method, however, that can lead to severe loss of statistical power.

A better method is to apply a randomization test to the vector of outcomes. Randomization tests are easy to carry out since all that is required is to repeatedly reassign subjects to treatment and control using random numbers generated by a computer to make the reassignments. The test statistic is recalculated for each

computer-generated random reassignment. This process produces an approximation to the 'exact' distribution of the test statistic under the null hypothesis that
group assignment made no difference in the study outcomes. The approximation
can be made as close as desired to the 'true' distribution by increasing the number
of random reassignments. If complete enumeration of all possible outcomes of the
test statistic is possible (as is often the case when the number of possible outcomes
is small), then an exact P-value is obtained. In the simple 2×2 table case, the randomization test is known as Fisher's exact test and has been widely recognized as
the most conservative way to statistically analyze binary data. The advantage of
this method over the Bonferroni adjustment is that it preserves the correlations
among the measurements.

ESTABLISHING CAUSALITY

The biggest outstanding question in the field of distant healing is 'Do distant healing efforts modify biological systems'. Trials exploring this question will be
successful only if they avoid the two central research errors: 'false-positive' and
'false-negative' conclusions. Avoidance of the false-positive result has been the chief
focus of researchers and critics of distant healing research; however, to the extent
that we are trying to sort one type of consciousness effect (distant healing) from
another (hope and expectation), the false negative also presents a significant pitfall.

Avoiding the false-positive result

Hope and expectation are the chief confounders in studies of distant healing.
While it is likely that hope and expectation effects would be synergistic with any
true non-local healing effects, the focus of distant healing experiments is exploration of the role of healer intentionality in modifying subject outcomes. The gold
standard for limiting the role of hope and expectation is the double-blind
randomized clinical trial (RCT). It has been well established, for example, that
there is a significantly higher likelihood of seeing an improvement with a new
therapy in a non-randomized trial than in a randomized one (Colditz et al 1989)
and that blinded studies with inadequate concealment and randomization protocols are also more likely to show positive results (Shulz et al 1995).
    The formula for the double-blind RCT requires that:

• patients are assigned to treatment group at random
• patients do not know which treatment they are receiving
• evaluators of treatment efficacy do not know which treatment the subject is
  receiving.

In doing research in distant healing the old admonition applies: 'extraordinary
claims require extraordinary proof'. The purpose of the double-blind RCT is to
eliminate mediators of experimenter bias or subject hope or expectation. Most clinical trials begin with open-label pilot studies and progress step-wise to definitive
double-blind methodology. In the field of distant healing, we find the 'open-label'
trials to be of limited utility unless the outcome being measured is entirely
objective, not susceptible to autonomic effects and not treatable by other means.

Double-blind RCTs

We assume that readers are familiar with standard double-blind RCT methodology. Specific points relevant to trials of distant healing are emphasized below. The purpose of blinding in the RCT is to minimize any elements of hope, expectation or belief that might mediate a differential outcome.

Blinding protocols. Adequate blinding is essential. For a definitive test of efficacy of a distant healing modality, it is required that:

- patients do not know of their group assignment
- no research staff member may know of subject group assignment
- no outside treating personnel may know of group assignment.

The only person who may know a subject's group assignment is the healer. Ideally, the healer and patient never meet and the healer has insufficient information about the patient to describe or contact him or her (e.g. first name or photo only).

This type of blinding can be accomplished using a series of lists and codes. Randomization should always be performed using a random number generator or randomization table. Use of chart numbers, admission order or patient birthday is not acceptable. In addition, randomization should be performed after the patient is enrolled in the study (i.e. it is not appropriate to randomize a subject and then decide he or she does not meet criteria). The following example describes how this could be done for a study in which subjects are randomly assigned to receive treatment from a healer or to be in a no-treatment group. Investigator 1 is identified as the subject contact person, Investigator 2 is identified as the healer contact person.

1. Subjects are recruited by Investigator 1 (I1). Initial assessment is done and subject is enrolled if he or she meets inclusion criteria.
2. I1 assigns non-sequential, randomly chosen enrollment numbers to each subject chart and creates a photocard for each subject with his name. He puts the photocard in an opaque sealed envelope and puts a removable sticky tag on the outside, with each subject's enrollment number. I1 then gives a list of the enrollment numbers, without names, to Investigator 2 (I2).
3. I2 uses a random algorithm to assign study numbers to each of the enrollment numbers. He then writes the appropriate study number on each patient envelope and removes the sticky label. The code-key is stored in a sealed envelope. He then uses a random algorithm to assign subjects to either the treatment or the control group. In the event where stratification or pair matching is required, key data such as subject age or CD4 count could be transferred along with the code lists for use by I2. I2 then locks the envelopes assigned to the control group in a drawer and returns the treatment group envelopes (with their new numbers) to I1.
4. I1 then gives the envelopes to the healer according to whatever schedule has been determined. I1 has no further communication with the healer for the duration of the study. Any staff communication with the healer must be handled by I2. If there is a need to interact with a subject during the course of the study, this will be done by I1.
5. Data collection from the subjects is done by I1 who enters data using the enrollment numbers. After all data has been entered, analysis is begun

6. Ideally the assignment codes are broken after the main group comparisons have been completed.

Use of sham control conditions. Under some conditions, for example when the healing treatment requires that the healer be present in the room with the patient, alternative blinding schemes can be used. In studies of non-contact therapeutic touch, Quinn (1989) used a sham condition in which for control patients the healer was present, made hand-passes over the patient's body but did not 'hold a healing intention'. Instead she performed mental arithmetic. This protocol has the advantage of preserving the integrity of the intervention as it is performed in the community but raises concerns, either that the healer may not be able to 'turn off' her healing ability (leading to a false negative) or that the patient might perceive in the healer's affect whether or not healing is being performed (false positive).

In studies in which the principal outcome measure is believed to be objectively stable, e.g. stroke-related paralysis that has been documented stable for years, tests of in-person healing can be done, if subject condition is documented over an initial waiting period of 1 or 2 months, then an intervention or sham intervention is performed and an investigator blind to the condition makes a second assessment. Both these types of protocols allow testing of hands-on healing or healing in which the healer believes he or she must be in the room.

It is not recommended that investigators use a control condition that does not mimic the healing condition, as the expectation effect for prayer and distant healing may be presumed in certain individuals to be the guiding principle of their lives.

In vitro trials. In in vitro trials it is also important to create sham treatment conditions for control samples. Any control sample should travel to the same room on the same schedule as treatment samples, be handled in the same way, and position in test tube racks or incubators should be the same as for treatment samples. To further assess mechanical and environmental factors, in laboratory comparison studies, it is also useful to use systematic negative controls (Walleczeck et al 1999). In this methodology, some trials compare a treated sample with a sham-treated sample whereas others compare sham treatment with sham treatment. This allows assessment of baseline variability in the treatment system. Many investigators have also used thermistor devices to ensure that healer hand temperatures do not affect treatment samples.

Avoiding the false-negative result

While most of the attention in distant healing studies is on eliminating the false-positive or type I error, there are a number of ways in which a positive result could be ignored or washed out by the experimental protocol. This mostly applies to situations where subject self-report of symptoms is a primary outcome or where outcomes are known to be modified by a subject's emotional state. This type of potential confounder has been seen in studies of distant healing in blood pressure (Beutler 1988), asthma (Attevelt 1988) and depression (Greyson 1996) in which patients were required to make regular clinic visits for interviews or attend sessions of relaxing in an empty room while blind to a treatment condition.

Subject study-related activity should be minimized, e.g. it is preferable that subjects do not come to the lab or clinic for regular study-related activities, that they do not keep a study-related journal, that they are not instructed to mediate once a day to make them 'more receptive' and that they are not telephoned by staff members to 'see how they are doing'. Any such activity has the potential to alter (usually reduce) symptoms. This symptom reduction will be equally present in both the treatment and control groups and may wash out a possibly more subtle treatment effect. Unless the healing intervention is thought to require the immediate presence of the healer, it is best that, once enrolled in the study subjects, have little or no contact with study personnel and that outcome measurement activities be kept to a minimum.

Effects of social pressure and expectation are well known in the social sciences (e.g. Hawthorn effect). Kiene (1996) has pointed out that such effects may also create type I errors. If subjects in double-blind experiments are overly encouraged to think an effect may occur, if they feel they have to 'please' the experimenter by showing improvement or if they interact with other study subjects who may be receiving the treatments, the effects of psychological pressure may lead to patients either psychophysically self-generating improved symptoms or simply inflating improvement scores on assessment tools. This 'pleasing' or 'peer pressure' effect is an equal risk among control or treatment subjects. These factors too could wash out a potential distant healing effect. For this reason it is recommended that subjects do not interact with each other and that at study enrollment, investigators limit their enthusiasm for the treatment.

Treatment outside the study creates an additional potential risk of false-negative results. This was discussed above under the heading of 'extraneous prayer'. Unlike trials of new pharmacological agents, patients have easy access to many forms of distant healing and cannot ethically be discouraged from seeking them out. Therefore, it is important to document patient use of or knowledge of sources of distant healing efforts on their behalf that may be occurring outside the study.

Experimenter effects

Experimenter effects have been widely documented and discussed in the literature (Kiene 1996). They can lead to either false-positive or false-negative results. Careful application of the double-blind RCT methodology with additional attention to experimenter equanimity in contact with subjects should minimize such effects. However, research in distant healing presents a special case in which the assumptions underlying the RCT are challenged. The RCT depends on the assumption that the beliefs or desires of the investigator and the subjects will not have unmediated effects. This presumes that the wishes of the investigator will not cause subjects to show improvement and that the wishes of the investigator or subject will not influence random assignments. If distant healing effects are shown to be robust, until it is known how they are mediated, there will always be a risk that the experimenter or the subject may also be in some way influencing the course of the study.

In fact, this issue was raised in the context of studies of the ability of research volunteers to influence the electrodermal activity of subjects in the next room (Braud & Schlitz 1983). This double-blind randomized study was replicated in numerous laboratories in the United States but failed in the laboratory of a skeptical investigator, Richard Wiseman, in England. After repeated failures of the protocol in his laboratory, Wiseman invited a successful experimenter (Marilyn Schlitz) to replicate the experiment in his laboratory. In alternating trials, when Schlitz functioned as chief investigator the positive results were found, when Wiseman was chief investigator the experiment failed (Wiseman & Schlitz 1999). A first possible explanation for this disparity is that some aspect of the experimenter manner, personality or instructions may have altered subject performance. However, this study also highlights the point that in studies investigating effects of consciousness over distance, all sources of influence must be considered. It does not preclude the possibility of meaningful double-blind RCTs; if an investigator's non-local influence on an experimental population is minimal, neutral or equal then it is possible to determine whether or not the experimental treatment is effective. Theoretically it would be possible for an investigator's non-local influence to wash out an effect, dampen an effect or be responsible for a differential effect. If a difference between the two groups is seen, therefore, it can still be concluded that the effect is non-local but theoretically it is impossible to know whether it was caused by the experimenter or by the healer. These questions suggest, first, the importance of the experimenter's interaction with subjects, especially with regard to whether he or she appears encouraging or discouraging. Second, it may be important in the future to conduct trials comparing outcomes by investigators with different levels of belief.

INTERPRETATION OF DATA

Because the implications of experimental claims for the efficacy of distant healing are so profound, the experimenter is obliged to hold his or her studies up to the most rigorous statistical scrutiny and maintain the highest methodological standards.

Evaluation of baseline factors

It is especially important when analyzing data from distant healing trials to discover whether there are interactions among relevant baseline variables and outcome measures. It has been our experience that differences which suggest a distant healing effect will be attributed by the scientific community to differences in baseline variables rather than the healing intervention, even when these baseline differences do not achieve statistical significance. Unless these baseline–outcome correlations are measured and understood, the study will be open to criticism that other factors could have led to the observed effect rather than the treatment. It is therefore important to run correlation analyses between all baseline differences and all outcome measures. Appropriate controls for multiple testing can then be used.

Of course, it is impossible to rule out all baseline differences as possibly explaining the result since it is impossible to think of or test all of them. But the importance of postulating factors that could have an effect on outcomes and measuring them at the start of the study cannot be overemphasized. Specific baseline and independent variables which should be examined include: baseline psychological status, other sources of distant healing, beliefs about distant healing, and the subject's guess as to whether he or she was in the treatment group or the control group.

Statistical power

There has been a recent trend in metaanalyses to report data not only in terms of *P*-value but also to calculate an effect size. The reason for this is that in a trial with small numbers of subjects the power to detect treatment effects may be small, even if an effect is present. The use of effect size measurement in addition to standard analysis may assist in evaluation of pilot studies and may allow comparisons between degree of efficacy between treatments that have not yet been evaluated in direct comparison trials.

OTHER RESEARCH APPROACHES

Although the double-blind RCT is the gold standard for establishing causality in clinical trials, qualitative patient and healer interviews (Cooperstein 1992) and descriptive survey studies (Krippner & Villoldo 1976) yield important information which may help define future controlled trials looking at mechanism, comparing interventions and understanding the healing process.

ETHICAL ISSUES

Research in distant healing raises the usual ethical issues involved in testing a treatment with unknown effects. One could argue that scientists have an ethical obligation to study distant healing as it is a modality for which important claims have been made, it is widely available and some people are choosing it over conventional therapies. Others argue that such research is not ethical because of a potential negative impact on subject belief systems as well as concerns as to possible negative uses of information from trials.

Informed consent

As for all trials of an untested intervention, it is required that informed consent be obtained under the guidance of a certified human subjects safety review committee. Some investigators have argued (Harris et al 1999) that because there has not been definitive evidence of harm to patients in distant healing trials, informed consent is not required. We disagree. There is considerable evidence already in the published literature for the modification of biological states via the mechanism of distant healing (see Benor 1992). Some of these data include the possibility of negative effects (Dossey 1993). As with all studies, potential loss of confidentiality should be considered a risk. As evidenced by the 14% refusal rate in the Byrd study, not all subjects wish to participate. As evidenced by the negative outcome for alcoholics who knew they were prayed for by relatives in the Walker study (1997), there is clearly at least some psychological risk. An additional risk includes the possibility of severe anger and disappointment in subjects after they learn they have been in the control group, as occurred in one of our studies. Lastly, in psychiatric populations there may be an additional risk of paranoia or delusions associated with the idea of an unknown person at a distance attempting to influence one's body.

For the protection of the subjects, as well as of the investigators, informed consent should be obtained. Subjects should be told the probability of their being assigned to a treatment or a control group and that it is not known whether the treatment will be beneficial, neutral or harmful. They should be offered psychological or medical consultation if distress occurs as a result of participation in the trial.

MECHANISM OF EFFECT

This chapter has focused on methodology for establishing whether or not an effect is occurring, rather than exploring possible mechanisms of action. One reason for this is that one cannot investigate mechanisms before the effect is known to occur. Nevertheless, investigators who feel they have established replicable protocols may wish to pursue studies of mechanism. These trials can proceed in many ways, probably principally by identifying limits on efficacy, such as studying whether certain techniques or certain individuals show a more reliable effect, or examining potential shielding of targets or looking at a cellular or molecular level to understand what systems are being affected at a microscopic or chemical level.

Theoretical physicists are working on models of consciousness and information transfer that may relate to distant healing, while experimental physicists are attempting to build devices that may detect or replicate energies which some people believe could be associated with distant healing (Rubik 1995). Clearly the distant healing effect is complex and multifactorial. Even the concept of looking at mechanism will mean different things to different people. At the same time as the embryologist describes the mechanism of human development as beginning with an exchange of DNA, the religious philosopher describes it as caused by the will of God. The discrepancy between these two points of view does not prevent meaningful and useful information from coming out of the work of both of these approaches.

BARRIERS TO RESEARCH

The primary current barriers to research in distant healing are lack of funding and of public acceptability of researching this field. To date, relatively few federal grants have been awarded to support a study of distant healing. This despite the hundreds of thousands of dollars required for a formal clinical trial.

Until recently, a frequent objection to distant healing research was that it simply could not be done. With the recent publication of several large clinical trials, this objection has been tested. More recently, questions have been raised as to the utility of information regarding distant healing. An extremely high scoring distant healing proposal from our laboratory was recently turned down by the Department of Defense with the comment 'it has no translational potential'. Other reviewers have objected that even if healing worked in a particular study, one would be unlikely to find other healers with this type of ability. Obviously, future research will have to determine the prevalence of healers in the population but meanwhile, it is incumbent upon researchers to suggest how healing abilities might be used, if they are in fact shown to have a clinical efficacy.

An additional barrier to research is caused by the existence of a social and academic stigma toward researchers who engage in studies of what many consider to be an implausible or laughable treatment. The only place in the medical literature where paranormal abilities are currently indexed, for example, is within psychiatry under the definitions for psychosis and schizophrenia. It is therefore not surprising that many experimenters feel uncomfortable about expressing an interest in pursuing studies in the area of conscious influence at a distance.

Another, somewhat surprising source of resistance has been religious communities. Some religious people have understandably objected to scientists equating 'intentionality' with prayer. This has led to the concern that testing distant healing is a form of 'testing God' and therefore interfering with the sacred and highly personal relationship of faith.

WHY DO DISTANT HEALING RESEARCH?

Prayer and distant healing have been part of nearly every culture since the dawn of civilization. If research determines that it has a measurable effect, under double-blind conditions, on any group of physical or psychological findings, this might encourage health-care practitioners of all descriptions to include distant healing modalities as part of their treatment plans. If no effects are measured, research should focus on understanding the ways in which the culture around prayer or healing activities serves to lift the spirits and enrich the lives of patients.

Without evidence from rigorous trials, it is not appropriate for physicians to either recommend or discourage distant healing; with such evidence, they will be in an informed position from which to usefully guide their patients.

Future research will help define the conditions (medical, psychological, physical) under which effects are most likely to be measurable, mechanisms by which healing may occur, target systems that are most amenable, the common denominators and necessary factors for distant healing interventions, the relationship between spiritual issues and distant healing outcomes and whether individuals can be trained to improve their distant healing abilities.

SUMMARY

- The double-blind randomized clinical trial is the gold standard for trials of prayer and distant healing.
- Adequate blinding and randomization procedures should be followed and documented.
- The intervention must be well defined (include frequency, amount of time and training and/or experience level of healers).
- Subjects should have risks and benefits of study participation explained to them and sign informed consent before enrollment.
- Populations should be homogeneous. Consider stratification for smaller samples.
- Baseline information, including psychological status, beliefs about prayer and healing and other sources of prayer and healing, should be collected from subjects in clinical trials. This should be examined as part of the final data analysis for contribution to outcomes.

- Objectively measurable outcomes with adequate variability should be chosen.
- Subject study participation activities such as clinical interviews, traveling to special sites, journaling or meditation should be minimized to avoid washing out a small effect.
- In clinical trials subjects should be asked if they *believed* they were in the treatment group and this information should be entered as a co-variate for data analysis.
- Healers/pray-ers should be treated in a collegial and respectful way. Their healing efforts (time, location, method) should be documented in a log and they should be periodically contacted and encouraged by experimenters if the study is taking place over an extended period of time.
- Observational and outcomes research can add an important dimension to healing research.
- Qualitative studies may also make an important contribution and help guide development of future controlled trials.

REFERENCES

Attevelt JTM 1988 Research in paranormal healing. Doctoral dissertation, State University of Utrecht, The Netherlands

Baumann S et al 1986 Preliminary results from the use of two novel detectors for psychokinesis. In: Weiner DH, Radin DI (eds) Research in Parapsychology. Scarecrow, Metuchen, NJ

Benor DJ 1992 Healing research. Helix Editions, Deddington

Beutler JJ 1988 Paranormal healing and hypertension. British Medical Journal 296: 1491–1494

Braud W 1989 Distant mental influence on rate of hemolysis. In: Berger RE, Henkel LA (eds) Research in parapsychology. Scarecrow, Metuchen, NJ

Braud W, Schlitz M 1983 Psychokinetic influence on electrodermal activity. Journal of Parapsychology 47(2): 95–119

Brennan B 1987 Hands of light. Bantam, New York

Byrd RC 1988 Positive therapeutic effects of intercessory prayer in a coronary care unit population. Southern Medical Journal 81(7): 826–829

Colditz G, Miller JN, Mosteller F 1989 How study design affects outcomes in comparisons of therapy. Medical Statistics in Medicine 8: 441–454

Dossey L 1993 Healing words. Harper Collins, New York

Dossey L 1997 Running scared: how we hide from who we are. Alternative Therapies in Health and Medicine 3: 8–15

Grad BR 1965 Some biological effects of laying-on of hands: a review of experiments with animals and plants. Journal of the American Society of Psychical Research 59: 95–127

Greyson B 1996 Distance healing in patients with major depression. Journal of Scientific Exploration 10(4): 447–465

Halifax J 1979 Shamanic voices: a survey of visionary narratives. Arkana Books, New York

Harris WS et al 1999 A randomized, controlled trial of the effects of remote, intercessory prayer on outcomes in patients admitted to the coronary care unit. Archives of Internal Medicine 159: 2273–2278

Kiene K 1996 A critique of the double blind clinical trial: part I. Alternative Therapies in Health and Medicine 2(1): 74–80

Krieger D 1975 Therapeutic touch: the imprimatur of nursing. American Journal of Nursing 7: 784–787

Krippner S, Villoldo A 1976 Spirit healing in Brazil. Fate (March)

O'Laoire S 1997 An experimental study of the effects of distant, intercessory prayer on self-esteem, anxiety and depression. Alternative Therapies in Health and Medicine 3(6): 38–53

Quinn JF 1989 Therapeutic touch as energy exchange: replication and extension. Nursing Science Quarterly 2(2): 79–87

Rauscher EA, Rubik B 1983 Human volitional effects on a modal bacterial system. Psi Research 2(1): 38

Rubik B 1995 Energy medicine and the unifying concert of information. Alternative Therapies in Health and Medicine 1(1): 34–36

Schmeidler GR 1998 Parapsychology and psychology. McFarland, Jefferson, NC

Sicher F 1998 A randomized double-blind study of the effect of distant healing in a population with advanced AIDS – report of a small scale study. Western Journal of Medicine 169(6): 356–363

Shulz KF 1995 Empirical evidence of bias. Journal of the American Medical Association 273: 408–412

Snel FWJ, Hol PR 1983 Psychokinesis experiments in casein-induced amyloidosis of the hamster. Journal of Parapsychology 5(1): 51–76

Snel FWJ, Van der Sidje PC 1995 The effect of paranormal healing on tumor growth. Journal of Scientific Exploration 9(2): 209–221

Targ EF 1997 Evaluating distant healing: a research review. Alternative Therapies in Health and Medicine 3(6): 74–78

Thomson KS 1996 The revival of experiments on prayer. American Science 84: 532–534

Vickers A, Cassileth B, Ernst E et al 1997 How should we research unconventional therapies? International Journal of Technology Assessment in Health Care 13(1): 10–15

Walker SR 1997 Intercessory prayer in the treatment of alcohol abuse and dependence: a pilot investigation. Alternative Therapies in Health and Medicine 3: 79–86

Watkins GK, Watkins AM 1971 Possible PK influence on the resuscitation of anesthetized mice. Journal of Parapsychology 35(4): 257–272

Wiseman R, Schlitz M 1999 Experimenter effects and the remote detection of staring: an attempted replication. Parapsychological Association Conference, Stanford, CA

Yanklovich Partners Inc 1998 Telephone poll of 1,004 adult Americans. Time/CNN

Yount GL, Quian C, Smith H 1997 Cell biology meets chi gong. Proceedings of the 16th Annual Meeting of the SSE

FURTHER READING

Colditz G, Miller JN, Mosteller F 1989 How study design affects outcomes in comparisons of therapy. I. Medical Statistics in Medicine 8: 441–454

Dossey L 1995 How should alternative therapies be evaluated: an examination of fundamentals. Alternative Therapies in Health and Medicine 1(2): 6–9

Dossey L 1997 The return of prayer. Alternative Therapies in Health and Medicine 3(6): 10–15

Kiene HA 1996 Critique of the double-blind clinical trial. Alternative Therapies in Health and Medicine 2(1): 74–80

Rubik B 1995 Energy medicine and the unifying concept of information. Alternative Therapies in Health and Medicine 1: 34–36

Schmeidler GR 1988 Parapsychology and psychology. McFarland, Jefferson, NC

Thomson KS 1996 The revival of experiments on prayer. American Science Journal 84: 532–534

Vickers A, Cassileth B, Ernst E et al 1997 How should we research unconventional therapies? International Journal of Technology Assessment in Health Care 13(1): 111–121

20

Clinical research in naturopathic medicine

Carlo Calabrese

INTRODUCTION

What is naturopathic medicine?

Naturopathic medicine is a worldwide profession with concentrations in the US, Germany, Canada, UK, Australia and India. There are differences between these national breeds but some of the approach to research presented here would apply to any of the traditions. In description, this chapter will focus on the US and Canadian lineage which the authors know best.

In the US and Canada, naturopathic medicine is a primary health-care profession which functions to promote health and to prevent, diagnose and treat disease. It is generally considered to be one of the complementary and alternative medical (CAM) practices and, in fact, is practiced as either a complement or an alternative to conventional medicine under different circumstances. A naturopathic physician must be licensed to practice in 11 states and three Canadian provinces. The license typically is broad, allowing naturopathic doctors (ND or, in some jurisdictions, NMD) to diagnose any disease and treat using any natural means. In Arizona and British Columbia, acupuncture is a part of the regulated practice; elsewhere, naturopathic physicians must obtain an additional license to practice acupuncture. Prescription drugs of natural origin are permitted in some jurisdictions and minor surgery and midwifery in most. The term 'naturopathic physician' is used to describe a practitioner in most licensed jurisdictions. Though a distinction may be made between the terms 'naturopathic medicine' and 'naturopathy' on the basis of disease focus or other theoretical considerations, the terms will be used interchangeably here.

There are perhaps 2000 licensed naturopathic doctors in the US who have been trained in accredited in-residence 4-year post-baccalaureate institutions. There may be several thousand more unlicenseable naturopaths whose training is highly variable. Licensed naturopathic physicians are considered by many to be the most broadly trained in CAM practices and by some to be the best prepared for integration into the mainstream health-care system due to their preparation in the basic and diagnostic sciences of biomedicine and their broad range of practice.

The practice is guided by its own principles, articulated by the American Association of Naturopathic Physicians in 1989.

- First, do no harm. Utilize methods and substances that minimize harm. Apply the least force for diagnosis and treatment.
- Nature heals (*Vis medicatrix naturae*). Organisms are inherently self-organizing. It is the physician's role to support this process by removing obstacles to health and contributing to the creation of a healthy internal and external environment.
- Identify and treat the cause. Symptoms may represent the body's attempt to defend itself and to adapt and recover. The physician's optimal approach is to seek and treat the causes of disease rather than suppress the symptoms.
- The doctor is a teacher. The physician's role is to educate the patient and emphasize self-responsibility.
- Treat the whole person. The multifactorial nature of health and disease requires attention to the physical, mental, emotional, spiritual, social and ecological aspects of our nature. Diagnosis and treatment which are constitutional and holistic are among the foundations of naturopathy.
- The prevention of disease by the attainment of optimal health is a primary objective.

Treatment modalities include, among others, botanical medicines, diet, nutritional supplements, homeopathy, physical medicine (physiotherapy, hydrotherapy, manipulation), counseling and psychotherapy. A naturopath, as part of a vitalistic tradition, may arrive at a functional and constitutional assessment as well as a disease diagnosis. Treatment is individualized for the particular patient's condition and capacities rather than for just a disease entity. Typically, a combination of treatments are applied and are continuously adjusted over time as the patient's condition changes.

Modern clinical research

Modern clinical research is primarily comparison and extrapolation. Research provides prediction by comparing what has happened under certain circumstances and concluding that the same is likely to happen in the future. Medical uncertainty persists because no two 'cases' can possibly be alike. A generalizable approach to human degeneration and injury, such as modern biomedical science, most economically prefers patients, practitioners, disease and remedies to display as little variation as possible from each other, as if all were engineering materials. Its gold standard of evaluation is the statistically guided blinded randomized controlled trial (RCT) – a brilliant invention but one with its own epistemological limitations. It is best used to answer narrow questions, e.g. 'Is one particular remedy better than another for people with a particular presentation of symptoms?'. The symptom array is often presumed to be the result of a unitary disease which ideally has a unitary cause which will be modified by a 'magic bullet'. The remedies are competing options within one theoretical system. Subjects who are at risk for adverse events or for whom the remedy is unlikely to work are eliminated (via inclusion and exclusion criteria). Outliers along some parameters, those who are not remedy adherent or for whom insufficient data have been collected may be discarded from the data before analysis (protocol violations, data 'cleaning'). The volunteer subjects are either desperate or altruistically devoted to medical progress or both, a special population with potentially distinct psychosomatic signatures. Only recently are treatment arms of 'no treatment' being more frequently added to trials for observation of the natural course of the condition. This can provide evidence on the effect of doing as close to nothing as possible in a trial which sometimes proves to be not statistically different from 'effective' treatment. Each of these issues should be understood when using the single drug and single disease pharmaceutical research model to evaluate alternative systems of medicine (or even in evaluating conventional medicine).

The RCT is very useful and should not be discarded in the evaluation of naturopathic medicine but, because of the necessarily fine specificity of the questions that the RCT can answer and the alterations of practice that the method may require, the questions need to be very carefully framed and its limitations respected. The best it can do is to treat naturopathic interventions as a 'black box'. The method will not provide broad answers about the medical system being evaluated. In fact, it is quite difficult to answer questions related to whole practices as opposed to small components of the practice unless the trial is large and comes to an accommodation with the issues addressed here. The lack of precedent research in whole practices is in part due to these difficulties. Economic issues in the constraints of naturopathic research are also contributory but those are left for another venue.

THE PROMISE

In the anticipations of its adherents, naturopathic medicine may offer a different dimension which will affect health-care outcomes in ways not anticipated with conventional bioactive single molecular agents used in a single disease-oriented approach. How could this possibility be evaluated? Because of the methodological and logistical obstacles touched on above and elaborated below, this has yet to be demonstrated in a way that is both internally and externally valid.

Despite the lack of demonstrations of efficacy of the whole practice, there are numerous studies and clinical trials that yield positive results in evaluating the effect of individual naturopathic treatments. Since single large studies have not yet been designed or performed to assess naturopathic medicine as a whole, a matrix of evidence that may suggest the possibility of marked efficacy in naturopathic medicine as a system is useful. For example, there is positive evidence for a number of naturopathic medicine's modalities tested in RCTs in preventing and treating many diseases. Identifying treatments for which evidence is strongly positive would give a sense of the possible magnitude of benefit with naturopathic medicine if it were practiced under a treatment selection criterion of randomized trial evidence. One may find a range of treatments used in naturopathic clinical practice which are well supported by trial evidence. These can be reviewed in the context of an orthodox disease classification. Such a method of analysis would involve reviewing the medical literature of randomized trials for all the naturopathic modalities for a given condition, primarily diet therapy, nutritional supplementation, botanical medicine, homeopathy, physical medicine (physical therapy, hydrotherapy, manipulation) and counseling/psychotherapy.

The criteria for selection of the treatments used here is whether there have been clinical trials of acceptable design for them and for which there is no significant evidence from other studies controverting the hypothesized effect. In asthma, for example, an array of positive results across the naturopathic treatment modalities is very promising. In the absence of studies looking at the whole practice as an entity, the RCT literature can give a good suggestion of the potential benefit. To gain an overall sense of the generalized efficacy of naturopathic medicine as a health-care system, different diseases which span the range of age, gender, chronicity, severity and mortality can be chosen for review in this manner.

The extant RCT literature typically, though not necessarily, demonstrates the efficacy of one substance at a time and generally neglects the possibilities of combinations of agents. It may seem self-evident that combination therapy with several interventions, each of which is supported by good evidence and which work via different pathways, is more likely to work than a single agent. Combination remedies are very common among naturopathic physicians. Combinations are often recommended in naturopathic education as more effective than single agents and, in fact, form an important part of the naturopathic formulary. The combinations' components are usually designed to work through widely differing mechanisms with the hypothesis that the therapeutic effects will be at least additive, if not synergistic. The specific therapeutic actions of each of the relatively benign components may be small, making the detection of clinical effect more difficult than a single agent trial, with the smaller sample sizes usually seen in natural medicine. The possibilities of polytherapy are increasingly recognized in intractable conditions, as in conventional AIDS treatment or natural treatment of recurrent migraine (Peroutka 1998).

MAJOR RESEARCH PROBLEMS IN NATUROPATHIC MEDICINE

Clinical research properly done in conventional medicine is a demanding discipline encompassing study design, ethics, clinical care, careful definition and precise measurement of diseases and outcomes, data management and statistics, analysis and interpretation. In addition, there are a number of special challenges which need to be taken into account in doing research in naturopathic medicine if the promise of the practice is to be evaluated. For some of these problems, there is no immediate solution. For others, a few suggestions are offered in the concluding section.

Research problems related to lack of preliminary data and methods

The accumulated scientific literature is thin in many of the practices and procedures that characterize naturopathy. While it may seem useful to determine if CAM systems are effective as a system in comparison to other forms of practice, the body of such evidence on the whole practice of naturopathic medicine is as vanishingly small as it is for other non-dominant whole systems of practice, such as Oriental medicine and Ayurveda. All these approaches are characterized by treatment through multiple modalities with a global approach to individuals and their unique constellation of physical and mental stressors and symptoms. The tools for such research are not well established or well known.

In part, the paucity of naturopathic literature is due to past publication bias against alternative medicine. Peer review boards are composed of conventionally trained scientists who, of course, reject submissions which present as a contradiction of the orthodox scientific knowledge base. Orthodoxies as systems are necessarily well organized to resist evidence of theoretically aberrant experiences. Simultaneously there has sometimes been little resistance to the publication of anecdotes and poorly designed studies which deny benefits and overemphasize the dangers of alternative approaches. While this prejudice may be overcome by several lines of evidence cogently presented to editors, such a scientific campaign is unlikely for most CAM professions which have not heretofore had the scientists needed to design and perform the many experiments that may be necessary to overcome resistance. The research tradition among naturopaths has largely been informal and unpublished. Lack of economic incentive due to unpatentability of the medicines and the failure to regulate naturopathic practice have retarded the development of journeyman program evaluators and researchers among naturopathic agencies.

A much more favorable publishing environment has arisen in the past few years among conventional peer-reviewed publications (Anonymous 1999), with the establishment of an increasing number of journals devoted to the CAM field, and at the NIH with the founding of the National Center for Complementary and Alternative Medicine (NCCAM). Even research in whole practices is gaining interest at the NIH with the articulated strategy of the NCCAM (Straus 2000). New study tools for whole-practice research are beginning to be accepted with the development of methodology in practice-based and outcomes research. Thus, an increasing number of relevant studies can be expected in the future but the data are not yet available for dissemination.

Problems related to the lack of research infrastructure

Though publication bias may have retarded the availability of preliminary data on naturopathic medicine, a more constraining circumstance has been the lack of research infrastructure within the profession. Sensitivity to the complexities of naturopath practice is certainly more available in the practitioner community, yet research is only a small portion of naturopathic professional activities. For most of the 20th century, much of the quite small professional community's energies were taken up with survival. From the late 1970s, as the profession was being revived, rebuilding educational institutions and professional standards has taken priority. While empirical physician and patient experience were sufficient to sustain practice, NDs are just beginning to evolve a fit with a socioeconomic model that either requires or can generate the resources needed for scientific documentation and evaluation of their whole practice as the pharmaceutical industry has done over the past six or seven decades. Thus, naturopathic medicine has lacked both research resources and the scientists who understand both the medicine and modern evaluative methods.

The revival of the profession on a more scientific foundation has finally begun to yield scientific output with at least a few scientists working at most naturopathic schools. The first clinical trials at naturopathic colleges (on single agents) were performed in the 1980s (Barrie et al 1987, Blair et al 1991). Only in the 1990s were the first data and statistics unit and research laboratory established and the first NIH grant provided to a naturopathic academic institution at Bastyr University. Clinical trials from the naturopathic schools have become increasingly frequent (e.g. Calabrese et al 1999) and collaborations with conventional academic and provider agencies are now common at the accredited naturopathic schools (e.g. Taylor 2001). However, as indicated above, simple trial capacities are not the only tools that need to be acquired for whole-practice research.

The fundamentals of descriptive and qualitative work in the whole practice (Melanson et al 2001, Standish et al 1992) are just beginning with observational studies at some naturopathic colleges. Observation of outcomes in a public health clinic in which naturopathic physicians are adjunctive practitioners is under way in the Seattle area. Some primarily descriptive pilots for longitudinal outcomes studies have been done or are planned at naturopathic teaching clinics. Also important is current descriptive work on community naturopathic physicians in licensed states on the model of the National Ambulatory Medical Care Survey. This study will describe the practice content of a representative sample of regulated acupuncturists, chiropractors, massage therapists and naturopaths in several states.

Since the number of licensable naturopathic physicians is small and they typically have solo or small group practices, clinical research networks to recruit subjects and gather data are needed. More skills in data management and analysis and statistical consultation will also be needed for both local preliminary studies and the more complex clinical research that will ultimately be required. Additional laboratories to increase the breadth of abilities for treatment standardization and effect are also needed. But more important than facilities is fostering the investigative inclinations of young naturopaths and inculcating the habits of mind that the documentation of practice results and methodological invention for whole-practice research will require.

Methodological problems

Research problems related to the indications

As with other whole practices, naturopathic disease nosology (its classification of human distress) is not always congruent with that of Western molecular biomedicine. This is not as great a problem with naturopathy as with some other alternative medical systems. Licensed naturopathic physicians have little difficulty in assigning an International Classification of Disease (ICD-9) code to their patients. Their view of etiologies, however, might cause concentrations in code numbers which would be unexpected by conventionally trained doctors.

As with other whole practices, primary variance in efficacy is more likely to vary with the conditions of a practice's native nosology than with a foreign one. Since different diseases are being treated, treatment response would be expected to have a different profile. Thus, the speed to healing as well as the disease being treated may be confounded in evaluating one system by the other's definitions and rules.

Some naturopathic conceptions may no longer have or may never have had a biomedical equivalent. These include, for example, the 'constitution' (a patient's given biological potential, tendencies, patterns of longstanding psychophysical strengths and weakness which are genetically and embryologically determined), the 'biological terrain' (background physical health and the individual context for the medical problem of immediate concern) or the 'vital force' (the motive plan or spirit animating mind and body expressed as physiological and psychological functionality and adaptability). In other parameters, biomedical equivalents exist for naturopathic system control concepts but they will be exploited therapeutically more thoroughly by naturopaths. Such concepts include 'balance' (as in the immune system, among microbial symbionts, hormonal, neurotransmitter, etc.), deficiency (not just nutritional but organ deficiencies, e.g. hypochlorhydria, hypothyroidism), constitution, functional reserves, endogenous and exogenous toxicities and dysmetabolisms (e.g. syndrome X). An important concept is that a disease syndrome may be an attempt by the body to adapt to ecological stress and should not be unnecessarily suppressed. This will not only be of interest as an independent variable but will have an influence on the measurement of the dependent variable as well.

Research problems related to the treatments (interventions)

Leaving aside for a moment the difficulties of evaluating the entire practice as a system, testing the many individual naturopathic treatments presents a challenge in itself. Firstly, there are a great many treatments to be evaluated. There are likely to be some that translate into the modern biomedical culture while demonstrating effectiveness. Some may not be translatable from the naturopathic vernacular and setting. There is also likely to be considerable chaff, as there has been in conventional medicine. Selecting the 'low-hanging fruit', i.e. pursuing definitive evaluation where there is already strong evidence, for example saw palmetto for BPH, is a good strategy to start with. However, this would leave most of the field untouched. In evaluating naturopathic treatment, therapeutic regimens should be understood in light of the following issues.

Problems related to standardization Standardization is the great strength of modern medicine's pharmacotherapeutics. Since replicability is a hallmark of the scientific method, specifically what is tested – whether a substance, a treatment procedure or a system of practice – would need to be defined, described and stabilized so that it can be delivered reliably from patient to patient and study to study in order that one can make a generalization about results obtained with it. Funders of research reasonably wish to shape social policy using the results of their support and they need some assurance of replicability.

In the absence of a formal research tradition, definition of the breadth of the practice is just beginning. With the patchy regulation of different jurisdictions, there have been equally patchy public constraints and guidance. Naturopathy is also just beginning to interface with health-care corporations which will also tend to define the practice toward efficient services delivery and management. While the overall practice is poorly defined, the separate modalities also have difficulties in standardization.

Botanical medicine, as an example, represents the well-known problem of non-standardization among alternative medicines. With herbs, it is quite possible to perform a single-agent controlled trial in a specific disease. But numerous choices need to be made regarding the intervention. Problems in studies begin with verification of plant species used, conditions under which the plant is grown and harvested and the storage and stability of active compounds. There are choices of whether to use the whole plant, particular parts, various crude extracts or a specific chemical constituent which may be concentrated in various ways and to varying degrees of purity. Crude fresh extracts, to which many clinical herbalists are partial, are susceptible to deterioration. In the most sophisticated systems of botanical medicine preparation, a product is standardized for a number of ingredients – for some guaranteeing a minimum concentration and for others, a maximum concentration. This, for example, is true of the *Gingko biloba* extract (Egb761, Schwabe GmbH) which has been most researched. Standardizing on constituents may present complications. For instance, active ingredients in plants are often classes of molecules, like polysaccharides, saponins or terpenes which are difficult to distinguish in biological activity among their members. Different compounds in a single species may have similar, possibly complementary effects, such as the polysaccharides and isobutylamides in Echinacea spp. During in vitro assays which guide fractionation of the crude extract toward a single active molecule, it is not uncommon for activity to increase but then diminish as greater purity of an identified molecular species is reached, as was the case of the terpenes of *Andrographis paniculata* (Androvir, Paracelsian, Inc.) which have an influence in cell signaling. Some manufacturers are adding cellular assays in the effort to standardize for an effect rather than a chemical constitutent. When such problems are addressed, these levels of standardization lead to testing the industrialization of botanical medicine rather than its roots and do not answer the question of whether the more commonly used crude extracts or powdered herbs produce the hoped-for clinical benefits.

The problems in botanical research may be compounded in other naturopathic modalities. Nutrition, for example, can be divided into dietary practices and nutritional supplements. Studies in dietary interventions are demanding. The gold standard for dietary intervention is a residential facility to maintain adherence to the therapeutic regimen, an expensive solution and difficult to recruit. Other populations with controllable diets include the armed forces, prisons, retirement homes and schools but ethical review would need to be vigorous. Often in dietary studies, a long observation time is needed as diets are often intended as preventives or restoratives for which clinical outcomes would take time to observe. Finding an appropriate comparison control may also be difficult. Among nutritional supplements, there are the simple (e.g. individual nutrients such as vitamins and minerals or other single molecule agents) and more complex interventions. Individual nutrients are well known and have been evaluated in general human health for many years. When they may be efficacious, they are likely to work in a carefully selected clinical population with idiosyncratic genetically or environmentally determined needs. Therefore clinical study may typically call for either extensive diagnostic studies or very large numbers of subjects (as relatively few will show clinical response). Complex nutritional supplements are special foods like probiotics (live bacteria taken to normalize commensal bacterial populations) or algae. Studies in these types of interventions have complications similar to botanical medicine studies.

Problems related to combination treatments   Combination treatment is almost a rule among naturopaths who use multiple remedies individualized for a particular case. Combinations complicate by orders of difficulty the research problems of standardization, clinical indications, therapeutic targets and potential toxicities. Yet combination treatment may be critical to demonstrating the success of naturopathic medicine. Single natural agents may have a true effect so small that a very large patient sample size would be required to detect a treatment difference. Several agents acting together, however, especially if by different mechanisms, may have an effect size determined by cumulative or synergetic interactions. These larger effects may be more readily detectable in a clinical trial. What naturopaths may forego in powerful pharmaceuticals, they may gain in the breadth of physiological support in using combinations for treatment. Combination treatment may also afford the practitioner latitude in choosing the correct remedy for a patient's condition, thereby increasing the treatment responder rate.

The possibility of adverse events could theoretically rise with combinations. However, combinations of the often less bioactive natural products exert gentler effects (usually distributed over several physiological) mechanisms. This may reduce the likelihood of a more severe reaction with a powerfully bioactive focus on a single physiological link such as with some highly efficacious drugs. While the problems of additive and synergetic actions, inhibition and toxicity associated with multiple synthetic and novel pharmaceuticals in combination are formidable, the history of use of the natural agent candidates and the experience of clinicians in using combinations of natural products in various clinical populations mitigate these problems. For example, when using whole botanicals at a traditional dose, early toxicity is most likely to result in nausea and vomiting or diuretic action. More serious adverse events, such as anaphylactoid reactions, are rarer with nutrients and botanicals of traditional medicinal use than with novel drugs of a refined single molecular species.

Naturopaths also combine modalities, e.g. homeopathy and counseling or manipulation and herbs, which are extremely unlikely to lead to a deleterious interaction but which, if successful, could each stimulate improvement by a completely different mechanism. In the hands of specifically skilled practitioners who are aware of both the historical and ethnographic body of knowledge and of modern toxicology, combinations are likely to be safe and more effective than single remedies. However, it is not possible to cite direct comprehensive evidence of this contention until more study has been made of typical naturopathic combinations and their adverse effects relative to comparably efficacious drug therapies.

Combination treatments greatly exacerbate the research problem of the sheer number of possible treatments for a given condition. There are 5000 herbs in the world's botanical pharmacopeias and hundreds in common use; there are 2000 homeopathic remedies in multiple potencies, there are hundreds of manipulation approaches and hundreds of dietary practices and systems. Clearly, it will be impossible to thoroughly evaluate naturopathy in all its particulars in the foreseeable future. A system-oriented research approach is warranted. Early experimental successes would spur further research. Early failures would deter intensified work so care in study design is needed early on or true medical benefits may be unnecessarily discarded.

Problems related to non-material interventions Naturopathic treatments, like conventional ones, can be categorized into things given (drugs, remedies), things done (procedures) and things shared (interactions – verbal and behavioral medicine). The RCT test system is mostly easily applied with the evaluation of substances – the first category. In evaluating procedural and interactive interventions, limitations arise. In naturopathy, both botanical medicine and nutrition are material interventions which, while there are difficulties involved, frequently have well-accepted research models. Adaptations of pharmaceutical clinical research methods may readily be made. Non-material process interventions, like manipulation, exercise, acupuncture and other forms of point work or psychological and spiritual treatment, are more methodologically problematic, for example in the RCT desideratum of blinding.

For some therapies, accommodations may successfully be made to sustain blinding. For manipulative practices, blinding can be maintained by having separate treaters and raters independently seeing the subject. If treatment strategy depends on a system-specific evaluation, a rater with similar expertise to the treater may determine whether the treatment has been correctly applied: for example, two naturopaths both trained in the same approach to craniosacral therapy seeing the subject successively. One might treat the subject while the other determines if the subject has improved before the subject goes on to a non-system (non-ND) bio-psychosocial medical evaluation. While all the virtues of the pharmacological model RCT may not be completely preserved, methodological compromises will allow the method to detect large and specific treatment effects.

A naturopathic leitmotif is 'body, mind, spirit' and naturopaths have continuously attended to patients' spiritual dimension which is just coming back into awareness in conventional medicine (Post et al 2000). If psychotherapy is expanded to include spiritual interventions (such as personal prayer, meditation, religious practice or belief), an arena often of significant interest to naturopaths, the research record as to intervention is nearly nil. Operationalization of spiritual experience is likely to be idiosyncratic or culture specific. Definitions of spirituality in the medical literature may refer to hope and meaning, a personal relationship with God (Swanson 1995), serenity (Roberts & Whall 1996), connectedness – all perhaps related to states of consciousness of the patient. A number of thinkers bemoan the lack of definition in the area (Goddard 1995). Though efforts to present a cogent, broadly acceptable definition have been made (Dyson et al 1997, Pehler 1997), they have not been widely successful. It was only in the fourth edition of DSM-IV (1995) that the possibility of a religious or spiritual problem was even recognized (Turner et al 1995). In the medical literature, most references to spirituality come from nursing. With few but increasing exceptions (Harris et al 1999), there is relatively little interest displayed in the effect of different spiritual interventions on health.

Problems of therapy individualization A skilled naturopath expects success through individualization of treatment regimes. Individualization means that remedies are not prescribed solely on the basis of disease entities but also on other characteristics of the specific patient. Such characteristics may be transient or constitutional or may be representative of the entire constellation of the patient's health problems and strengths and their capacity for self-care. The lack of fit of a person's health syndrome with a conventional disease model – expressed perhaps in the inability or reluctance of a conventional practitioner to diagnose a particular health problem – may be the very reason a patient turns to naturopathic medicine. If a medical system does not recognize an entity, it is unlikely to have an effective therapy for it. The complaint will be managed as something else, resulting in ineffective treatment while nevertheless exposing the patient to its side effects. Conversely, a medical system that provides an adequate explanatory model for a patient's experience of symptoms, their origin, aggravators and ameliorators has a better chance of providing effective treatment or management for the condition.

Thus individualization of treatment is a strength of CAM rather than merely a research problem. If the need for individualization is neglected in research design, the design will fail to apply the medicine as practiced and will fail to evaluate its potential benefit. Compromises may be made to practice in order to make a trial of therapy possible but they may diminish therapeutic effect.

Issues of practitioner effects A confounder in a clinical trial is an apparent therapeutic effect that can be attributed not to the test treatment but to a factor associated with the treatment. This is a risk inherent in all research. These are reasons why randomization, blinding and 'hard' measures are valuable in distinguishing true differences in effect among medications. The most honest scientists may have conscious or unconcious behaviors which bias study results.

However, an important confounder that may be integral to treatment is intentionality. The potential therapeutic action of pure intention, which is not mediated by language or any well-known material force, might be espoused by only a small minority of naturopaths though it may actually be more widely practiced among them. This may be called 'psychic' healing or simply 'healing'. If the intent is to determine whether these techniques have an effect on disease, surprisingly there may be no particular difficulties to doing studies than are already addressed here. Trials of intercessory prayer may provide a model (Harris et al 1999). Design differences may be called for if the therapists were special (gifted) versus ordinary people or depending on whether the healing energy is directed/willed versus invoked (as from God or spirits). There is little written on the capacity of intention to influence physical outcomes; in fact, there is implicit rejection of the idea based on Cartesian mind–body duality. Nevertheless, there are a number of studies which indicate its existence (Benor 1993, Schlitz & Braud 1997). Studies of the effect of prayer may also be relevant here (Targ 1997) and raise the possibility that specific kinds of intentionality may make a difference.

Studies which blind the practitioner and patient decrease or eliminate the possibility that intentionality will contribute to a positive outcome yet CAM theories explicitly accommodate bonding and expectation as contributors to outcome (Wirth 1995). Intentionality, if it is effective at improving health outcomes, is a difficulty only for research. In clinical practice, therapist intention is a wholly non-toxic intervention exercised by all healers – is, in fact, the *sine qua non* of healers.

A similarly nebulous practitioner-associated quality which may have an influence on outcome is intuition. This might be thought to bear on diagnosis, as a source of data, or on therapeutics as a guide among possible alternative strategies. While intentionality and intuition are not listed in the educational catalogs of naturopathic academic institutions as requisite health-care skills, they are common concepts in the culture of naturopathy. They are not generally considered as anti-scientific concepts that should be expunged from the awareness of students. Indeed, they might be acknowledged and even honored as a possible source of data and therapeusis as long as their 'discoveries' are not contradicted by harder evidence. The informality of the inclusion of intention and intuition in naturopathic practice compounds the difficulty of including these concepts in some reproducible way in research protocols.

Issues related to the setting

Conventional medical care is also practiced within a culture, whereby practitioners and patients have roles and expectations which reinforce belief in expected outcomes. Some studies have indicated that good physician–patient communication results in better medical outcomes (Stewart 1995). Thus, some of the magnitude of effect may depend on the setting in which naturopathic care is offered.

Differences in outcome between medical practices may hinge on the difference between research versus non-research settings. For example, it is possible that those who refuse to be randomized have a psychological orientation that may work synergistically with the physical effects of the practices of a medical culture which they prefer or are native to. If this is true, the evaluation of systems of practice relative to each other would preclude simple randomization. Trials that should be of real interest to policy makers are not simply those which determine whether a practice 'works' for anyone to whom it is applied, as is the case with the RCT, but whether it works (and is cost effective) among those who choose it. A study design that could determine the added value of the availability of naturopathic care in those who choose it is to use groups randomized either to strict assignment of alternative or conventional care or to a choice of alternative or conventional care. Such a four-group trial would compare the effect of the different practices among those patients who actively select them versus those who are simply assigned to them.

Finer distinctions of outcome differences between naturopathic and conventional medical care in different settings would require answering a series of questions. These include whether naturopathic care leads to lower overall morbidity and mortality not only for those who are randomized to it versus not randomized but also for those to whom it is equally available on the basis of cost and access versus those to whom is not equally available and, finally, among those who would actively pursue it in the presence of health system structural resistance (e.g. devoted consumers) versus those who would only choose it if were equally available. The answers to these questions involve belief, motivation, cost and the restraint of use due to cost (from the consumer's side), the restraint of access due to cost (from the provider side) and compliance. The answers may be fundamental to determining both the efficacy and efficiency of the inclusion of naturopathic medicine in a rationally structured health-care delivery system.

Research problems related to measures and outcomes

The RCT, as usually but not necessarily performed, tends to neglect effects on diseases other than the target disease, not to speak of neglecting effects on the entire constitution of the patient. Naturopaths and their clients expect to see positive results not only in objective disease parameters but in general disease-related body functions (e.g. fatigue, pain, inflammation, digestion) at a perceptible level, as well as the reduction of risk factors for diseases of aging. Thus methods to assess the efficacy of naturopathic medicine should use holistic measures accounting for effects throughout the body systems and over the lifecycle, if possible. Beyond the effectiveness of medicine for the individual patient, measures of an entire practice should address public health, environmental and social and economic outcomes. Of course, this is ideally the way conventional medicine should also be assessed. When consistently applied to both, a comparison of the practices' comparative virtues could perhaps be done. Clearly this would require large and lengthy trials. In the past 25 years, substantial strides have been made in the development of measures which assess individual health globally. There has been progress with the development and wide adoption of instruments such as the SF-36 and of measures such as quality-adjusted life-years saved. However, there continues to be a lack of sensitivity to changes in disease at the upper levels of function where the burden of human suffering is great, given the number of 'walking wounded', and which has enormous societal costs, both medical and non-medical, in life quality, functional impairment and missed opportunity. This lack of sensitivity relates to the general absence of health measures in clinical trials as opposed to disease measures.

Measures have not so far been attempted for such concepts as the 'vital force' or other explanatory health models largely due to a lack of definition or demonstration of their correlation with other kinds of outcomes. Some measures are possible but not convenient, such as digestive capacity, bioavailability to the individual or markers of general toxicity.

The lack of sensitivity of measures is also an issue given the possibly smaller effect magnitude per time that may be expected from gentler natural treatments than with carefully engineered pharmaceutical and surgical interventions. Besides slower healing which may be common with some naturopathic treatments, the concept of the 'healing crisis', a temporary exacerbation of symptoms on the way to more definitive improvement, also calls for longer increments of time over which to make measurements in order to evaluate the response to treatment. The reluctance of naturopaths to 'suppress' symptoms while seeking and treating the cause may also lead to a lengthening of the assessment period in order to properly evaluate therapeutic impact. Ultimately, the possibility of superiority of naturopathic care in a few areas, such as longevity, the incidence of chronic disease in aging or the incidence and prevalence of disease in progeny, requires multi-decade evaluations.

TOWARDS SOLUTIONS

Solutions for some of these problems are available. For a solution to the lack of preliminary work, patience is required. However, the breadth of the valid literature relevant to naturopathic evaluation is now increasing. The entry of naturopathic physicians into health delivery systems in the past 20 years has generated data on utilization and cost which can be used for comparison with other professions, though these data remain, in large measure, unexplored. Descriptive study is under way. The lack of training and experience at the interface of modern clinical research and naturopathy is rapidly changing as the profession gradually attracts or trains skilled researchers who understand the medicine and as the modest research programs at the accredited naturopathic schools continue to grow. At a structural level, since the number of licensable naturopathic physicians is small and they typically have solo or small group practices, clinical research networks to recruit subjects and gather data are needed. More skills in data management and analysis and statistical consultation will also be needed for both local preliminary studies and the more complex clinical research that will ultimately be required. Additional laboratories to increase the breadth of abilities for treatment standardization and effect are also required.

But more important than facilities is fostering the investigative inclinations of young naturopaths and inculcating the habits of mind that the documentation of practice results and methodological invention for whole-practice research will require. It would be valuable to fund the development of research infrastructure directly at naturopathic institutions for research training, facilities and projects. Such investments will foster development of methods, experience and capacities which will continue, over time, to be devoted to the research opportunities. This would sustain the investigative machinery permanently, not merely in response to clinical or political fad. The good questions are deep and require extended programs of research.

While all components of valid and reliable methodologies are not yet fully available, wisdom would recommend the use of the clinical research methods where they are useful. One of the most important research methods to pursue is the single agent RCT. RCTs are usually what skeptics mean when they ask for evidence. The RCT is a brilliant invention which has the highest internal validity of any clinical research method. Studies with randomization to eliminate selection bias and blinding to reduce non-specific effects provide the strongest evidence, if results are significantly positive, that a well-defined medication should be preferred over its controls in the particular population selected. There are many research questions regarding naturopathic medicine which can and should be addressed by RCTs. Though the RCT is a gold standard, it is by now well accepted that it cannot answer all questions (Rabeneck et al 1992). In the evaluation of CAM, the RCT can be started too early, before the requirements for a valid RCT are accomplished, e.g. before the intervention is standardized and the right population is identified for sampling. They are also expensive; witness the $4.5 million the NIH awarded in 1997 for an $N = 300$ trial of St John's wort (Hypericum) for depression. Such expenditures, of course, cannot be made for very many interventions. While compromises to the practice may be necessary to perform a clinical trial, equally it must be understood that compromises to trial methodology may be needed in order to fairly evaluate the medicine as practiced. The methodology of the RCT itself is undergoing rapid evolution to accommodate, for example, patient preference (Feine et al 1998, Rucker 1989).

Given the number of clinical possibilities to be screened in naturopathic medicine, the value of small trials, open trials, case series and case studies should be recognized. A controlled trial generally requires four times the number of subjects that an open trial does to detect the same size therapeutic difference in an outcome measure. Open trials are especially valuable in many conditions where there are hard objective endpoints. While one cannot be as sure of the validity of the answer, for a rapid response to health questions, several open trials can be done for the expense of one randomized trial. Since what is needed is preliminary information to select the best possibilities for more stringent trials, such design compromises are reasonable in early screening studies.

Many designs are not frequently used but will provide good information early in investigational programs. Single-patient randomized trials have reached a high level of sophistication, minimizing risk to subjects (Barlow et al 1977, Guyatt et al 1990, Kiene & Von Schon-Angerer 1998) and allowing for individualized treatment. Time series studies have been developed for in-office practice and applied to CAM treatments (Keating et al 1985). When the medicine and mechanisms are not well defined, a 'best case' series method, such as has been adopted by the National Cancer Institute for novel therapies, will be of use. Careful investigation of remarkable cases, such as reports of retroconversion to seronegativity in HIV disease, may provide excellent leads for follow-up (Weibo et al 1995). Case controls on hardy patients may work back to beneficial characteristics and behaviors (Carson 1993). For treatments which call for adaptation of medication such as homeopathy, response-adaptive design theory may have a contribution (Rosenberger & Lachin 1993). Contrary to what many alternative practitioners believe, good designs are available even for non-material interventions (Vickers 1996). Of course, funding review committees need to be as open to the possibilities of alternative trial designs as naturopathic agencies need to be to accomplishing objective and appropriate evaluation. Innovative trial designs need a chance to be developed and tried.

Observational studies can track outcomes of a number of therapies simultaneously (Standish et al 1997). The essence of outcomes research is to evaluate the health status of individuals before and after different clinical interventions for a given problem and to compare the interventions with each other for relative effectiveness. Health status typically is determined by clinical measures of the particular health condition as well as an assessment of the patient's global physical and social functioning and sense of well-being. The therapeutic interventions are usually those of everyday treatment in the general clinic patient population. Despite earlier contrary evidence, observational studies have recently been shown not to overestimate effect size (Benson & Hartz 2000). For these reasons, the results are reasonably generalizable despite the number of possible confounders. Outcomes work is efficient in that it takes advantage of the natural experiment involved in ordinary care simply by keeping track of the results. The economic and ethical advantages of observational studies among patients who voluntarily associate with a particular health practice are an early and efficient means especially of answering questions which require many years or many subjects. Comparisons can be drawn to conventional care tracked with the same method if the restraints of differential cost of care and difficulty of access are reduced by a level playing field. In this way, observational models can incorporate change in effect due to setting.

Diagnostic and therapeutic algorithms – rule sets for programmed decision making – are clinical trial methods to address two of the so far unaddressed issues in naturopathic research: non-congruence of diagnoses with Western disease nosology and the need for individualization for best outcomes.

Algorithms may be derived from observation of practice, modeling of expert behavior or 'Delphi' panels of naturopathic clinical experts.

An alternative to decision-making algorithms may be to use the practitioner as the unit of intervention. Practitioners of a given education and experience would be allowed their own judgment for the fit between diagnosis and treatment, perhaps after patients with a specific Western diagnosis are referred to naturopathic care. The use of the practitioner as the unit of intervention also will include unknown practitioner effects as contributors to outcome.

In summary, research methods should be chosen which least interfere with the practice to be studied, rather than distorting practices to fit models of research intended for patentable drugs. Naturopathic medicine needs to be delivered in context and broad measures of health and well-being are required to evaluate its outcomes. For some studies in individualized medicines, treatment could be determined by algorithm but for others, using expert CAM practitioners for the more complex multimodality treatments may be a necessity on a case-by-case basis. For a trial of a medical system, the practitioner could be considered as the intervention. All the methodologies which may be appropriate to the evaluation of CAM practices have not been developed yet. Innovative designs which do not distort CAM practice will be needed rather than conventional designs which produce high-validity answers to the wrong questions. The right questions will surround whether the availability and use of naturopathic medicine lower lifetime morbidity and mortality cost effectively. This requires the capacity for whole-practice research. Comparison trials between different systems of practice are needed with holistic practices such as naturopathic medicine. Such comparisons, if correctly done, can answer the bigger questions on naturopathic medicine.

REFERENCES

Anonymous 1999 Alternative medicine: the AMA reviews scientific evidence. Clinician Reviews 9(2): 87–90

Barlow DH, Blanchard EB, Hayes SC, Epstein LH 1977 Single-case designs and clinical biofeedback experimentation. Biofeedback and Self Regulation 2(3): 221–239

Barrie SA, Wright JV, Pizzorno JE 1987 Effects of garlic oil on platelet aggregation, serum lipids and blood pressure in humans. Journal of Orthomolecular Medicine 2(1): 15–21

Benor DJ 1993 Healing research: holistic energy medicine and spirituality. Helix Verlag, Munich

Benson K, Hartz AJ 2000 A comparison of observational studies and randomized, controlled trials. New England Journal of Medicine 34(25): 1887–1892

Blair DM, Hangee-Bauer CS, Calabrese C 1991 Intestinal candidiasis, *L. acidophilus* supplementation and Crook's questionnaire. Journal of Naturopathic Medicine 2(1): 33–36

Calabrese C, Myer S, Munson S, Turet P 1999 A cross-over study of the effect of a single oral feeding of medium chain triglyceride oil vs. canola oil on post-ingestion plasma triglyceride levels in healthy men. Alternative Medicine Review 4(1): 23–28

Carson VB 1993 Prayer, meditation, exercise, and special diets: behaviors of the hardy person with HIV/AIDS. Journal of the Association of Nurses in AIDS Care 4(3): 18–28

Dyson J, Cobb M, Forman D 1997 The meaning of spirituality: a literature review. Journal of Advanced Nursing 26(6): 1183–1188

Feine JS, Awad MA, Lund JP 1998 The impact of patient preference on the design and interpretation of clinical trials. Community Dentistry and Oral Epidemiology 26(1): 70–74

Goddard NC 1995 'Spirituality as integrative energy': a philosophical analysis as requisite precursor to holistic nursing practice. Journal of Advanced Nursing 22(4): 808–815

Guyatt GH, Keller JL, Jaeschke R, Rosenbloom D, Adachi JD, Newhouse MT 1990 The n-of-1 randomized controlled trial: clinical usefulness. Our three-year experience. Annals of Internal Medicine 112(4): 293–299

Harris WS, Gowda M, Kolb JW et al 1999 A randomized, controlled trial of the effects of remote, intercessory prayer on outcomes in patients admitted to the coronary care unit. Archives of Internal Medicine 159(19): 2273–2278

Keating JC Jr, Giljum K, Menke JM, Lonczak RS, Meeker WC 1985 Toward an experimental chiropractic: time-series designs. Journal of Manipulative and Physiological Therapeutics 8(4): 229–238

Kiene H, Von Schon-Angerer T 1998 Single-case causality assessment as a basis for clinical judgment. Altern Ther Health Med 4(1): 41–47

Melanson SJ, Mykhalovshiy E, Kup R, McLeod D, Jaeger TV 2001 Combined medical and naturopathic services: a novel approach in HIV primary care. In press

Pehler SR 1997 Children's spiritual response: validation of the nursing diagnosis spiritual distress. Nursing Diagnosis 8(2): 55–66

Peroutka SJ 1998 Beyond monotherapy: rational polytherapy in migraine. Headache 38(1): 18–22

Post SG, Puchalski CM, Larson DB 2000 Physicians and patient spirituality: professional boundaries, competency, and ethics. Annals of Internal Medicine 132(7): 578–583

Rabeneck L, Viscoli CM, Horwitz RI 1992 Problems in the conduct and analysis of randomized clinical trials. Are we getting the right answers to the wrong questions? Archives of Internal Medicine 152(3): 507–512

Roberts KT, Whall A 1996 Serenity as a goal for nursing practice. Image: Journal of Nursing Scholarship 28(4): 359–364

Rosenberger WF, Lachin JM 1993 The use of response-adaptive designs in clinical trials. Controlled Clinical Trials 14(6): 471–484

Rucker G 1989 A two-stage trial design for testing treatment, self-selection and treatment preference effects. Statistics in Medicine 8(4): 477–485

Schlitz M, Braud W 1997 Distant intentionality and healing: assessing the evidence. Altern Ther Health Med 3(6): 62–73

Standish LJ, Guiltinan J, McMahon E, Lindstrom C 1992 One-year open trial of naturopathic treatment of HIV infection class IV-A in men. Journal of Naturopathic Medicine 3(1): 42–64

Standish LJ, Calabrese C, Reeves C, Polissar N, Bain S, O'Donnell T 1997 A scientific plan for the evaluation of alternative medicine in the treatment of HIV/AIDS. Altern Ther Health Med 3(2): 58–67

Stewart MA 1995 Effective physician–patient communication and health outcomes: a review. Complementary Medicine Association Journal 152(9): 1423–1433

Straus S 2000 Draft five-year strategic plan. NIH NCCAM, Bethesda, MD

Swanson CS 1995 A spirit-focused conceptual model of nursing for the advanced practice nurse. Issues in Comprehensive Pediatric Nursing 18(4): 267–275

Targ E 1997 Evaluating distant healing: a research review. Altern Ther Health Med 3(6): 74–78

Taylor J, Calabrese C, Sanders F, Standish L, Lee J 2001 A randomized trial of Echinacea for the treatment of colds in children. A collaborative study among the University of Washington, Bastyr University, and the Puget Sound Pediatric Research Network. Funded by NIH NCCAM

Turner RP, Lukoff D, Barnhouse RT, Lu FG Religious or spiritual problem. A culturally sensitive diagnostic category in the DSM-IV. Journal of Nervous and Mental Diseases 183(7): 435–444

Vickers A 1996 Methodological issues in complementary and alternative medicine research: a personal reflection on 10 years of debate in the United Kingdom. Journal of Alternative and Complementary Medicine 2(4): 515–524

Weibo L, Ruixing W, Chongfen G, Yizhe W, Shao J, Mshiu E, Mbena E 1995 A report on 8 seronegative converted HIV/AIDS patients with traditional Chinese medicine. Chinese Medical Journal 108(8): 634–637

Wirth DP 1995 The significance of belief and expectancy within the spiritual healing encounter. Social Science and Medicine 41(2): 249–260

FURTHER READING

Diet
Ogle KA, Bullock JD 1980 Children with allergic rhinitis and/or bronchial asthma treated with elimination diet: a five-year follow-up. Annals of Allergy 44: 273–278

Ninety-one percent of 322 children with negative inhalant and skin allergy tests showed significant improvement during trial.

Unge G et al 1983 Effect of dietary tryptophan restrictions on clinical symptoms in patients with endogenous asthma. Allergy 38: 211–212
Double-blind crossover in 18 patients treated with either a low tryptophan or normal tryptophan diet for one month showed subjective improvement and increases in PEF ($P < 0.02$).

Nutritional supplements
Anah CO et al 1982 High dose ascorbic acid in Nigerian asthmatics. The attenuation of exercise-induced bronchospasm by ascorbic acid. Annals of Allergy 49(3): 146–151
Forty-one children, 1000 mg/d vs placebo for 14 weeks, had $\frac{1}{4}$ as many and less severe attacks. One of several articles which indicate that C reduces sensitivity to various inducers of attacks.

Bray GW 1931 The hypochlorhydria of asthma in childhood. Quarterly Journal of Medicine 1881
In 200 asthmatic children, 80% showed gastric acid secretion was below normal. Treatment with HCl in these children before or during meals and exclusion of food allergens was associated with improved appetite, weight gain and sleep and ameliorated asthmatic attacks.

Botanicals
Gupta S et al 1979 *Tylophora indica* in bronchial asthma: a double-blind study. Indian Journal of Medical Research 69: 981–989
135 patients; 200 mg Tylophora vs placebo for 6 days of treatment demonstrated improvement in symptoms, FEV1, and PEFR. Side effects with Tylophora were less than placebo.

Homeopathy
Reilly DT et al 1994 Is evidence for homeopathy reproducible? Lancet 344: 1601–1606
In a placebo-controlled randomized trial in 28 patients with allergic asthma, 77% on homeopathy had improved symptoms vs 20% on placebo ($P < 0.003$), with similar trends in respiratory function and bronchial reactivity.

Physical medicine
Singh V et al 1990 Effect of yoga breathing exercises (pranayama) on airway reactivity in subjects with asthma. Lancet 335: 1381–1383
Placebo-controlled study in 18 patients who had practiced yoga breathing for one week, required a significantly increased dose of histamine to induce a 20% reduction in FEV1.

Girodo ME et al 1992 Deep diaphragmatic breathing: rehabilitation exercises for the asthmatic patient. Archives of Physical Medicine and Rehabilitation 73(8): 717–720
Sixty-seven asthmatic adults were randomly assigned to deep breathing, physical exercise or a waiting list. Deep breathing resulted in significant reductions in intensity of symptoms and medication use and a 300% increase in time spent in physical activities.

Counseling/Psychotherapy
Henry M et al 1993 Improvement of respiratory function in chronic asthmatic patients with autogenic therapy. Journal of Psychosomatic Research 37(3): 265–270.
Twenty-four patients were randomized to either autogenic training or supportive group therapy. The autogenics group showed a significant change in respiratory function.

Index